Every Decker book is accompan[ied by] a CD-ROM.

The disk appears in the front of each copy, in its own sealed jacket. Affixed to the front of the book will be a distinctive Bc̄D sticker **"Book *cum* disk"**.

The disk contains the complete text and illustrations of the book, in fully searchable PDF files. Additional resources have been added to the CD-ROM to make the learning experience more valuable. These include multiple choice questions that test students' comprehension of the subject matter as well as links to biomedical web sites that broaden the resource material available to students of biochemistry. The book and disk will be sold *only* as a package; neither will be available independently, and no prices will be available for the items individually. BC Decker Inc is committed to providing high quality electronic publications that will compliment traditional information and learning methods.

We trust you will find the Book/CD Package invaluable and invite your comments and suggestions.

Brian C. Decker
CEO and Publisher

PDQ SERIES

ACKERMANN
PDQ PHYSIOLOGY

CORMACK
PDQ HISTOLOGY

DAVIDSON
PDQ GENETICS

JOHNSON
PDQ PHARMACOLOGY, 2/e

KERN
PDQ HEMATOLOGY

McKIBBON
PDQ EVIDENCE-BASED PRINCIPLES AND PRACTICE

NORMAN, STREINER
PDQ STATISTICS, 2/e

STREINER, NORMAN
PDQ EPIDEMIOLOGY, 2/e

PDQ (Pretty Darned Quick)

PDQ BIOCHEMISTRY

R. ROY BAKER, PhD
Professor of Biochemistry

ROBERT K. MURRAY, MD, PhD
Professor Emeritus of Biochemistry

both of
University of Toronto Faculty of Medicine
Toronto, Ontario

with illustrations by
Erin A. Baker, BSc

2001
BC Decker Inc
Hamilton • London

BC Decker Inc
20 Hughson Street South
P.O. Box 620, L.C.D. 1
Hamilton, Ontario L8N 3K7
Tel: 905-522-7017; 1-800-568-7281
Fax: 905-522-7839; 1-888-311-4987
e-mail: info@bcdecker.com
website: www.bcdecker.com

01 02 03 04 / PC / 9 8 7 6 5 4 3 2 1

ISBN 1-55009-150-6

Printed in Canada

Sales and Distribution

United States
BC Decker Inc
P.O. Box 785
Lewiston, NY 14092-0785
Tel: 905-522-7017; 1-800-568-7281
Fax: 905-522-7839; 1-888-311-4987
e-mail: info@bcdecker.com
website: www.bcdecker.com

Canada
BC Decker Inc
20 Hughson Street South
P.O. Box 620, L.C.D. 1
Hamilton, Ontario L8N 3K7
Tel: 905-522-7017; 1-800-568-7281
Fax: 905-522-7839; 1-888-311-4987
e-mail: info@bcdecker.com
website: www.bcdecker.com

Japan
Igaku-Shoin Ltd.
Foreign Publications Department
3-24-17 Hongo, Bunkyo-ku
Tokyo 113-8719, Japan
Tel: 81 3 3817 5680
Fax: 81 3 3815 6776
e-mail: fd@igaku-shoin.co.jp

U.K., Europe, Scandinavia, Middle East
Harcourt Publishers Limited
Customer Service Department
Foots Cray High Street
Sidcup, Kent   DA14 5HP, UK
Tel: 44 (0) 208 308 5760
Fax: 44 (0) 181 308 5702
e-mail: cservice@harcourt_brace.com

Singapore, Malaysia, Thailand,
Philippines, Indonesia, Vietnam, Pacific
Rim, Korea
Harcourt Asia Pte Limited
583 Orchard Road
#09/01, Forum
Singapore 238884
Tel: 65-737-3593
Fax: 65-753-2145

Australia, New Zealand
Harcourt Australia Pty Limited
Customer Service Department
STM Division
Locked Bag 16
St. Peters, New South Wales, 2044
Australia
Tel: 61 02 9517-8999
Fax: 61 02 9517-2249
e-mail: stmp@harcourt.com.au
website: www.harcourt.com.au

Foreign Rights
John Scott & Company
International Publishers' Agency
P.O. Box 878
Kimberton, PA 19442
Tel: 610-827-1640
Fax: 610-827-1671
e-mail: jsco@voicenet.com

To Gail and Jean for all their love and support over the years,
and to Dr. Bill Thompson, an exceptional scientist
and a very courageous gentleman.

Preface

This book is an introductory overview of biochemistry, a text that emphasizes important features of the discipline in a concise and focused manner. It is meant as an economical, portable, and rapidly accessed companion rather than a costly, stationary, weighty, and comprehensive text. We have based this book on lectures given to undergraduate students at the University of Toronto within both the Faculty of Medicine and the Faculty of Arts and Science. As there are few biochemistry texts that serve medical undergraduates or students in related health disciplines, this book discusses many diseases and clinical applications as well as the basics of biochemistry. *PDQ Biochemistry* can serve as a refresher for those who have taken a biochemistry course before or as an introduction for those coming from non-science disciplines. These latter students are in need of a clear and easily understood text. At the same time, both medical students and students in the health sciences may benefit from a concise and well-mapped journey through the science of biochemistry as they will use it as a stepping stone they can revisit en route to a particular specialty. The student, like a visitor to Europe, Latin America, the Middle East, or Asia, will hopefully find this book to be similar to *Biochemistry on $25 a Day* in its ability to point out relevant sites on the journey and reasonably priced hostels within sight of the Acropolis.

The topics in *PDQ Biochemistry* follow the curriculum presented to our medical students in their first year. This text is divided into eight chapters, with proteins being a central theme running through each. Proteins are well beloved of biochemists, for they are the principal functional elements within the body. Proteins are, in many ways, not just molecules of living organisms but molecules that are "alive". However, as this text hopes to demonstrate the relevance of proteins within the body, we will show how the proteins participate within their surroundings and not simply as isolated molecules.

In Chapter 1, the biochemistry of muscle is presented with an introduction to amino acids and protein structure. This chapter features the structures of actin and myosin; the biochemical mechanisms of contraction; structural and functional differences between skeletal, cardiac, and smooth muscle; ion transport across membranes and membrane-based receptors; and the actions of nitric oxide as a vasodilator. Chapter 2 describes plasma proteins, the biochemical basis of edema, metal ion-transporting proteins, the important roles of iron and copper within the body, diseases associated with defects in the handling of these metal ions, and atherosclerosis. In Chapter 3, enzymes are described as dynamic proteins that catalyze reactions leading to the generation or destruction of molecules within the body. In addition, we discuss serum or plasma enzymes as markers for various diseases. The biochemical basis of hemostasis and thrombosis is discussed in Chapter 4, as are the hemophilias. In Chapter 5, we cover the structure and function of hemoglobin as well as the genetic defect responsible for sickle cell anemia. This chapter also describes the metabolism of the heme group and the biochemistry of jaundice and the porphyrias. The importance of vitamins B_{12} and folate is addressed in Chapter 6 in relation to megaloblastic anemias. Chapter 7 provides an introduction to metabolism: how enzymes cooperate within pathways and cycles that synthesize or degrade molecules. Hormonal regulation of metabolism, diabetes mellitus, and inborn errors of metabolism, such as phenylketonuria, are also discussed here. In Chapter 8, the use of molecular biology within medicine is outlined, along with an introduction to DNA and RNA and a description of methodologies used in the pursuit of disease genes.

In this text, you will find that we have not agonized unduly over chemical structures. In the end, it is important from a medical viewpoint to grasp quickly the overall picture and the important biochemical features. We shall be delighted if some of the material in this text is retained by medical graduates, and, to that end, we have added certain elements of humor and anecdotes that may serve as aide-mémoire. There are also historical notations of medical relevance that have been included as we believe that an interest in medical science should be balanced by an interest in the humanities.

R. Roy Baker
Robert K. Murray
May 2001

Acknowledgments

We wish to acknowledge the invaluable help of Dr. Margaret Rand of the Hospital for Sick Children in Toronto, who reviewed Chapter 4 and provided many helpful comments. We are also very grateful to Dr. Alex Marks, who for many years has coordinated the Biochemistry Seminar Program for Year One medical students at the University of Toronto.

Contents

PDQ
BIOCHEMISTRY

1

Proteins: Introduction to Proteins and the Biochemistry of Muscle

In this chapter, we will introduce proteins and some of their prominent features. The specific introductory example will be the proteins of muscle, with emphasis on those involved in muscular contraction. Comparisons will be made using skeletal, cardiac, and smooth muscle found in the vascular system. We will comment on ion transport, with particular emphasis on cardiac muscle cells, and the involvement of calcium in excitation events. Lastly, the role of nitric oxide as a vasorelaxant and the sources of energy for muscular contraction will be considered. The information presented is of importance to studies of cardiovascular physiology and health, but it will also pave the way for insights into other areas of protein function.

BASICS OF PROTEIN STRUCTURE

It is valid to ask why biochemists are so "hung up" about proteins. Are there no other molecules in the human body worthy of attention? Well, of course, there are many others, but proteins, like popular political figures, have charisma and glamour. And, unlike popular political figures, they actually get things done, and in a very dynamic manner. Most proteins are functional molecules that play very specific roles in your body, and, indeed, there are thousands of them, rather like all the possible occupations you may have considered in grade school: butcher, baker (pardon the pun), candlestick maker, stockbroker, scientist, newspaper vendor—virtually as many parts as you can find women and men playing in the real world (presumably, we are told, the realm outside the universities). Yet, if you remove the distinctive clothing or tools from each profession, you invariably find that people do have anatomic features in common. (You will also hopefully realize, upon this universal disrobing, that there are two major subdivisions, but this is perhaps a subject best left to PDQ Anatomy).

So what do proteins have in common? Well, they do consist of building blocks called amino acids, and true to their name, amino acids do have an amino group $-NH_3^+$ and an acid or carboxyl group $-COO^-$ (Figure 1–1A). Remember these two groups, as they are vitally important in the joining together of amino acids. What happens is that the carboxyl group of one amino acid is linked to the amino group of a second amino acid when a peptide bond is formed. You will see that water is liberated in this bond formation. Peptide bonds are true covalent bonds because there is a sharing of electrons between carboxyl C and amino N. The term **peptide** is used in the naming of these linked amino acids. Figure 1–1B shows the formation of a dipeptide from two amino acids, and 1–1C gives an oligopeptide formed from a small number of amino acids. Proteins (which are often referred to as polypeptides) are the largest and most commonly occurring of these amino acid polymers and may have thousands of amino acid building blocks, with the distinctive, repetitive peptide linkage. You can see, because of the end-to-end linkage of amino acids, that proteins have a dis-

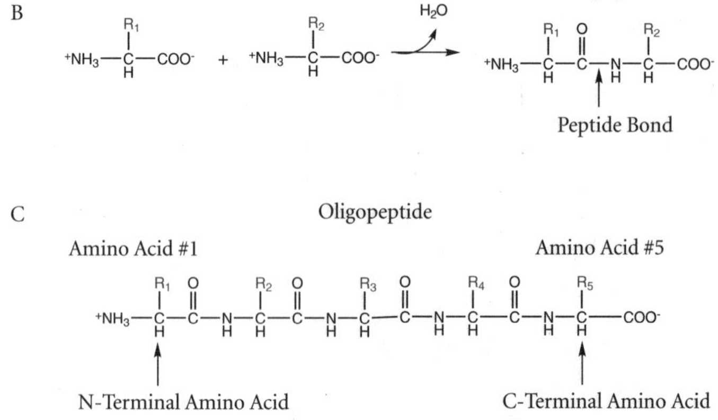

A   Amino Acid

$$^+NH_3-\overset{\overset{\displaystyle R}{|}}{\underset{\underset{\displaystyle H}{|}}{C}}-COO^-$$

B   H₂O   Dipeptide

$$^+NH_3-\overset{\overset{\displaystyle R_1}{|}}{\underset{\underset{\displaystyle H}{|}}{C}}-COO^- \ + \ ^+NH_3-\overset{\overset{\displaystyle R_2}{|}}{\underset{\underset{\displaystyle H}{|}}{C}}-COO^- \longrightarrow \ ^+NH_3-\overset{\overset{\displaystyle R_1}{|}}{\underset{\underset{\displaystyle H}{|}}{C}}-\overset{\overset{\displaystyle O}{\|}}{C}-\overset{}{\underset{\underset{\displaystyle H}{|}}{N}}-\overset{\overset{\displaystyle R_2}{|}}{\underset{\underset{\displaystyle H}{|}}{C}}-COO^-$$

Peptide Bond

C   Oligopeptide

Amino Acid #1   Amino Acid #5

$$^+NH_3-\overset{R_1}{\underset{H}{C}}-\overset{O}{C}-\overset{}{\underset{H}{N}}-\overset{R_2}{\underset{H}{C}}-\overset{O}{C}-\overset{}{\underset{H}{N}}-\overset{R_3}{\underset{H}{C}}-\overset{O}{C}-\overset{}{\underset{H}{N}}-\overset{R_4}{\underset{H}{C}}-\overset{O}{C}-\overset{}{\underset{H}{N}}-\overset{R_5}{\underset{H}{C}}-COO^-$$

N-Terminal Amino Acid   C-Terminal Amino Acid

Figure 1–1 Structure of an amino acid and peptide bonds. Amino acids have amino and carboxyl groups as well as characteristic side groups, R. *A,* A general amino acid structure. *B,* Two amino acids are joined by a peptide bond to form a dipeptide. *C,* An oligopeptide of five amino acids linked by peptide bonds.

tinctive orientation so that there is an N-terminus (with its free amino group) and a C-terminus (with its free carboxyl group). Amino acids in a protein are numbered in succession from the N-terminal amino acid, which is given the number 1.

Now, if amino acids had only an amino group and a carboxyl group utilized in peptide bond formation, you could get polymers of these building blocks that would be just about as exciting as plastic wrap. (Mind you, plastic wrap was a rather novel commodity back in the 1970s.) However, there are some 20 different amino acids in the human body because each has a distinctive R-group (see Figure 1–1). The letter R is used to indicate a variety of possibilities, extending from a simple H to rather complicated aromatic rings. These R-groups are important because they effectively determine how a long string of amino acids folds to give a protein its distinctive three-dimensional shape. And, indeed, the shape of a protein is vitally important to its function. Often, the analogy is used that amino acids in a protein are like different beads on a string or in a necklace. What is a better analogy is that the 20 amino acids are rather like 20 different charms on a charm bracelet. Each is connected to the bracelet by common fittings (to form peptide bonds), but the actual charm itself (the R-group) that extends out from the bracelet is remarkably different, be it a miniature pair of dice, a palm tree, a bottle of cola, Joe Carter, or a reduced replica of your local baseball stadium. It is the interaction of these "charms" or R-groups and their attraction to or repulsion by water that largely determine the folding of the protein into its three-dimensional shape.

An understanding of the amino acids is important because the sequence of these distinctive amino acids in a protein virtually constitutes a language. Each protein has a different sequence of amino acids, and it is this sequence that ultimately determines the protein's three-dimensional form. To ensure that a molecule of protein X made by your body on Monday is precisely the same as another molecule of X that is made on Friday, each protein X is carefully assembled using the 20 different amino acids by following a plan or blueprint. This blueprint indicates what the sequence of amino acids should be in protein X, and the blueprint is really a code that is constructed using DNA in the nucleus of each of your cells. Thus, the genetic material guides the synthesis of proteins. An error or change in the sequence of amino acids could lead to a loss of protein function. Just as there are many different ethnic backgrounds within any population, there can be variations in single amino acid identities at specific sites in a protein sequence. These are based on variations or mutations in the genetic code for a protein. Luckily, these changes often do not compromise the function of the protein, but when they do, they can bring about an inherited disease that can be passed from generation to generation.

For example, there was considerable consanguinity among many of the royal families in Europe at the end of the 19th and the beginning of the 20th centuries. This commonality could be traced to a lack of enthusiasm for the introduction of nonroyals into royal families, and indeed, at one time, Queen Victoria was grandmother to a variety of royal heirs. Queen Vic not only lacked amusement at many of the antics of her son Bertie (later King Edward VII) and others of the British aristocracy, she also passed on through her daughters to their male children a genetic defect that could result in hemophilia A. This disease is caused by a mutation in the genetic code for a protein called factor VIII (antihemophilic globulin), which is essential in blood coagulation. The gene coding for this protein is carried on the X-chromosome. Males have only one X-chromosome and will show the disease if their one gene coding for factor VIII is defective. Prior to World War I, the young Russian crown prince Alexis manifested this bleeding disorder. This prompted his mother, the Czarina Alexandra, to make use of the rather dubious abilities of the "mad monk" Rasputin to keep her son alive. (Although Rasputin was remarkably charismatic, his auxiliary advice in political matters certainly did not help to stem the tide of the Russian revolution.) While you may not have royal relations, it is nonetheless not a good idea to contemplate marriage with your cousin Sid or Surinder because of the expression of potential defects in children when dealing with a limited gene pool. (We will discuss disease genes in Chapter 8.)

To turn from the intrigues of the Russian court to the more important nature of amino acids, it is not our objective to pause at this point while readers commit to memory all the 20 amino acids. For simplicity's sake, let's try to group the amino acids on the basis of the nature of their R-groups and hit some of the more prominent amino acids. These amino acids will pop up at key points throughout the various topics dealt with in this text.

First, the simplest R-group is H, and the corresponding amino acid is glycine (Figure 1–2A). Some of the amino acids have aliphatic R-groups. Leucine serves as an example. Aromatic R-groups are found in phenylalanine, tyrosine, and tryptophan, and these R-groups are characterized by cyclic ring structures. Note that tyrosine also carries an –OH group. Sulfur-containing R-groups are exemplified by methionine and cysteine. Cysteine has an –SH or thiol group that can be used to form cross-links in proteins when the R-groups of two cysteines interact to form an –S–S bridge (Figure 1–2B). Serine and threonine are examples of amino acids carrying an alcohol group –OH. Negatively charged or acidic R-groups (carrying –COO⁻) are found in aspartate and glutamate. Glutamate is also known as the flavor enhancer monosodium glutamate (MSG). Glutamate can serve as a neurotransmitter, a chemical that stimulates the propagation of nerve impulses. A proportion of the population is sensitive to MSG, developing headaches after ingesting food treated with this amino acid (hence the rising

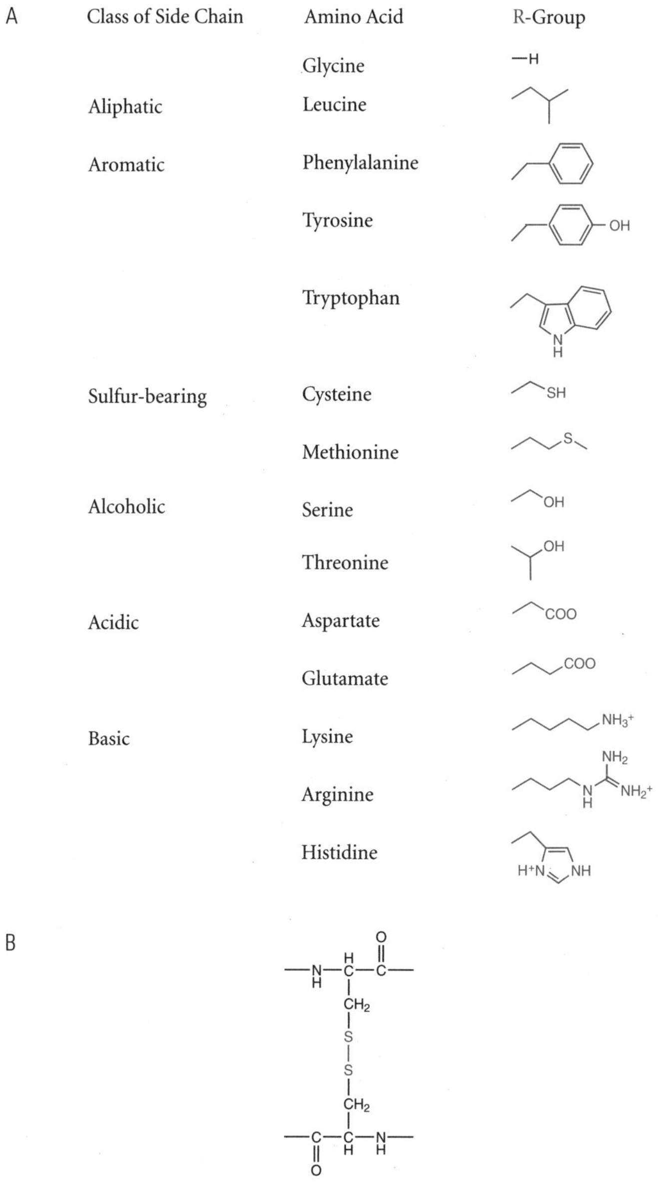

A

Class of Side Chain	Amino Acid	R-Group
	Glycine	—H
Aliphatic	Leucine	
Aromatic	Phenylalanine	
	Tyrosine	OH
	Tryptophan	
Sulfur-bearing	Cysteine	SH
	Methionine	S
Alcoholic	Serine	OH
	Threonine	OH
Acidic	Aspartate	COO
	Glutamate	COO
Basic	Lysine	NH_3^+
	Arginine	
	Histidine	

B

Cross-bridge between cysteine residues formed by disulfide bridge

Figure 1–2 *A*, R-groups of selected amino acids. These can be classified by the nature of the R-groups, as these groups are of particular importance in protein structure. Some are hydrophobic (e.g., phenylalanine, leucine, methionine) and will seek the interior of the protein during protein folding, while the charged and polar groups interact with water at the protein surface. *B*, The disulfide bridge formed using the side chains of cysteine residues found within protein sequences.

popularity of restaurants that do not use MSG and are denoted ⌐MSG⌐). Positively charged or basic R-groups are found in the amino acids lysine, arginine, and histidine (see Figure 1–2A).

While the aliphatic side groups, the aromatic side groups of phenylalanine and tryptophan, and the side group of methionine are hydrophobic (they tend to avoid contact with water), the polar side groups (e.g., those of serine, threonine, and tyrosine) and charged side groups are hydrophilic and readily interact with water.

You should realize that once amino acids are linked by peptide bonds within proteins, the peptide bonds themselves are not charged, although there is a definite polarity to each peptide bond. Polarity means that a bond shows an uneven distribution of charge so that atoms associated with the bond may have a partial-negative or -positive character. More important contributors to the distinctive charge and polarity of a protein are the various R-groups containing alcohol, thiol, carboxyl, and amino groups (as well as the N-terminal and C-terminal amino acids in a protein that have a free amino and a free carboxyl group).

Protein structure is a large area of investigation that is being pursued by advanced technologies, such as x-ray crystallography and nuclear magnetic resonance (NMR). A variety of different structures are associated with proteins. Each protein does have a distinct, overall three-dimensional shape. However, when you look inside this large protein structure, you will be able to identify smaller component substructures that can be found in many other proteins. One analogy would be "faces" that children could build using different kinds of dry pasta. The faces would likely be very different, but on close examination, you would see that each face contained elements of macaroni, rotini, linguini, and so on. One of the simplest of the component substructures is the α-helix (Figure 1–3A). In this structure, often shown as a cylinder, a number of amino acids linked in sequence by peptide bonds within the protein form a coil (a little like a spiral staircase). In this structure, the R-groups of component amino acids are oriented to the outside of the helix. Another simple structure is the β-sheet, which is an extended, open expanse of amino acids in sequence, often represented by a flat arrow (see Figure 1–3B). Both the helix and the sheet are stabilized by interactions between the N–H and C=O groups found in different peptide bonds. These interactions are known as H-bonds. The ability to form these helical or sheet substructures is often dictated by the nature of the amino acids in linear sequence within the protein. Proteins can have varying contents of these two types of substructure.

The overall three-dimensional shape of the protein comes from the bringing together of different substructures from all over the protein linear sequence so that different helices or sheets may associate with each other. Often, this overall folding pattern is driven by water, as amino acids with nonpolar R-groups are forced together toward the inside of the protein to

A

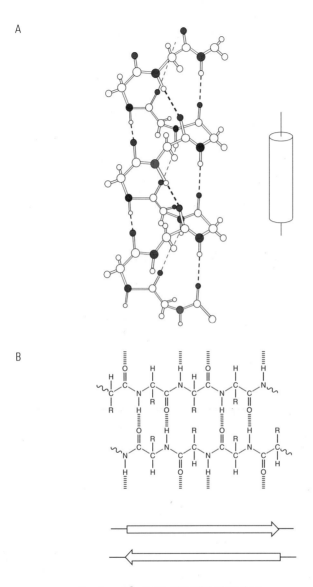

B

Structure of β-sheet (antiparallel orientation)

Figure 1–3 Component substructures seen within the three-dimensional structure of proteins. These structures are formed by sequences of amino acids and are stabilized by noncovalent bonds (H-bonds shown by dotted or hashed lines) that utilize the C=O and N-H components of peptide bonds. *A*, The α-helix, a coil of amino acids (often represented by a cylinder). Here, R-groups of amino acids are oriented to the outside of the coil. *B*, The β-sheet, an open structure often represented by a flat arrow, and bonding between sheets is often found. The orientation of the β-sheet is shown by the direction of the arrow, so that → indicates a direction from N to C, or from amino to carboxyl group of each amino acid.

avoid contact with the aqueous environment, while charged and polar amino acid residues localize themselves on the protein surface for interaction with water. One image might be that of a single line of dogs (six huskies and six poodles) harnessed to a sled that was to transport you across the Arctic. Each dog could represent a different amino acid. Imagine what would happen if the huskies (dogs numbered 1, 3, 6, 7, 9, and 12 in harness) loved the snow, while the poodles were deadly afraid of it. After a period of re-arrangement (folding) just as you begin your journey, you would find an interesting configuration (three-dimensional shape) where all the huskies were still in contact with the snow, while the poodles were balanced on top of you and the sled. Hopefully, there is an obvious moral here for your next land trip to Dawson Creek/Juneau/Murmansk.

On the basis of their overall shapes, proteins can be classified into two large classes. The globular proteins are those that are water soluble, folded approximately into compact spheres with a classic hydrophilic surface and hydrophobic interior. The globular proteins are particularly dynamic and can bind a variety of specific biologic molecules. An example of a globular protein is myoglobin, the oxygen-binding protein of muscle (Figure 1–4). In myoglobin, you can see the component α-helices within the overall three-dimensional structure. The second class comprises the fibrous proteins. These are elongated, thread-like, and water insoluble and usually play structural roles as mechanically tough proteins found in teeth, bones, tendons, and skin. They often consist of a purely helical structure that continues through the whole expanse of the protein (see Figure 1–4). Examples of fibrous proteins are collagen and α-keratin (found in hair, skin, and fingernails). At Thanksgiving and the December holidays, you may have close encounters with these fibrous proteins constituting the tough and rubbery

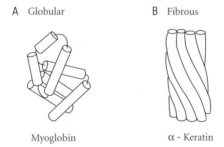

A   Globular   B   Fibrous

Myoglobin   α - Keratin

Figure 1–4 Structures of globular and fibrous proteins. *A*, The globular protein myoglobin that has eight different α-helices, folded to give a roughly spherical shape. *B*, The fibrous protein α-keratin. Fibrous proteins are often considered cables of helical structure, and often the cables interact with each other.

linear connections between the muscle and bone found at the ends of turkey drumsticks. Alternatively, if there is no large poultry at hand, you may take your own hand, place it flat on a surface, palm down, and, moving each of your fingers upward, observe the tendons that facilitate this process. You can certainly try these activities at home, although after weeks of human anatomy you may find these observations only too familiar.

There are some proteins that are tough but are not based on helical structure. Silk, for example, is made up of the protein fibroin that consists of interlocking arrays of sheets. Besides being a desirable fabric (for pajamas and handkerchiefs), silk is remarkably strong. In the days of the American Old West, when gunfighters carried out their deadly duels, it was the habit to sport a silk handkerchief in a jacket breast pocket. The breast pocket also served, apparently, as your opponent's target of choice in a gunfight. Fast forward to the present day when certain researchers began to look into gunslinger graves in various old "Boot Hills." They did unearth a number of mortal remains that showed evidence of death by gunshot wounds. Within some of the mouldering chest cavities of these individuals, they found silk handkerchiefs, intact, and bearing within them the slugs that killed the gunfighters; the handkerchiefs were virtually pushed unbroken into the chest.

Proteins can be made up of both β-sheet and α-helical structures, brought together by the process of protein folding, which occurs as the protein is being assembled using constituent amino acids. You should also remember our earlier comments on the dynamic nature of proteins, as the shape or conformation of proteins can be altered by interaction with other molecules. Because of this ability to modify their form, proteins seem to be almost alive, responding to the ever-changing environment within cells, blood, or extracellular fluid.

PROTEINS OF MUSCLE

Now we have the opportunity to look at some specific proteins in detail. Obviously, muscle makes up a considerable portion of the human body and is of particular interest in skeletal muscle, heart, and blood vessels, and in the study of cardiovascular physiology. Let's start with skeletal or voluntary muscle, which was one of the first areas for intensive biochemical study of proteins in the mid-1960s.

Skeletal muscle is designated as striated because of its characteristic repetitive banding pattern. This can be seen in the element of structure called the **myofibril** (Figure 1–5), which itself is a unit of the muscle fibers, which, in turn, make up the muscle fasciculus. Each myofibril is composed of a series of functional units called **sarcomeres**. Considering the striated appearance, each sarcomere is delimited by two Z lines within the I bands

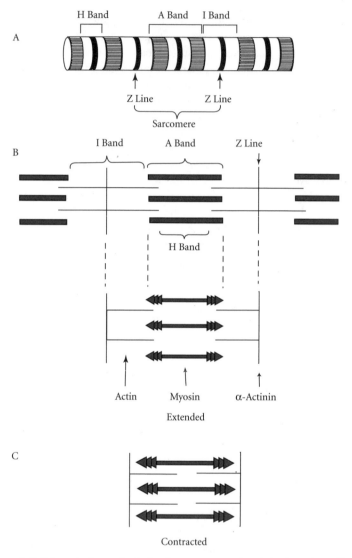

Figure 1–5 Schematic diagram for the banding patterns seen in a skeletal muscle myofibril and the corresponding protein filaments. *A*, Myofibril showing the sarcomere unit. *B*, Banding patterns in the extended muscle. *C*, Myosin–actin interactions in muscle showing the arrow-like head groups of myosin interacting with actin to give the contracted state.

and each sarcomere has an H band. The smaller H band is contained within the A band that runs between the I bands. So much for the histologic framework. However, the banding pattern is important to consider because it results from the positioning of the muscle proteins within the sarcomere.

Thick filaments are found in the A band and are principally made of the protein myosin (see Figure 1–5). Thin filaments are found within the I band and also continue into the A band; the proteins actin, tropomyosin, and troponin are found in these filaments. Actin is the predominant of these three proteins. In cross-section, each thin filament is surrounded by three thick filaments, and each thick filament is surrounded by six thin filaments. The various bands show the nature of the overlap of thick and thin filaments. The Z line (composed of the protein α-actinin) links the thin filaments of actin. Thick and thin filaments interact by cross-bridges, indicated by the "arrowheads" on the thick filaments (see Figure 1–5).

Actin and myosin are the two principal proteins of muscle. G-actin is a monomer (a single protein or polypeptide) that makes up 20 to 25% of the weight of muscle. Monomers of G-actin can polymerize to form F-actin, although the bonds between the G-actin monomers are not covalent (Figure 1–6). F-actin has a double helical configuration and makes up the backbone of the structure of the thin filament. Also associated with the F-actin are the proteins troponin and tropomyosin, which play a role in muscle contraction.

Myosin makes up some 60 to 70% of muscle protein. Unlike F-actin, myosin is not constructed of small monomers but, rather, is composed of two long polypeptide chains (the heavy chains) and four associated light chains. As such, myosin can be referred to as a hexamer of subunits. The heavy chains are remarkable because they are largely made up of intertwining helical structures (rather like fibrous proteins), but each ending in a globular head (Figure 1–7). Associated with each globular head are two light chains, which have the ability to bind calcium ions. The globular heads of the heavy chains effectively form noncovalent cross-bridges with F-actin, and this interaction is really the basis of skeletal muscle contraction. Myosin and F-actin bind together to form the actin–myosin complex.

The interesting hybrid-like structure of myosin was revealed by the biochemical dissection of the myosin molecule. Rather like William Harvey,

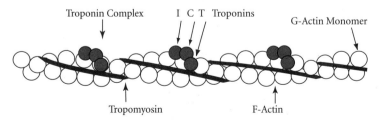

Figure 1–6 Schematic diagram of F-actin with its associated proteins. F-actin is shown as a double helix of G-actin monomers, with shorter tropomyosin strands and the troponin complex (I-, C-, and T-subunits). Adapted from Murray RK, Granner DK, Mayes PA, Rodwell VW. Harper's biochemistry. 25th ed. Stamford (CT): Appleton and Lange; 2000.

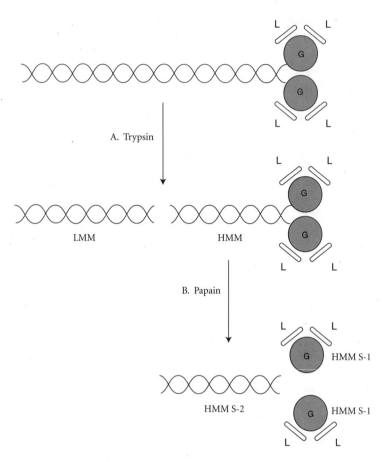

Figure 1–7 Biochemical dissection of myosin. Myosin can be hydrolyzed by the enzyme trypsin to give heavy meromyosin (HMM) and light meromyosin (LMM). In turn, HMM can be broken by the enzyme papain to yield S-1, containing the globular head groups (G) associated with myosin light chains, and S-2. The location of myosin ATPase in the globular heads could thus be shown. Adapted from Murray RK, Granner DK, Mayes PA, Rodwell VW. Harper's biochemistry. 25th ed. Stamford (CT): Appleton and Lange; 2000.

who in the 17th century postulated the mechanism of blood flow through the body by actual experimentation and dissection, it was necessary for biochemists to attempt to break down the myosin molecule to study its component parts and understand how they might play a role in muscle contraction.

This biochemical dissection of myosin was carried out using a class of proteins called **enzymes**. We shall discuss enzymes in detail in Chapter 3. At this point, we need to know that enzymes accelerate chemical reactions and are very specific in the biochemical reactions they catalyze. For example, when you eat and digest a steak, enzymes work in your intestine to break down these muscle proteins to their constituent amino acids. If a steak is not your preferred source of dietary protein, you would perhaps be better picturing yourself digesting tofu or a veggie-dog. At any rate, the digestion of plant or animal protein is carried out by enzymes that are secreted by your pancreas and are activated within your intestine. One of these enzymes is called **trypsin**, and it specifically cleaves or hydrolyzes peptide bonds in proteins at arginine or lysine residues. In this enzyme-catalyzed reaction, a water molecule is used to break the peptide bond. Trypsin is called a **protease** because it degrades protein, and the suffix -ase is often used to denote enzymes. As lysine and arginine have positively charged side chains (or R-groups), you can appreciate that trypsin has a three-dimensional structure that accommodates either of these interesting side chains so that the nearby peptide bond can be broken.

When the heavy myosin chain is mixed with trypsin, it is broken into two parts, one called **heavy meromyosin**, containing the globular head of the molecule and about a third of the helical chain, and the other part designated **light meromyosin**, containing the rest of the helical chain (see Figure 1–7). As this experiment was rather a success, the biochemists were encouraged to attempt another enzyme dissection. For these experiments, they used another enzyme called **papain**. You may have encountered it if you have made sorties into the culinary world, that is, if you actually have some experience in preparing your own steak. Papain is also known as a meat tenderizer and can be used on tougher cuts of meat once you have subjected them to a certain amount of physical abuse. Papain comes from papaya, and if you have eaten fresh forms of this fruit (and, parenthetically, are able to tolerate the smell), you may also feel the effects of its constituent enzyme, which can begin to hydrolyze proteins in the lining of your mouth. When papain is added to heavy meromyosin, it very effectively hydrolyzes another peptide bond and releases the globular head groups. These globular units are referred to as S-1. Papain is less selective than trypsin in the peptide bonds that it can break. The fact that papain so neatly cleaved the globular units suggested that there could be an area at the junction of the globular unit and the helical chain that was structurally more susceptible to cleavage by this enzyme. It was later appreciated that this susceptible region operated rather like a hinge to allow movement of the globular unit within the myosin molecule.

The whole point of producing these fragments from heavy meromyosin was to help determine the functions of individual fragments. For example, it was found that both heavy meromyosin and, more specifically, S-1 possess an enzymatic activity. This activity was not that of a protease but, rather, the activity of an enzyme called **ATPase**. ATP (or adenosine triphosphate) will also be described in more detail when we come to Chapter 7, but in the meantime, you should know that ATP is a molecule that possesses substantial chemical energy. In other words, there is considerable energy stored in certain chemical bonds of ATP. Thus, when there is a need for energy, say within a muscle cell, ATP is degraded, usually with the release of inorganic phosphate. Indeed, the action of the globular ATPase accomplishes this precise degradation, and the energy released is used in muscle contraction. The S-1 fragment was found to bind ATP as well as the light myosin chains. Interestingly, S-1 could also bind F-actin, and the S-1 fragments actually looked like arrowheads on the surface of the F-actin (remember the arrowheads shown in Figure 1–5). However, this binding to F-actin occurred only when ATP was absent. Apparently, the binding of ATP to myosin results in a change in the shape of myosin so that the binding of F-actin is greatly reduced. Remember our comments that proteins seem to be almost living molecules, responding very profoundly to the presence of other molecules. As we shall see, these binding and structural features of myosin are very important in the mechanism of striated muscle contraction.

BIOCHEMISTRY OF MUSCLE CONTRACTION

On the basis of the biochemical nature of the S-1 fragment and the very characteristic histology of striated muscle, a theory for muscle contraction founded on actin–myosin interactions emerged from these studies. Initially, myosin binds with ATP, and the ATP is subsequently hydrolyzed by the globular ATPase (Figure 1–8). As a result, myosin changes conformation and is able to bind F-actin with increased affinity. This is the basis of the genera-

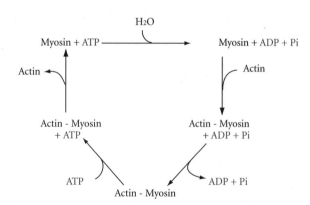

Figure 1–8 Biochemistry of muscle contraction. A cycle in which myosin ATPase converts ATP into ADP and inorganic phosphate (Pi), allowing actin to bind to myosin. The loss of ADP and Pi initiates the power stroke in which myosin pulls the actin light chains and produces the contraction event. Subsequently, ATP interacts with the actin–myosin complex, facilitating the release of actin and relaxation.

tion of the cross-bridges between the thick and thin filaments. Following the binding of actin, there is a release of the products of hydrolysis of ATP from myosin. These are inorganic phosphate and ADP (adenosine diphosphate). This release initiates another change in the conformation of myosin, effectively pulling the actin closer to the center of the sarcomere. This is known as the **power stroke**. Remember the hinge region between the globular head and the helical parts of myosin? This region allows the globular head to move along the F-actin, pulling the F-actin, as the main helical portion of myosin remains immobile. It is believed that the globular head moves by rotation (Figure 1–9). The series of interactions of the globular head with F-actin constitute the formation of cross-bridges within the actin–myosin complexes.

To simulate this (something you can try at home), place your hand on a table so that the "heel" of your palm (close to your wrist) is in contact with the table, while the rest of your palm and fingers and thumb are in the air. Think of your hand as the movable globular unit of myosin and your wrist and arm as the helical part of myosin. Arrange a shoestring (the F-actin) so that one end is held under the part of your palm contacting the table and the length of the string runs in a straight line below your outstretched palm and fingers. Now curve the rest of your palm and outstretched fingers and bring them down in sequence like a crescent onto the shoe-string while pulling the string toward your wrist. Your wrist rises up above the table but does not move along the table. Thus, the globular head rotates along F-actin and pulls on it. This is the basis of the contraction of striated muscle.

To complete the cycle, ATP now binds to the actin–myosin complex at the globular head and in so doing reduces the affinity of myosin for actin.

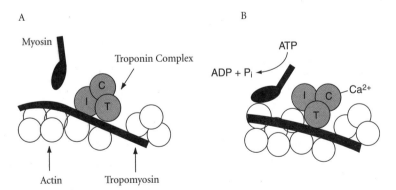

Figure 1–9 Troponin complex and tropomyosin involvement in contraction. *A*, In the absence of free calcium ions, the troponin complex effectively blocks myosin from making contact with actin. *B*, With rising levels of free Ca^{++}, Ca^{++} binds to troponin C and in so doing removes the block to actin–myosin interaction so that a contractile sequence can be initiated. Only one G-head for myosin is shown to simplify the diagram. Adapted from Ganong WF. Review of medical physiology. 17th ed. Norwalk (CT): Appleton and Lange; 1995.

F-actin is released, and this is the relaxation phase, which depends on the binding of ATP. As ATP is once again hydrolyzed by myosin ATPase, the contraction phase begins anew and can result in further motion of the F-actin toward the center of the sarcomere. Presuming that you have not irreparably damaged your hand carrying out the last series of acrobatics, you can think of a series of arc-like motions of your palm and fingers along the actin shoestring, first coming down onto the string pulling it toward the wrist, then releasing the string, dropping the heel of the palm onto the string (fingers up in the air again) and going through the arc movement over again. Each time you may pull the string several inches along. You might ask: what prevents the F-actin from slipping back to its original position? The answer is that there are very many globular head groups in association with the thin filaments (a little like many hands on one rope in a tug of war). Thus, dissociation of one set of globular head groups can be balanced by others still pulling on the filament. The general mechanism of striated muscle contraction is known as the "sliding filament cross-bridge model" and was first proposed independently by Henry and Andrew Huxley on the basis of initial electron microscopic observations of muscle.

You can see the importance of energy generated by the breakdown of ATP in the cycle. Also apparent is the need for ATP to enter the relaxation phase (when myosin disengages from actin). Here, we can consider the physician in the role of coroner (a part that has had singular success in television, likely because of the forensic aspects and our interest in mystery and mayhem). When someone dies, levels of ATP in the body decrease rapidly. ATP is made during the breakdown of fuel compounds, such as glucose, when oxygen is available to cells. Death precludes circulation; thus, oxygen (and glucose) supplies dwindle. In the absence of ATP, the actin–myosin complex in its contracted state cannot dissociate; thus, there is a gradual stiffening of muscles, called **rigor mortis**. Following death, calcium levels within cells also increase, and as we shall see, this promotes the contractile response. As this information may possibly come your way near Hallowe'en, it makes it that much more difficult to explain the human kinetics associated with "night of the living dead" films or equally ancient Michael Jackson videos that are popular at this time of year.

Tropomyosin and the Troponin Complex

One issue that may have come to mind during the discussion of this contractile mechanism is how do you control it? Leaving behind the concept of walking cadavers, if you are breathing normally and there is a healthy supply of ATP, why are you not in a continuous series of contractile responses? The answer simply is that there are various regulatory features imposed on muscular contraction. Rather like the 8-year-old who realizes that (1) the candy store is open, and (2) the piggy bank is close at hand, the inevitable factor (the parent) steps in between the young hero and the front door to moderate any rash spending impulses.

As can be seen in Figure 1–6, F-actin is not alone in the thin filament. Draped around the F-actin polymers are paired chains of a protein called **tropomyosin**. Also found on the F-actin chain is troponin, or more precisely the troponin complex, composed of three different protein subunits. These subunits are called T, I, and C. The T-subunit binds to tropomyosin, the I-subunit can play a role in blocking the binding of myosin to F-actin, and the C-subunit binds calcium ions. Subunit C is similar to a well-known and ubiquitous calcium-binding protein called **calmodulin**, which can bind as many as four calcium ions per protein molecule.

The troponin complex is the "brain" behind the control of striated muscle contraction. In muscle that is not excited or activated, the I-subunit prevents the binding of myosin to F-actin. It has been proposed that the troponin complex can deploy tropomyosin to block the actin–myosin interaction. Thus, ATP cannot trigger a contractile event on its own. However, when muscle is excited, another regulatory player enters the scheme. This is the calcium ion, which enters the muscle cell on excitation. You should appreciate that levels of free calcium ions are very low within the cellular cytoplasm before muscular excitation. Calcium, bound to other molecules, is present, but it is the rising level of *free* calcium that triggers a variety of interesting responses in activated or stimulated cells. In striated muscle, calcium will bind to the C-subunit of troponin, and this promotes an interaction between the C- and I-subunits, which effectively disengages the troponin complex from F-actin, permitting a myosin–actin interaction. When muscle recovers from the stimulation or excitation, levels of *free* calcium drop back to normal, and the inhibition of muscle contraction controlled by the troponins can be established once again.

Calcium and the Control of Muscle Contraction

While the troponin complex is the agent that directly regulates contraction, the complex, in turn, relies on calcium levels within the cell. Skeletal muscle is under nervous control, and there are neuromuscular junctions in which nerves interface with muscle. As shown in Figure 1–10, the nerve ending at the neuromuscular junction carries the neurotransmitter acetylcholine within the synaptic vesicles. Upon nerve stimulation (e.g., when you wish to raise your arm), acetylcholine is released into the narrow gap (the synaptic cleft) between the nerve ending and the muscle membrane. Acetylcholine is used to relay a message from one excitable cell (the nerve) to another (muscle). In the muscle membrane at the neuromuscular junction are proteins called **acetylcholine receptors** (yet another example of protein

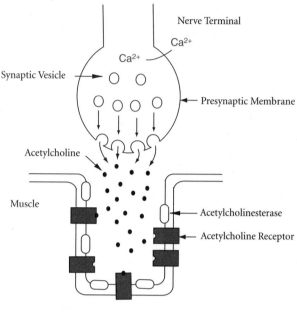

Junctional Fold

Figure 1–10 Events following the release of the neurotransmitter acetylcholine at the neuromuscular junction. With nerve excitation, the nerve terminal is depolarized, calcium enters the terminal, and synaptic vesicles carrying acetylcholine release their contents into the synaptic cleft. Acetylcholine can interact with acetylcholine receptors in the muscle plasma membrane and initiate a depolarization of this membrane. Acetylcholine can also be hydrolyzed by acetylcholinesterase to inactive components, thus removing excess acetylcholine and limiting the stimulatory power of the neurotransmitter. Adapted from Murray RK, Granner DK, Mayes PA, Rodwell VW. Harper's biochemistry. 25th ed. Stamford (CT): Appleton and Lange; 2000.

function). Each acetylcholine receptor is composed of five distinct proteins called **subunits**. Each subunit spans the plasma membrane, and the five subunits come together to construct a central pore that serves as the ligand-gated channel. The acetylcholine receptor in the muscle plasma membrane (or sarcolemma) binds the ligand (released acetylcholine) in a noncovalent manner and undergoes a conformational change.

This change in the structure of the acetylcholine receptor results in the opening of the channel that permits the movement of ions across the membrane. Most cells have an unequal distribution of sodium and potassium ions across the plasma membrane so that there is a high concentration of sodium ions outside the cell and a high concentration of potassium ions inside. A resting cell has what is called a **membrane potential** because of the unequal numbers of positively charged ions on either side of the membrane. When acetylcholine binds to its receptor and the channel opens, there is an inrush of sodium ions into the cell. The acetylcholine receptor is a ligand-gated channel, whose action is depicted in Figure 1–11. This entry of cations leads to a loss of membrane potential, which is called **depolarization**. This depolarization of the sarcolemma generates an electrical impulse that spreads along the plasma membrane throughout the component sarcomeres. The acetylcholine receptor can be blocked by the drug curare, a natural compound used by certain tribes along the Amazon as an arrow poison. Blocking the acetylcholine receptor results in paralysis of muscles and death.

The sarcolemma also contains an enzyme called **acetylcholinesterase** (see Figure 1–10). As suggested by its name, acetylcholinesterase effectively breaks acetylcholine into its two component parts: acetate and choline. Neither component can trigger depolarization. Thus, acetylcholinesterase clears the synaptic cleft of excess acetylcholine so that there will not be prolonged stimulation of the acetylcholine receptor. In this way, the depolarization initiated by the release of acetylcholine is controlled by this enzyme. There are poisons that can very effectively and irreversibly inhibit acetylcholinesterase

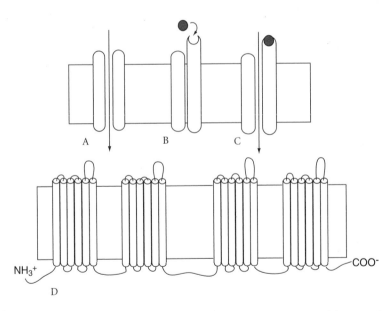

Figure 1–11 Schematics of channels found within plasma membrane. *A*, Voltage-gated channel, which opens with depolarization and allows the passage of cations. *B, C*, Ligand-gated channel, such as the acetylcholine receptor, that opens in response to ligand (●) binding, allowing cation movement. *D*, The α-subunit of the Na⁺ channel. This is made up of 24 membrane-spanning protein regions, organized in four sets of six regions each. The loops represent intracellular or extracellular areas of protein sequence that link the transmembrane regions. The structure, as shown, is spread out, but the various transmembrane regions come together in the membrane to form a pore or channel for Na⁺ ions.

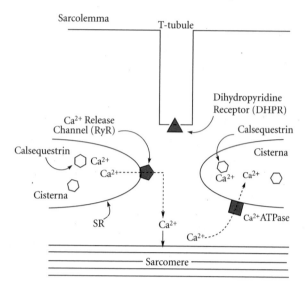

Figure 1–12 Depolarization of skeletal muscle and the fate of calcium. With depolarization spreading over the muscle plasma membrane and the T-tubule system, the dihydropyridine receptor (DHPR), a channel for calcium ions, opens. The DHPR is in close proximity to the ryanodine receptor (RyR), which is activated following DHPR opening. RyR provides Ca^{2+} from the cisterna of the sarcoplasmic reticulum (SR), initiating contractile events. Ca^{2+} released by the RyR channel is quickly moved back into the cisterna by the action of Ca^{2+}-ATPase. Adapted from Murray RK, Granner DK, Mayes PA, Rodwell VW. Harper's biochemistry. 25th ed. Stamford (CT): Appleton and Lange; 2000.

and cause death because of continuous stimulation of muscle cells. These poisons can be used as insecticides (such as parathion) to protect crops. However, such is the nature of evolution that insects and humans both have acetylcholinesterase, and both can be killed by exposure to these poisons. We shall consider the chemical action of these inhibitors of acetylcholinesterase in Chapter 3, but you should be very aware of the substances, potentially dangerous to young children, kept in garages or in the garden sheds of gardening enthusiasts. Garages also often contain more mundane substances that are also toxic. For example, a mouthful of methanol-based windshield wiper antifreeze can be deadly.

Let's return to our normal example of muscular excitation, removed from the influences of rose dust or aphid spray. The spreading depolarization that begins with the neuromuscular junction travels along the transverse tubule (T-tubule) system, a system of channels connected to the sarcolemma and permitting communication with the filaments of the component sarcomeres (Figure 1–12). The depolarization of the T-tubule system can open up what is termed a **slow calcium voltage channel** in the membrane of the T-tubule. This channel also goes by the name **dihy-**

dropyridine receptor and is a protein that (like the acetylcholine receptor) spans a membrane. Dihydropyridine is a very effective inhibitor that binds to the receptor, and channels can be given names for the ligands or chemicals that bind and influence their function. Thus, calcium ions enter into the cytoplasm (or sarcoplasm) via the dihydropyridine receptor, although the quantity of calcium coming from this voltage-gated channel does not play a major role in muscle contraction. The dihydropyridine receptor in the T-tubule membrane is in very close proximity to another receptor, which is located in the membranes of the intracellular sarcoplasmic reticulum (SR) and controls the release of calcium ions from the SR. The SR is a system of tubules surrounding cisternae that function as intracellular stores of calcium ions sequestered from the sarcoplasm and the contractile filaments.

The calcium channel in the SR is known as the **ryanodine receptor** (RyR) because it binds a plant alkaloid called ryanodine, which can control the function of this channel. The dihydropyridine receptor acts as a voltage sensor so that with depolarization, the dihydropyridine receptor can activate the RyR and facilitate a robust release of calcium ions from the store of calcium within the SR. The rise in sarcoplasmic free calcium ions is from a very low resting concentration (10^{-7} M) upward to 10^{-5} M. This calcium interacts with the C-subunit of the troponin complex, allowing myosin–actin interaction as the prelude to muscle contraction.

As you are perhaps beginning to appreciate, any of these dramatic events, such as the activation of the acetylcholine and ryanodine receptors and the activation of the muscle contraction cycle by calcium, must inevitably have control mechanisms that allow a return to the resting state. Otherwise, all our voluntary muscles would be seized in contraction following a stimulus. With the entry of calcium ions into the sarcoplasm, there are compensating mechanisms that operate to pump calcium ions back into the cisternae of the sarcoplasmic reticulum. This is a little like water coming into a basement during a storm—it triggers a prompt response, particularly if you happen to live in the basement. The response requires energy, either you mopping up the water and relaying it to a drain (hoping, of course, that the water did not enter through the drain in the first place!), or the involvement of a pump, which will pump water to the outside.

Just as a pump can push water outside your basement dwelling, so too does a protein, called a calcium pump, that spans the membrane of the sarcoplasmic reticulum and functions to drive calcium ions into the cisterna (see Figure 1–12). As the cisternae have higher levels of calcium than does the sarcoplasm, this pump does require energy in the form of ATP, the molecule that supplies energy for muscular contraction. You can see how ATP is really a currency that can be used in a variety of biochemical circumstances that require energy—somewhat like a MasterCard for your cells. Perhaps a better analogy is your library card that has a chip in it. You need, of course, to activate the card using money (e.g., generate ATP during the breakdown of fuel compounds) to allow you to carry out a variety of activities, such as making photocopies, paying fines, or even purchasing snack food. The calcium pump is, thus, called a Ca^{2+}ATPase, as the pump has an enzymatic function that degrades ATP to provide energy for the movement of the calcium ions into the cisternae of the SR.

CARDIAC MUSCLE COMPARED WITH VOLUNTARY MUSCLE

The heart is a rather specialized muscular pump that excites a great deal more interest than voluntary muscle simply because the effects of malfunction of cardiac muscle are more immediately spectacular and life threatening. Portrayals of emergency room procedure rarely, if ever, show the application of the electric paddles to the forearm, for example. Cardiac muscle has certain similarities to voluntary muscle, in that it is striated and also relies on the interaction of actin and myosin for contraction and the troponin system for regulation of the contractile cycle. Unlike voluntary muscle, cardiac muscle relies more heavily on the entry of extracellular calcium ions for contraction, as this calcium entry appears to stimulate the ryanodine receptor and facilitate a larger release of calcium ions into the sarcoplasm.

Amazingly, heart muscle has its own rhythmicity and will continue to beat on its own, provided that the heart is supplied with extracellular calcium ions. Another interesting feature not seen in voluntary muscle is that the heart has a number of different receptors located at its sarcolemma (or plasma membrane), such as **α- and β-adrenergic receptors** that respond to adrenaline (also known as epinephrine). Adrenaline released into your bloodstream will increase your heart rate (by interaction with β-adrenergic receptors) and cardiac output. Thus, if you are watching a particularly frightening movie, your heart rate could easily increase, as would your blood pressure.

To return to the heart, there are certainly situations where the effects of adrenaline can be deleterious. Patients who have experienced myocardial infarction can have erratic heart rhythms that are exacerbated by adrenaline. Thus, drugs can be used to block the β-adrenergic receptors on the plasma membrane of the cardiac myocytes. You may see patients who have increased blood pressure as a result of stress (quite possibly brought on by a trip to your office!). It is important to determine the nature of the hypertension, but a β-blocker, such as propranolol, may effectively treat hypertension caused by a stressful lifestyle. Cardiac muscle is responsive to adrenaline, noradrenaline, and acetylcholine, while only the last compound controls contraction of voluntary muscle.

THE HEART AND ION TRANSPORT

We have mentioned briefly the use of proteins as channels and pumps. Now, here, we must consider the chemistry of transport across biological membranes in greater detail. Membranes function as hydrophobic barriers around cells and organelles so that water-soluble compounds and ions do not pass readily across them. Thus, there is a need for transporters to regulate flow into and out of cells and for organelles within cells. Indeed, this is one of the important rationales for a membrane: to maintain a specific microenvironment by controlling the entry and exit of molecules and inorganic ions. A cell is not simply a bag of components. Rather, it is a highly organized collection of interacting compartments, whose separation optimizes efficiency. For example, mitochondria are sites of oxidation-reduction reactions that result in the generation of chemical energy in the form of ATP. It would be unreasonable to try to run these oxidative cycles in the same environment that you wish to synthesize molecules (such as proteins) and polysaccharides (such as glycogen).

Transport can be divided into a number of types, depending on the transporter and the nature of the transport itself. For example, there is simple diffusion, in which there is no transporter, and ions or solutes simply diffuse across the membrane. The rate of this diffusion is inversely related to the polarity of the molecule. Thus, a hydrophobic drug may readily diffuse through a membrane, while it takes longer for glucose to enter by simple diffusion and even longer for sodium ions to enter by this mechanism. Simple diffusion is driven by a concentration gradient, as molecules or ions move into areas of low concentration. Once the concentration is the same inside and outside a cell, for example, the diffusion across the plasma membrane will cease.

Of course, relying on simple diffusion across a membrane to supply your cellular and organelle needs would be like waiting in January for a bus to take you into the city, a bus whose frequency, as we all know, varies directly with the ambient temperature. Thus, within membranes, there are specialized proteins that facilitate the passage of molecules and ions. We have already considered one of these: the acetylcholine receptor. The receptor actually controls a channel or pore that allows ions, such as sodium, to run down their concentration gradients. This channel permits rapid entry of sodium ions into the cell from the extracellular fluid, provoking a rapid depolarization of the cell membrane. The acetylcholine receptor is a ligand-gated channel (see Figure 1–11), responding to the binding of acetylcholine. Ligand-gated channels are often associated with intracellular proteins called **G-proteins**. The activation of G-proteins by the activation of the receptor leads to a variety of intracellular metabolic events that we will consider in Chapter 7. The dihydropyridine receptor of the T-tubule system is a voltage-gated channel (see Figure 1–11), opening up in response to depolarization events and allowing the passage of calcium ions into the cell.

There are voltage-gated channels for sodium, potassium, and calcium ions. The sodium channel comprises three different types of protein subunits. The largest is the α-subunit, which has four major domains that can form a pore for the movement of sodium ions (see Figure 1–11). Each of these domains consists of six membrane-spanning regions. Thus, the sodium channel is considered an integral membrane protein with 24 sequences of amino acids that can interact with the hydrophobic core of the membrane. The pore of the voltage-gated sodium channel can be blocked by tetrodotoxin or saxitoxin. The first toxin comes from the puffer fish, which you are unlikely to encounter outside Japanese restaurants (and then, hopefully, with its toxic organs removed). However, saxitoxin poisoning is commonly associated with marine shellfish, which can accumulate the toxin after consuming certain dinoflagellates. This is the so-called "red tide" (presumably the color associated with these microorganisms when they occur in considerably high numbers, although the color is not often readily seen from the shore), and warnings are often posted along the marine coasts proclaiming the dangers of eating shellfish. The sodium channel responds to depolarization spreading out from the neuromuscular junction and promotes further depolarization by allowing rapid entry of sodium ions.

Uptake of calcium from the sarcoplasm can occur via the calcium pump (Ca^{2+}ATPase), but a more important ion transporter in cardiac muscle is the Na^+-Ca^{2+} exchanger. This protein is a transporter but not a pump, as ATP is not required for its action. Instead, the large sodium ion gradient from outside to inside the cell is used to drive the removal of calcium ions from the sarcoplasm to outside the cell. Technically, this type of transport is known as **antiport** (Figure 1–13), since the one transporter protein handles the passage of both sodium and calcium ions, but in opposite directions. The exchanger moves three sodium ions into the cell for each calcium ion expelled from the cell. The Na^+-Ca^{2+} exchanger can operate in the reverse direction. For example, directly following the inrush of sodium ions into the cell in depolarization, the exchanger can effectively move sodium ions out of the cell and bring in calcium ions that can contribute to cardiac contraction. The Na^+-Ca^{2+} exchanger and other membrane transport proteins are shown schematically in Figure 1–14.

As we have noted earlier, resting cells have low concentrations of sodium ions (5 to 15 mM) in comparison with an extracellular concentration of about 145 mM, while there is also a high concentration of potassium ions (140 mM) within the cell, in comparison with 5 mM outside. This gradient of cations is accomplished by Na^+, K^+-ATPase, which is both a transporter and an enzyme. This transporter in the plasma membrane is a pump that uses ATP to drive sodium ions out of the cell while bringing potassium

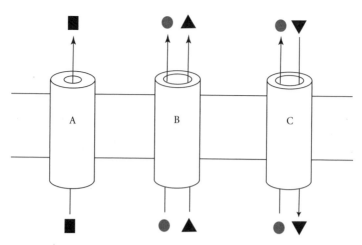

Figure 1–13 Types of membrane transport making use of membrane transport proteins. *A,* Uniport: when a single solute moves across the membrane. *B,* Symport: when two solutes are moved by a transporter in the same direction across the membrane. *C,* Antiport: when two solutes are moved in opposite directions across the membrane. For symport and antiport, at least one of the solutes is moving down its concentration gradient.

ions into the cell. In both cases, the movement of the ions is against a concentration gradient (Figure 1–15). The transport facilitated by Na$^+$, K$^+$-ATPase is a good example of **active transport**, using energy to drive the passage of solutes. This active transport mechanism is extremely important in establishing the membrane potential because the mechanism involves the outward passage of three sodium ions for every two potassium ions entering the cell. Na$^+$, K$^+$-ATPase accounts for the utilization of a considerable portion of the ATP of the cell. This is particularly true in nervous tissue, where up to 70% of cellular ATP can be expended in maintaining the sodium and potassium gradients across a relatively large cellular surface area. Brain is particularly at risk in ischemia (when blood supply is compromised in hemorrhage or stroke). This occurs because levels of ATP cannot be maintained without an adequate supply of glucose and oxygen, and existing cellular ATP concentrations are very quickly depleted by the ion pumps.

Na$^+$, K$^+$-ATPase establishes the sizeable sodium gradient across the cell that is important in the transport of calcium out of the cell (Na$^+$- Ca^{2+} exchanger) and is also involved in the transport of other compounds (e.g., the entry of amino acids into the cell for use in protein synthesis). As both amino acids and sodium ions move into the cell, this transport is called **symport**.

There is also a Na$^+$-H$^+$ exchanger in the plasma membrane that facilitates the outward movement of protons in exchange for the movement of incoming sodium ions down the sodium ion concentration gradient. Such an

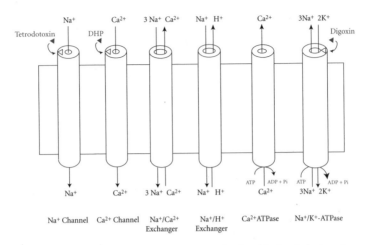

Figure 1–14 Schematic of various transporter proteins found in the plasma membrane of cardiac muscle. Filled triangles indicate inhibitors for individual transporters.

exchanger is important in the maintenance of cellular pH. Na⁺, K⁺-ATPase can be inhibited by the drug digoxin extracted from the plant *Digitalis purpurea* (purple foxglove). Given in appropriate doses, digoxin can provoke a rise in cellular sodium ion concentration, which via the Na⁺, Ca²⁺-exchanger elevates intracellular calcium to increase the strength of cardiac contractions.

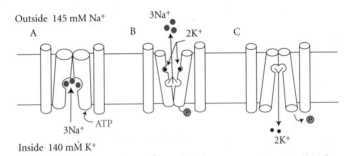

Figure 1–15 Biochemical mechanism of Na⁺, K⁺-ATPase at the plasma membrane. This enzyme facilitates active transport of Na⁺ ions out of the cell and K⁺ ions into the cell. By this process, large Na⁺ and K⁺ gradients are established across the plasma membrane. *A*, Three Na⁺ ions are bound to sites on the enzyme that are accessible to the cytoplasm. *B*, ATP is used to phosphorylate the enzyme, promoting a conformational change in the protein that now exposes the Na⁺ ions to the outside and facilitates their release. K⁺ ions now bind at the extracellular surface to K⁺ binding sites. *C*, Dephosphorylation of the enzyme permits a return to the original conformation with K⁺ ions released inside the cell.

SMOOTH MUSCLE: COMPARISON WITH STRIATED MUSCLE

Smooth muscle contains myosin, actin, and tropomyosin but lacks the tro-ponin complex. Thus, smooth muscle has a mechanism of contraction that differs from that found in skeletal and cardiac muscles. Contraction of smooth muscle is indeed a very important topic, as smooth muscle is found in the vascular system, gastrointestinal system, lung, and elsewhere. Thus, smooth muscle has considerable importance in a variety of diseases, includ-ing stroke, myocardial infarction, intestinal disorders, and asthma.

While smooth muscle does have myosin, the light chain of its myosin dif-fers from that found in striated muscle. Here, the interaction of F-actin with the myosin head group is prevented by the myosin light chain. The ATPase activity of the head group is thus inactive. This block to contraction can be removed by the phosphorylation of the light chain by an enzyme known as **myosin light chain kinase** (MLCK) (Figure 1–16). When the word "kinase" is used to describe an enzyme, it indicates that ATP is either used or produced by the enzyme-catalyzed reaction. In this case, MLCK uses ATP to phos-phorylate the hydroxyl side chains on serine and threonine amino acid residues in the light chain. Essentially, the enzyme is creating phosphate esters at these R-groups. When the light chain is phosphorylated, a confor-mational change in the protein allows the interaction of smooth muscle F-actin and myosin. The action of MLCK is regulated by calcium, so this ion once again is involved in the control of contraction, although with a differ-ent mechanism in smooth muscle. When calcium ions enter smooth mus-cle cells, they bind to a protein called **calmodulin**. Remember, earlier, we compared troponin subunit C of skeletal muscle with calmodulin. Calmod-ulin has four binding sites for calcium ions and basically functions as a cal-cium sensor in the cell. The calcium–calmodulin complex activates MLCK, thus facilitating contraction. However, to return to a relaxed state, calcium levels fall, and so do levels of calcium–calmodulin, and the MLCK activity declines. Naturally, there is also a mechanism to remove phosphate from the phosphorylated myosin light chain, and this is catalyzed by a phosphatase enzyme that has no reliance on calcium for its activity. Thus, a cycle of light-chain phosphorylation and dephosphorylation can be achieved with the ris-ing and falling levels of free calcium ions in the cell.

Like cardiac muscle cells, smooth muscle cells also have receptors at the plasma membrane so that the cells can respond to hormone binding. For example, the binding of adrenaline to a β-adrenergic receptor leads to the activation of G-proteins (similar to the case for the acetylcholine receptor in voluntary muscle), and this, in turn, stimulates the production of what is called a **second messenger** (Figure 1–17). Thus, the hormone does not, in this case, enter the cell but, rather, stimulates within the cell the produc-tion of a molecule called **cyclic adenosine monophosphate** (or cAMP)

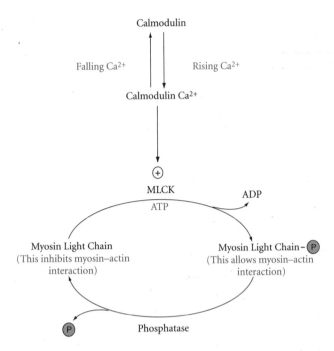

Figure 1–16 Mechanism of smooth muscle contraction. When levels of free Ca⁺⁺ increase within smooth muscle cells, Ca⁺⁺–calmodulin complexes are formed that activate myosin light chain kinase (MLCK). The phosphorylation of the myosin light chain facilitates the interaction of myosin and actin, and muscle contraction is promoted. With falling levels of free Ca⁺⁺, the MLCK activity declines and myosin light chains can be dephosphorylated by a phosphatase. Myosin light chains once again block myosin–actin interaction, and muscle relaxation is promoted.

from ATP by the enzyme adenylate cyclase. cAMP is the second messenger, and it triggers a sequence of biochemical events within the cell that leads to a definite physiologic response.

This situation may be compared to your reaction to a friend who telephones you in your hotel room to wake you in the morning. (Picture yourself in some luxurious Hilton Hotel in Cancun, if you will.) The telephone call triggers a series of responses from you (rising, showering, dressing, eating, leaving for a day's trip to the Mayan pyramids) that would possibly not happen should your friend forget to call you. The telephone call is like the second messenger (cAMP) that is initiated within your room by your friend's action from the outside.

cAMP was discovered in the 1950s by Earl Sutherland, who won the Nobel Prize for this novel finding of a second messenger. The generation of cAMP within the smooth muscle cell following adrenergic stimulation leads to the activation of an enzyme called **protein kinase A** (PKA) (see Fig-

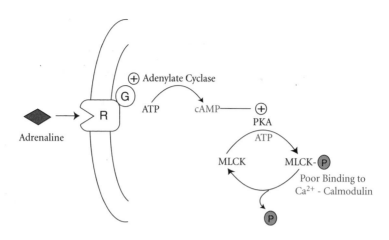

Figure 1–17 Action of adrenaline on smooth muscle. Binding to its receptor (R), adrenaline promotes the formation of the second messenger cAMP via G-protein activation of the enzyme adenylate cyclase. cAMP activates protein kinase A (PKA), which, in turn, phosphorylates MLCK (myosin light chain kinase). This form of MLCK has a much lower affinity for Ca^{2+}–calmodulin and cannot be as easily activated, promoting smooth muscle relaxation.

—or produces ATP 😊)
(see p. 21)

ure 1–17). In turn, this protein kinase (an enzyme that phosphorylates other proteins) will phosphorylate the enzyme MLCK. This phosphorylation of MLCK diminishes the affinity of the enzyme for the calcium–calmodulin complex and, thus, decreases the phosphorylation of the myosin light chain. In this manner, adrenergic receptor binding and generation of cAMP effectively reduce smooth muscle contractile responses to rising levels of cytoplasmic calcium. The response of smooth muscle to β-adrenergic stimulation is muscle relaxation.

There is another control mechanism of smooth muscle contraction that is not shared by voluntary or cardiac muscle. This involves the protein caldesmon. In resting muscle, caldesmon binds to actin and tropomyosin and prevents the myosin–actin interaction. However, caldesmon can bind the calcium–calmodulin complex, and so, with rising cytoplasmic calcium within the smooth muscle cell, the caldesmon interaction with actin is diminished, allowing contraction by the actin–myosin interaction. It is also possible to phosphorylate caldesmon using a protein kinase, and this modified caldesmon will also be unable to prevent actin–myosin interaction (Figure 1–18). *2 mechanisms to disable*

As you are perhaps beginning to understand, there is a variety of controls for smooth muscle contraction, underlying the importance of having diverse ways of regulation of smooth muscle. Indeed, there is one more, and before you may start saying "enough already," we might note that this mechanism involves a gas, made within your body, and whose absence figures largely in what is coyly referred to as ED (erectile dysfunction).

NITRIC OXIDE

what name would you think is not coy? Broken prick?

If you have a parent or grandparent with a heart condition, you may be aware that these patients are often prescribed nitroglycerine pills. These are generally taken for the onset of angina, pain caused by insufficient blood flow to the heart. The use of nitroglycerine pills leads to vasodilation and is of particular importance at the coronary arteries.

Nitroglycerine can serve as a source of nitrate for your cells, and certain of these can generate nitric oxide (NO) from the conversion of nitrate to nitrite and nitrite to NO (Figure 1–19). As it is a gas, NO can travel into cells and does not make use of a receptor at the cell surface. NO acts as a vasodilator that is involved in the control of blood pressure. Initially, it was observed that acetylcholine acted as a vasodilator in blood vessels. However, when this effect was studied further, it was noted that the effect of acetylcholine was not exerted directly on the smooth muscle of the vessel itself. When endothelial cells of the vessel were removed from the smooth muscle, there was no direct vasodilatory effect of acetylcholine. It appears that acetylcholine, interacting with its receptor on endothelial cells, triggers a rise in intracellular calcium and a formation of NO in the cytoplasm of the endothelial cell from the amino acid arginine, by the action of the enzyme NO synthase (NOS) (see Figure 1–19). NO diffuses from the endothelial cell and enters the underlying smooth muscle cells, where it stimulates the production of cyclic GMP (cGMP, a compound similar in structure to cAMP). cGMP

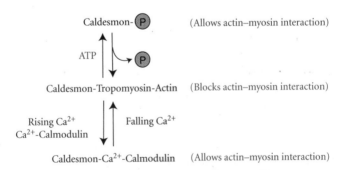

Figure 1–18 Role of caldesmon in smooth muscle contraction. Caldesmon is a protein that binds to tropomyosin and actin and prevents myosin–actin interaction. With rising levels of Ca^{2+}, Ca^{2+}-calmodulin binds to caldesmon, permitting access of actin to myosin and muscle contraction. A similar result follows the phosphorylation of caldesmon, as the phosphorylated protein does not bind actin. A phosphatase returns caldesmon to its original conformation, permitting interaction with tropomyosin–actin.

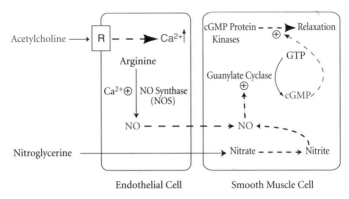

Figure 1–19 Formation of nitric oxide (NO). Acetylcholine interacts with its receptor (R) on the surface of an endothelial cell lining a blood vessel. This promotes the formation of NO from arginine by the action of NOS (nitric oxide synthase) activated by rising intracellular Ca^{2+}. NO can diffuse into nearby smooth muscle cells and activate guanylate cyclase to produce cyclic GMP (cGMP). This second messenger promotes muscle relaxation by the action of cGMP protein kinases. Nitroglycerine can provide nitrate leading to the formation of NO in muscle cells. Adapted from Murray RK, Granner DK, Mayes PA, Rodwell VW. Harper's biochemistry. 25th ed. Stamford (CT): Appleton and Lange; 2000.

(cyclic guanosine monophosphate), which also acts as a second messenger, can, in turn, activate certain cGMP-dependent protein kinases. The action of these kinases ultimately leads to smooth muscle relaxation. NO, thus, has the roles of vasodilator (and can relieve angina) and hypotensive agent, but it is also involved in penile erection. Thus, deficiencies in NO synthesis can be associated with erectile dysfunction. NO also inhibits platelet aggregation (an event important in the formation of thrombi, which can be formed as aggregates of platelets and fibrin following injury of blood vessels). Because of its chemical reactivity, NO has a very short half-life (about 3 to 4 seconds) in tissues of the body.

ENERGY SUPPLIES AND MUSCLE CONTRACTION

When you consider the contraction of voluntary, cardiac, or smooth muscle, there is a definite need for ATP that is used to power contraction. Thus, the supply of blood to muscle is of great importance, as it provides fuel substrates (such as glucose and fatty acids) and oxygen, which are vital for the formation of ATP. If a coronary artery (which, sad to say, is not a particularly large vessel) is blocked, heart muscle cells will die if they are totally deprived of these vital components for a certain length of time, and an infarct can be formed at the area of interruption of blood supply.

Thus, the generation of ATP is critical to cardiac and other muscle function. ATP can also be used in a wide variety of other reactions that support many different synthetic processes within the cell. In the process of generation of ATP, glucose or another fuel enters the cells from the blood and is broken down. The energy that is released is conserved, in part, by the formation of ATP. The breakdown of glucose initially involves a process called **glycolysis** (meaning splitting of sugar), which we shall deal with in more detail in Chapter 7. Muscle cells also have supplies of glycogen, a polymer of glucose, that can be broken down to supply the compound glucose-6-phosphate for glycolysis (Figure 1–20).

Glycolysis supplies some ATP for cells, and the end product of glycolysis (pyruvate) can enter into mitochondria and be further broken down, supplying energy for a process called **oxidative phosphorylation**. In this process, considerable ATP is made and travels back into the cellular cytoplasm. This ATP, in turn, can serve as a substrate for the enzyme creatine kinase, which phosphorylates a compound called **creatine**. Creatine phosphate represents a stored form of chemical energy within cells. In times of need, creatine phosphate is used in the formation of ATP from ADP by creatine kinase, and the ATP is used in muscle contraction. In turn, the ADP generated during contraction is recycled back to ATP in the mitochondria by ongoing oxidative phosphorylation. We shall consider these processes in more detail in Chapter 7, but it is important that you have an overview of how energy is supplied for ATP synthesis and how ATP serves as a carrier of chemical energy between the mitochondria or creatine phosphate stores and the muscle filaments, which are the sites of muscle contraction.

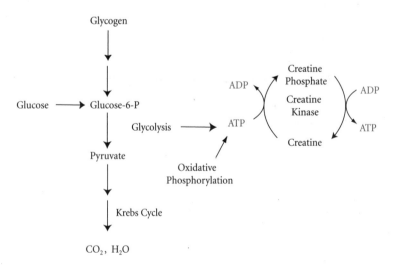

Figure 1–20 Muscle contraction and the supply of energy. Muscle glycogen and glucose can provide substrates for glycolysis. Glycolysis and the Krebs cycle (via oxidative phosphorylation) provide ATP that can be used in muscle contraction or in the formation of creatine phosphate. The latter acts as an energy store that can be used to reclaim ATP.

This chapter has provided an introduction to proteins and many of the functions associated with these dynamic molecules. Table 1–1 summarizes the functions of the proteins that we have discussed here and some examples of each. Some proteins can play multiple roles. The ryanodine receptor is considered a receptor because it can bind calcium, but it is also a ligand-gated channel for calcium ions coming from the sarcoplasmic reticulum into the cytoplasm of the muscle cell. Similarly, the acetylcholine receptor binds acetylcholine and also functions as a ligand-gated channel. Na^+, K^+-ATPase certainly has enzyme properties but also facilitates active transport. These multiple roles of proteins emphasize that proteins may have different regions or domains that can carry out distinct functions. Proteins that carry out these various functions will be the prominent features of this book and will appear in each of the subsequent chapters.

Table 1–1
Functions of Proteins

Function	Examples of Proteins
Contraction and regulation of contraction	Actin, myosin, tropomyosin, troponins, calmodulin, caldesmon
Structural	Collagen, α-keratin
Enzymes (catalysis of reactions)	Myosin ATPase, myosin light chain kinase, phosphatase, acetylcholinesterase, nitric oxide synthase (NOS), protein kinase A (PKA), cGMP-activated protein kinases, Na^+, K^+-ATPase
Receptors (at plasma membrane)	Acetylcholine receptor, α- and β-adrenergic receptors (for adrenalin)
Receptors (T-tubule and intracellular)	Dihydropyridine receptor (DHPR), ryanodine receptor (RyR)
Channels: Voltage-gated	Dihydropyridine receptor, Na^+-channel
Ligand-gated	Acetylcholine receptor, ryanodine receptor
Transporters (membrane bound, at plasma membrane)	Na^+, K^+-ATPase, Na^+-Ca^{++} exchanger, Na^+-H^+ exchanger
Transporters (intracellular)	Ca^{2+}-ATPase

ATP = adenosine triphosphate; cGMP = cyclic guanosine monophosphate.

2

Biochemistry of
Plasma Proteins

The preceding chapter gave an overview of the variety of roles for proteins, including contractile and motile functions (e.g., actin and myosin), enzymes that facilitate chemical reactions, receptors that bind hormones or neurotransmitters, and channels and transporters that move ions from one side of a membrane to another. This was essentially a big-picture introduction to proteins. In this chapter, we will consider the soluble proteins in the blood, particularly those that act as transporters for certain molecules and ions that can be delivered to or picked up from various tissues in the body. Unlike transporters that act like quickly opening or rotating doors in membranes, the soluble protein transporters of the blood are more like transport trucks that travel long distances to bring you lobster from the Canadian or American maritimes or steel goods from Hamilton or penicillin from Indianapolis.

Blood is composed of several types of blood cells, including red cells that carry the oxygen-transporting protein hemoglobin (this protein will be covered in Chapter 5), a variety of white cells (or leukocytes) that play important roles in immune defense and immune reaction, and the numerous, smaller platelets that are vital to the formation of hemostatic plugs that stop up severed vessels to prevent blood loss. These cells are suspended in a protein-rich fluid called **plasma**. If you draw blood from a patient, you often do so into tubes that contain an anticoagulant, such as citrate or the chelator ethylenediaminetetraacetic acid (EDTA). These anticoagulants bind calcium ions to prevent blood coagulation. This anticoagulated blood can be subjected to centrifugation (spinning the blood in tubes) to pellet the cells, leaving the plasma above. One can also allow the blood to clot, spin down the clot and any free cells, and leave above a fluid called **serum**. Serum differs from plasma, as coagulation promotes the removal or modification of a number of proteins involved in the clotting process, as well as the secretion of various cellular constituents from platelets, including certain proteins and smaller molecules. Serum and plasma are useful, accessible fluids that can be used in the diagnosis of disease, as we shall see in Chapter 3.

Proteins are the major solutes in plasma, although this fluid also carries vital electrolytes, such as sodium, potassium, calcium, magnesium, chloride, and bicarbonate ions. Also in plasma are various nutrients, such as glucose and amino acids, as well as the metabolite of glucose, lactate, and a variety of circulating hormones, such as adrenaline, glucagon, and insulin, whose actions we shall analyze more closely in Chapter 7.

The plasma proteins occur at concentrations of 7 to 7.5 g/dL (one decilitre [dL] = 100 mL). The dL is a unit of volume often used by health-care professionals, although you may not have encountered dL before even if you have a background in the basic medical sciences. Plasma proteins are a very diverse group with respect to their functions, although many, indeed, are involved in transport. Fibrinogen, which can be converted to fibrin, is a protein used to stabilize blood clots during coagulation. Other proteins of the coagulation system are also found in plasma, mostly as inactive or zymogen forms. Many kinds of antibodies, or immunoglobulins, can be found in plasma and reflect exposure to foreign materials, organisms, or disease. Generally, these are called γ-globulins. There are also enzymes in plasma, such as acetylcholinesterase (we noted the action of acetylcholinesterase at the nerve–muscle interface, discussed in Chapter 1), as well as a number of enzymes that can be released from cells. This release can occur either during normal processes of cell death or during accelerated cell damage in pathologic conditions, such as the leakage of enzymes from heart muscle cells following a heart attack and myocardial infarction. We shall talk of these in the section on diagnostic enzymology in Chapter 3.

The plasma proteins that act as transporters are also a varied lot, as noted in Table 2–1. There is albumin, the principal plasma protein, which is a veritable bus that picks up and delivers many different ions and compounds to many different destinations. Haptoglobin is a plasma protein that binds hemoglobin found outside the red cells. Transferrin is an important protein that carries iron ions, and ceruloplasmin binds copper ions. Lipoproteins are also important constituents of plasma and represent lipid particles with a coat containing proteins: they circulate as transporters of triglycerides (or triacylglycerols, which is a more modern term) and cholesterol esters. Triglycerides are often referred to as "fat" and serve as an efficient storage form for fatty acids that can be used as fuel compounds. The lipoproteins are classified on the basis of their density: going from the least dense to the densest, there are chylomicrons that are assembled at the small intestine, following digestion of dietary fats, and the very-low-density lipoproteins (VLDLs) and the high-density lipoproteins (HDLs), both made by liver. HDLs and low-density lipoproteins (LDLs, made during the catabolism of VLDL) are important carriers of cholesterol. The above

Table 2–1
Constituents of Plasma (Serum)

Component	Concentration in Plasma (Serum)
Electrolytes (meq/L) *+Platelet Secretions* *Hormones* *Metabolites* *Enzymes*	
Na$^+$	132–145
K$^+$	3.4–5.2
Ca^{2+}	2.25–2.59
Mg^{2+}	1.7–2.3
Cu^{2+}	0.008–0.021
Cl$^-$	101–111
HCO$_3^-$	21.3–28.5
Glucose (mM)	3.5–5.5
Amino acids (mM)	2.4–3.6
Proteins (g/dL)	
Albumin	4.2–5.4
γ-Globulins *— Immunoglobulins*	0.88–1.5
Transferrin	0.24–0.51
Ferritin (mg/dL)	0.003–0.030
Ceruloplasmin	0.020–0.036
Fibrinogen (plasma) *Haptoglobin*	0.22–0.58
Cholesterol (mg/dL)	130–260 (3.7–7.2 mM)
LDL cholesterol *+VLDL*	88–214
HDL cholesterol *Chylomicrons*	27–68
Triglycerides mg/dL	60–302

Data from Diem K, Lentner C, editors. Scientific tables. 7th and 8th eds. Basle, Switzerland: JR Geigy Publications; 1970, 1984.

plasma proteins are some of the major players, but there are numerous other plasma proteins that serve specialized transport roles in blood.

While proteins can be purified from plasma for study, for diagnostic purposes, they are usually separated by electrophoresis. This allows quantitation of different proteins or groups of proteins. Cellulose acetate electrophoresis is commonly used to analyze plasma samples. The degree of separation of the plasma proteins is not remarkable, as many different proteins migrate together, but it is inexpensive and relatively quick and gives evidence of pathologic conditions that have major effects on plasma proteins. In this procedure (Figure 2–1), a small sample of plasma is loaded onto a cellulose acetate sheet and the sheet placed within an electric field in buffer at pH 8.6 so that plasma proteins can migrate on the basis of their charge. A buffer is simply a solution of a weak acid or base that holds the pH at a certain value. Albumin has a net negative charge and travels farthest toward the positive pole, while γ-globulins travel farthest toward the neg-

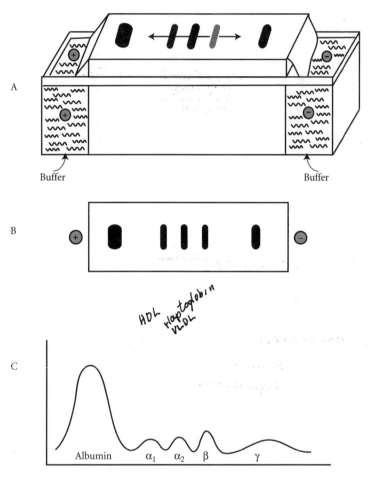

Figure 2–1 Cellulose acetate electrophoresis of plasma proteins. *A*, A sample of plasma is applied to the strip. Within an electrical field (as shown by the + and − terminals), proteins migrate at characteristic speeds toward either of the two terminals, depending on their net charges. *B*, Protein bands are visualized by staining the strip. *C*, Result of scanning the stained strip using a densitometer to measure the size and intensity of staining of each band.

ative pole, reflecting a net positive charge on these proteins at pH 8.6. The intermediate protein bands are called α_1-, α_2-, and β-globulins, and each contains several plasma proteins. The positions of the bands are seen by staining the cellulose acetate sheet using a dye and determining the intensity of each stained band by scanning densitometry. This gives an indication of the quantity of the proteins in the bands. The α_1-band contains several proteins, including HDLs, and the α_2-band contains haptoglobin, ceruloplasmin, and VLDLs. We shall discuss each of these proteins in more detail later in this chapter.

Five bands are visualized on the cellulose acetate sheet, and often, ratios are constructed of band intensities as potential indicators of disease. For example, liver disease may be reflected by a decreased production of albumin so that the albumin/γ-globulin ratio will decline. Analbuminemia (careful, you should pronounce that an-albuminemia!) is reflected by an absence of serum albumin in patients. This is not as devastating as it might sound, as the production of other plasma proteins can be increased in an effort to make up this albumin deficit. Similarly, a child suffering from recurrent infections may show a high albumin/γ-globulin ratio, indicating low levels of immunoglobulins. If you have suspicions about individual plasma proteins, other than albumin, their levels can be tested by forms of electrophoresis that facilitate better resolution of proteins, such as sodium dodecylsulfate (SDS)–polyacrylamide electrophoresis (SDS-PAGE). In this form of electrophoresis, proteins are unfolded in the presence of the negatively charged detergent SDS, which also binds to proteins, so that each has a uniform negative charge density. The proteins are then placed within a gel matrix that acts like a molecular sieve to precisely separate the proteins on the basis of their molecular weight (in contrast to cellulose acetate electrophoresis, where separation is simply based on charge).

CHARACTERISTICS OF PLASMA PROTEINS

The liver is a very important organ that regulates many components of the blood and sees to the needs of many other tissues and organs in the body. The liver functions rather like a conscientious and highly organized mother, father, or designated grandparent, who ensures that other family members take their homework, lunches, and medications before leaving the house each morning.

Most plasma proteins, with the notable exception of the immunoglobulins, are made by the liver. As shown in Figure 2–2, this is done using protein synthetic machinery centered on particles called ribosomes associated with the endoplasmic reticulum. In Chapter 1, we noted how a genetic blueprint was used to ensure high fidelity in the sequential assembly of amino acids into a specific protein. Remember that the sequence of amino acids determines the three-dimensional shape of the protein, and shape is essential for protein function. The genetic blueprint is also known as messenger ribonucleic acid (mRNA), and it contains the genetic code for the protein found within nuclear deoxyribonucleic acid (DNA). The process of transcription of DNA genetic sequences into mRNA will be described in Chapter 8. Using mRNA that codes for the amino acid sequence of a protein, such as albumin, amino acids are carefully assembled in precise sequence, linked by peptide bonds. These plasma proteins made by the liver are secretory proteins and follow a path that differs from that of soluble proteins destined

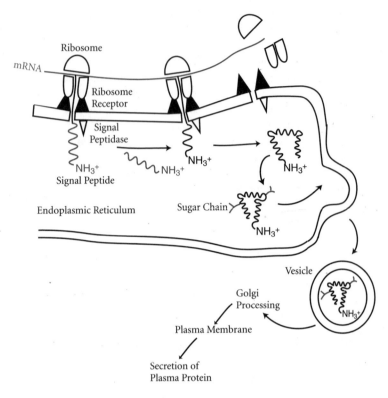

Figure 2–2 Production of plasma proteins in the liver. At the endoplasmic reticulum, a complex of messenger RNA and ribosome subunits translates the genetic code in mRNA, resulting in the assembly of amino acids into protein. The signal peptide at the N-terminus of the protein is the first to emerge from the ribosome and assists the passage of the protein into the lumen of the endoplasmic reticulum. The signal peptide is removed, and the protein undergoes processing (e.g., sugar or oligosaccharide additions) at the endoplasmic reticulum and the Golgi apparatus. The mature protein travels from the Golgi apparatus to the plasma membrane where it is released from the cell.

to remain in the liver cell. Initially, these secretory proteins are made as larger precursor proteins, or **preproteins**. The preprotein moves through the membrane of the endoplasmic reticulum into the lumen. This movement is guided by the N-terminal sequence of about 16 to 30 amino acids that emerges first from the ribosome. This leading sequence is called the **signal peptide**, and it is removed by the action of signal peptidase on the luminal side of the membrane. The protein is further modified by the stepwise addition of sugars to form chains or by the addition of preformed sugar (oligosaccharide) chains. These chains can be modified within the endoplasmic reticulum and later within the Golgi apparatus. Indeed, most plasma proteins, with the exception of albumin, are designated glycoproteins. This is because they have covalently bound sugar chains linked to the side chains of serine and threonine or to the side chain of the amino acid asparagine (similar to aspartic acid, but with the carboxyl group in the side chain taking part in a simple amide, -CO-NH$_2$).

The mature proteins move from the Golgi apparatus, in vesicles, to the plasma membrane, where membrane fusion events permit the secretion of these plasma proteins from the liver cell.

Most molecules in the body do not last forever but, rather, must be replenished as they lose their function. Plasma proteins can be degraded within the circulation or removed from the blood and degraded within cells. Thus, the liver is continuously making plasma proteins for secretion. Individual plasma proteins have characteristic half-lives in the circulation. This simply represents the time taken for the loss of 50% of the molecules of a specific protein, measured from the time they reach equilibration within the blood and other extracellular spaces. This can be evaluated following the injection of radioactively labelled plasma protein and observing radioactive peaking and then loss from the blood. For example, haptoglobin has a half-life of 5 days, while that of albumin is longer at 15 to 20 days. There are pathologic conditions that accelerate the loss of plasma proteins, and these would lower the corresponding half-lives. In Crohn's disease (an intestinal inflammatory disease), plasma proteins can be lost into the intestine, thus drastically reducing the half-lives of plasma proteins. The synthesis of certain proteins, including fibrinogen, haptoglobin, and one we have not previously mentioned, called C-reactive protein (CRP), is stimulated in tissue damage or inflammation. These are known as acute-phase proteins, and their levels can be elevated in various diseases, including cancers.

ALBUMIN, ONCOTIC PRESSURE, AND EDEMA

Albumin is the major plasma protein, accounting for 60% of the total, at about 4 to 5 g/dL. Albumin is also found in the interstitial space, and indeed, 60% of the total albumin is found in this extracellular fluid, while 40% is in plasma. Liver dedicates considerable energy in making albumin, as some 12 g of albumin are synthesized per day (approximately 25% of the total protein production of the liver), representing about 50% of the liver's output of secretory protein.

Albumin has a molecular mass of 69 kDa. The kDa signifies kilodaltons, with the dalton representing an atomic mass unit of 1. Albumin in human plasma is made up of 585 amino acids linked in sequence. There is also a number of disulfide bridges linking the R-groups of cysteine residues in the protein. These were discussed briefly in Chapter 1, when amino acid structures were outlined. The formation of these -S-S- bridges can assist the stabilization of the three-dimensional structure of the protein. As a protein folds, it assumes a three-dimensional shape, largely on the basis of hydrophobicity and hydrophilicity of the component amino acid side chains (i.e., how they respond to an aqueous environment). In the formation of the preferred shape of an individual protein, the generation of -S-S- bridges between nearby cysteine residues may be considered similar to spot welding, as these covalent bonds can support the overall configuration that is initially dependent mainly on noncovalent forces.

One of the major roles of albumin, which we have not discussed, is the part it plays in osmotic or oncotic pressure (sometimes represented as π). Osmotic pressure is simply a measure of the number of particles that are in a specific volume. For example, an aqueous solution with a high concentration of sodium chloride (NaCl) also has a high osmotic pressure, with both Na^+ and Cl^- ions contributing to this. The effect of high osmotic pressure in the medium surrounding cells is to draw water from the cells. Thus, a piece of celery can go relatively limp when placed in a concentrated salt solution. Albumin has a relatively modest molecular mass (69 kDa), compared with other plasma proteins. Albumin is also the protein in the highest concentration in plasma, and thus, it plays a major role (on the basis of the number of albumin molecules per milliliter of fluid) in the osmotic or oncotic pressure of plasma and of the interstitial fluid.

At the capillaries, there is a delivery of fluid and solutes, such as glucose, to interstitial fluids and also, of necessity, a drawing back of fluid and waste products from the tissues to the capillaries to make up the venous return that eventually comes back to the heart. As shown in Figure 2–3, the force with which fluid enters the interstitium from the capillaries or returns into the capillaries from the interstitium is based on the net force of the hydrostatic pressure (depending on blood pressure) driving fluid out from the capillary and the oncotic pressure pulling fluid back into the capillary. There are much smaller oncotic pressures and hydrostatic pressures associated with the interstitial fluid. When normal cardiovascular function is occurring, it is the hydrostatic pressure in the capillary that can show substantial change. With a relatively high hydrostatic pressure, there is a net delivery of fluid to the interstitial space. However, with a significant decrease in hydrostatic pressure, there is a recovery of fluid back into the capillary from the interstitial fluid. It is believed that fluid returns to the capillary when the capillary sphincter closes (see Figure 2–3), reducing the hydrostatic pressure so that the oncotic pressure of plasma is sufficiently high to facilitate fluid recovery by the capillary. The pressure numbers and calculations are included in Figure 2–3.

This simple fluid loss and fluid retrieval system can be confounded in a number of ways, which result in poor fluid recovery. This leads to accumulation of fluid in tissues and a condition known as **edema**, which can occur as a result of a number of different pathologic conditions. For example, the main venous return is into the atrium on the right side of the heart.

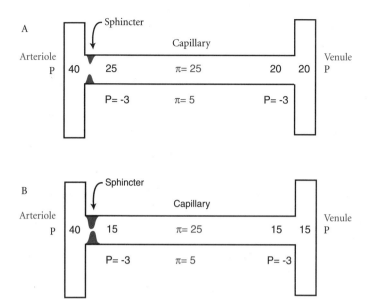

Figure 2–3 Fluid departure from and return to a capillary. "P" represents the hydrostatic pressures (mm Hg) found in the capillary and surrounding tissue; "π" represents the osmotic or oncotic pressures (mm Hg) exerted by solutes such as the protein albumin within the capillary or surrounding tissue. *A*, Fluid leaves the capillary as the net outward pressure is the difference of the net hydrostatic pressure (25-[-3]) mm Hg and the net oncotic pressure (25-5) mm Hg, giving an outward pressure of 8 mm Hg driving fluid into the tissues. *B*, With the arrest of capillary blood flow and reduction in capillary hydrostatic pressure to 15 mm Hg, there is a corresponding net inward pressure of (15-[-3]) - (25-5) or -2 mm Hg, which promotes the return of fluid into the capillary.

Should there be right heart failure, the hydrostatic pressure will increase on the venous side, and this will oppose the recovery of fluid into the capillaries and lead to peripheral edema.

In another manner, a decreased oncotic pressure in the plasma will also lead to poor return of fluid to the capillary. Thus, any disease that decreases the production of albumin by the liver can potentially drop the oncotic pressure of plasma, as albumin is the greatest contributor to this osmotic pressure. In liver disease associated, for example, with chronic alcoholism or hepatitis C, liver malfunction can be seen in diminished production of albumin. Kwashiorkor is a disease caused by dietary insufficiency of protein and is commonly seen in developing countries. It is particularly apparent in children (who are no longer breast fed) and is manifested by a swollen abdomen. Because protein is required for growth, deficiency of it is more apparent in children than in adults who are maintaining an adult body mass. Dietary protein deficiency means a poor supply of essential amino acids needed for the assembly of proteins. You can synthesize certain amino acids from other molecules supplied by other foods, such as glucose from carbohydrates. However, there are so-called essential amino acids that must be supplied by proteins in the diet. It is important to obtain a good variety in dietary protein and not to rely on one source of protein (say, gelatin, to keep our naming generic) that might have deficiencies or low quantities of certain essential amino acids. Poor supply of dietary protein can result in diminished production of albumin by the liver, low plasma oncotic pressure, and edema that is apparent in the swelling of the abdominal cavity because of fluid accumulation. Fluid that accumulates in the abdominal cavity is called **ascites**. Another potential location of fluid accumulation is the lung. In left heart failure, there are difficulties with the return of blood from circulation in the lungs. This is commonly seen in myocardial infarction, and fluid may accumulate rapidly in the alveoli of the lungs. This is called **acute pulmonary edema** and is a very serious condition, as the patient can essentially drown in his or her own body fluid.

Other causes of edema include the following:

- Hypoproteinemia resulting from renal disease (albuminuria) or from bowel disease (gastroenteropathy)
- Retention of sodium ions (e.g., high sodium intake and increased renal absorption of sodium ions)
- Obstruction of lymphatics (e.g., as a result of neoplasm, inflammation, or elephantiasis, in which certain parasites obstruct the lymphatics)
- An increase in capillary permeability mediated by the action of histamine, for example, in allergic responses

TRANSPORT FUNCTIONS OF PLASMA PROTEINS

Albumin is a principal transporter in the blood. If you are fasting or perhaps involved in strenuous activities that last for a prolonged length of time (say, a long distance run), you will need to make use of the fat stores in your body to provide yourself with fuel compounds as substrates for energy production. Recall our description of the production of adenosine triphosphate (ATP) using glucose as a fuel compound in muscle, in Chapter 1. ATP can also be made during the breakdown of products derived from fat. When you need to mobilize your fat reserves (and most of our readers are likely only too aware of their locations in the body), the complex stored fats are broken down within the fat or adipose cells that make up fat tissue. Breakdown products, called **fatty acids**, are released into the bloodstream. Because they are hydrophobic compounds, fatty acids are not readily soluble in water. Albumin has a number of binding sites for these hydrophobic compounds and can readily carry them to tissues, such as muscle and heart, that can use these fatty acids as fuel substrates. Albumin can also carry other hydrophobic molecules, such as steroid hormones, bilirubin (a hydrophobic breakdown product of heme, the iron-bearing constituent of hemoglobin), certain drugs (such as aspirin, the anticoagulant dicoumarol, penicillin, sulfonamides, digoxin, and barbiturates) and the amino acid tryptophan, as well as calcium and copper ions. The transport potentials of albumin are remarkable, and it can function to both supply materials to various sites in the body and remove compounds from these sites.

Another plasma protein with transport function is haptoglobin. Haptoglobin, like a number of proteins, can exist in polymorphic forms. Humans have at least three forms of haptoglobin, the simplest (Hp 1-1) having a molecular mass of 90 kDa. These polymorphic forms carry out similar functions but differ in size because these proteins are made using genetic blueprints that come from more than one gene for this plasma protein. Haptoglobin functions to bind hemoglobin that is extracorpuscular (i.e., hemoglobin that is outside red cells). Hemoglobin is a protein packaged within the red cells of blood, and its principal function is to transport oxygen from the lungs to the various tissues of the body. We will discuss hemoglobin, its synthesis, and breakdown in Chapter 6. Hemoglobin can be lost from the red cells directly into blood, and this free hemoglobin is destined for degradation, following its binding to haptoglobin. This accounts for about 10% of the hemoglobin that is degraded on a daily basis. The rest is broken down when older red cells are removed by cells of the reticuloendothelial system (e.g., histiocytes and certain splenic cells). Haptoglobin can bind hemoglobin in a 1:1 ratio, as noted in Figure 2–4, forming a complex of 155 kDa. This complex can be rapidly taken up by the liver and broken down, thus preserving the iron (Fe) found in hemoglobin. Hemoglobin that is not complexed can pass through into the kidney and precipitate in the kidney tubules or enter into urine (hemoglobinuria). In contrast, the haptoglobin–hemoglobin complex is too large to pass through the glomerulus. The half-life of the hemoglobin–haptoglobin complex (90 minutes) is consider-

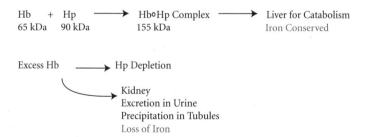

Figure 2–4 Haptoglobin binds extracellular hemoglobin. The complex of haptoglobin (Hp 1-1) and hemoglobin, because of its size, is not lost in urine. Instead, it is catabolized, following uptake of the complex by the liver. In certain pathologic conditions (e.g., fragile red cells in certain of the anemias), excess free hemoglobin can deplete or exceed haptoglobin levels and can appear in the urine.

ably shorter than the half-life of free haptoglobin (5 days). Thus, haptoglobin levels are depressed in the hemolytic anemias, as the release of hemoglobin from the red cells is accelerated in these diseases. Remember that haptoglobin is an acute-phase protein whose levels can be elevated with inflammatory disease. Certain snake venoms also contain an enzyme that will attack the membranes of the red cells, releasing hemoglobin into blood. Thus, a snake bite (depending on the extent of the venom delivered) can also lead to the appearance of hemoglobin in the urine. Before you jump to dire conclusions during your first daily excursion to the washroom, remember that beets eaten the night before (possibly as an associated dietary penance for consuming that excess animal fat) can also color urine.

Transferrin (80 kDa), as its name suggests, is a plasma protein that transports iron (at saturation, 2 molecules of Fe^{3+} per molecule of transferrin). Iron is a very important inorganic component of a number of proteins, including hemoglobin, myoglobin (a protein related to hemoglobin that binds oxygen and facilitates its diffusion within muscle cells), and the cytochromes. Certain cytochromes are important constituents of the electron transport chain, whose operation powers the production of ATP in mitochondria (see Chapter 7). Each of these proteins depends on iron for its function; iron is delivered to the various cells and tissues of the body by the transport protein transferrin.

Iron is supplied by the diet, largely in red meat, eggs, and liver. Cooking in iron frying pans (apparently the utensil of choice among discerning specialists in the preparation of grilled-cheese sandwiches, pancakes, and other like delicacies) will also serve as a significant source of iron. One word (several, actually) of caution: avoid exposure of metal surfaces to acids, as metallic ions may be liberated as a result. You can certainly be poisoned by the ingestion of too much iron or excess of other metallic ions, such as zinc, copper, cobalt, or aluminum, to give a few examples. The metallic ions may interact with proteins (other than their transporters) and even interfere with enzyme function. Going back a number of years, there was a Sunday school picnic (rather a highlight of existence in the 1950s, as it allowed you to leave school early), where an unfortunate choice of container was made for the preparation of lemonade. Because of the volume of drink needed, a new garbage pail was employed. Now, this was not a plastic garbage can that many of our readers are familiar with; rather, it was a galvanized (i.e., zinc-coated) metal garbage can that was a dominant feature of waste disposal in the largely preplastic era of the 1950s. The citric acid in the lemonade mobilized the zinc ions from the galvanized coating of the garbage pail and poisoned a number of the participants at the picnic.

There are certainly other examples of metal ion poisoning. In the 1970s, it was discovered that cobalt in small quantities could stabilize foam, preventing its dissipation in freshly poured glasses of beer. As a good "head" in a glass of beer is considered a desirable feature, traces of cobalt were sometimes added to these beverages in the belief that the small quantities of cobalt would not be harmful. It was estimated that an individual would have to consume several dozens of bottled or poured glasses of beer to encounter toxicity. After this beer product was released, there were reports of increasing occurrences of cardiomyopathy concentrated in northern Quebec mining towns. Cobalt can cause this heart problem, and indeed, there were miners and others who could consume a remarkable quantity of beer within an evening. This foam-stabilized beer was therefore withdrawn.

The corresponding risk with metals that you are much more likely to encounter outside mining towns is the poisoning of young children with vitamin pills fortified with iron. Evolving from this risk was the development of the safety cap on bottles of vitamins and other drugs and the quite reasonable, subsequent protests of those suffering from arthritis who could not then open their medications (such as aspirin), until a compromise cap could be developed. If the body is subjected to an iron overload or overdose, iron will bind to a variety of proteins besides those designed to act as its transporter, and this can compromise the functioning of these vulnerable proteins quite severely. Iron can also promote deleterious oxidation reactions within the body. Toxicity due to iron can be treated in several ways. Following efforts to remove iron from the stomach, iron ions may be picked up therapeutically using compounds called **chelators** that bind the iron so that the complexes can be diposed of in urine. Different chelators function to remove different cations, and the chelators can differ in their efficiency in ion sequestration. A degree of caution should be exercised in the use of chelation therapy, as other essential ions besides the ones in excess may be removed as well. It is also important not to place a patient in essential mineral deficiency, and this is a possibility in the treatment of Wilson's disease (to be covered later within this chapter).

Should you feel that chelators are relatively exotic compounds, check the ingredients on a bottle of salad dressing (not the fat-free type), and you may find that one of the ingredients is EDTA, a chelator that can bind calcium or magnesium ions. The structure of EDTA is shown in Figure 2–5. These chelators act as sequestering agents and prevent the deleterious effects that ions, such as iron, can have on foodstuffs. You may also find chelators in radiopaque dyes used for injection during angiography (i.e., to outline the blood vessels in the body); these chelators remove traces of the divalent cations present in the dye solution itself. Parenthetically, these dyes can pose some risks to certain patients (e.g., allergic response).

This being said about metal poisoning, dietary deficiencies in essential minerals also have serious consequences. Iron is a very important mineral micronutrient in the diet. Other important minerals (classified as mineral macronutrients because they are required in quantities that exceed 100 mg/d)

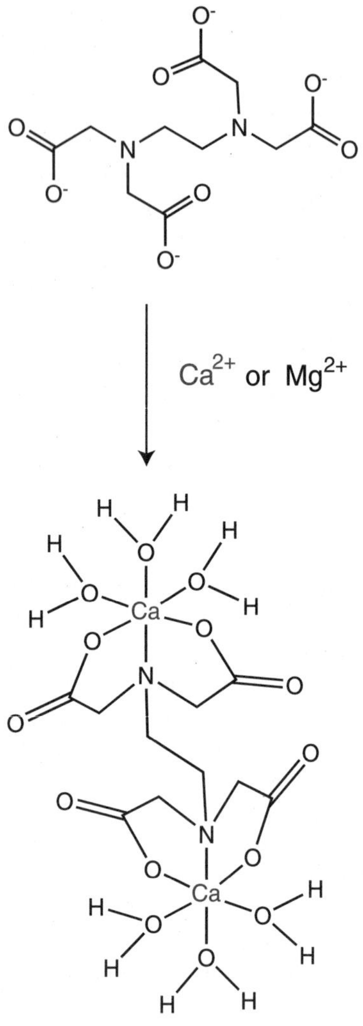

Figure 2–5 Chelation of Ca^{2+} and Mg^{2+} ions by the chelator EDTA (ethylenediamine-tetraacetic acid).

include calcium, phosphorus, and magnesium for bones and teeth (and other functions including nerve and muscle regulation, synthesis of ATP, and enzyme operation) and sodium, potassium, and chloride, which are very important electrolytes. Within medicine and the related health sciences, you ignore nutrition at your peril, as poor diet can account for many of the signs and symptoms that your patients may present to you. Iron intake is of consequence, as we do lose iron on a daily basis. In adult males, this is about 1 mg/d, and in adult females, the loss of iron can be considerably higher because of menstruation. Iron is largely used in the synthesis of hemoglobin, the oxygen-transporting protein of red blood cells that has iron bound to the protein at the center of a specialized heme group. Iron plays a very central role in the oxygen-binding properties of hemoglobin. Women and those suffering from gastrointestinal bleeding are more prone to iron deficiency anemia, in which the functioning of the red cells in oxygen transport is compromised. In this form of anemia, the red cells are small in size (microcytic) and hypochromic (not as intensely colored as normal red cells). Pregnant women also have increased requirements for iron, minerals, and other nutrients.

Also, at the risk of being taken to task by those inside and outside our families who do not eat red meat (and without attempting to classify these individuals, another foolhardy venture for the carnivore), doctors and associated health professionals should be aware that their patients who do follow these diets can be at greater risk of iron deficiency anemia. Plants are not remarkable sources of iron. Spinach does have some, but this iron is not readily available when spinach is ingested. (Cartoon characters should adjust their lifestyles accordingly.) Also at risk of iron deficiency are infants and adolescents experiencing growth spurts.

Another group to watch out for is the elderly, particularly men and women living alone, who may show remarkably little variety and scant nutrition sense in what they eat (e.g., a diet of tea and toast). As our readers may largely be in their second and third decades, it is very worthwhile to point out that there is a glut of individuals (born in the baby boom following World War II) who are approaching retirement and old age within the next 10 to 30 years, and it is inevitable that this group will be the dominant one within your patient population (unless you specialize in obstetrics/gynecology, pediatrics, or sports medicine).

If you wish a short crash course in both minerals and vitamins in nutrition, you should purchase a bottle of vitamin pills recommended for expectant mothers and read the detailed label on the bottle. You may find it enlightening. A smaller education in vitamins may be gleaned at the breakfast table reading certain breakfast cereal boxes that list the various nutrients added to these products (presumably after many of these vitamins were removed in processing).

Between 10 and 20 mg/d of iron is taken into the body in foods. Cooking can increase the breakdown of links between iron and foods (e.g., muscle protein). The acidic environment of the stomach and the presence of vitamin C (ascorbic acid) as a reducing agent promote the conversion of oxidized iron (Fe^{3+}) into reduced iron (Fe^{2+}). In this reduced form, iron ions can be absorbed within the small intestine (principally at the duodenum). One potential limitation to iron absorption is the secretion of bicarbonate by the pancreas and the resulting neutralization of intestinal contents that favors iron oxidation. The fate of iron in the body is shown in Figure 2–6. Iron (Fe^{2+}) taken up by the mucosal cells that line the duodenum can be passed on to the blood capillaries. In circumstances where the body is already loaded with iron, a protein called **apoferritin** can be synthesized within the mucosal cell to bind the iron tightly and prevent its passage into the capillaries. In iron deficiency, this protein is not present in significant quantities in mucosal cells.

Now that we are (figuratively) inside the body and the bloodstream, we should point out the places where iron is found. This is shown in Table 2–2. In a 70-kg male, there is, on average, 3.5 to 4.0 g of iron. About two-thirds of the body's iron is in hemoglobin (2.5 g), found in red blood cells. Myoglobin, the protein that promotes oxygen diffusion in muscle, and iron in cytochromes and enzymes accounts for 300 mg or 8.0%. Transferrin is the iron transport protein of plasma and contains 3 mg (0.1%), while ferritin (a protein that binds and stores iron) accounts for 1 g (26%).

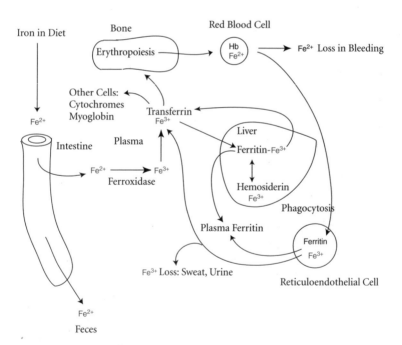

Figure 2–6 Iron absorption and use within the body. Dietary iron is absorbed at the intestine and, following oxidation to Fe^{3+}, is bound and transported by transferrin. Iron can be used in the synthesis of hemoglobin in bone (ultimately, hemoglobin appears in the red blood cells in the circulation) and in the synthesis of myoglobin and cytochromes. Iron can be stored by the protein ferritin in the liver and the reticuloendothelial cells.

Transferrin and Iron Transport

While iron is absorbed as Fe^{2+}, it must be oxidized to enable binding to transferrin. The oxidation of iron to Fe^{3+} is carried out by an enzyme activity called **ferroxidase** found as a distinct plasma protein, and in the plasma protein, ceruloplasmin, which also functions to bind copper ions (we shall discuss ceruloplasmin at a later point in the chapter). Transferrin carries iron to various sites, for example, the liver and bone marrow, where it is used in synthesis. This is noted in Figure 2-6. Equally importantly, transferrin picks up iron released following the catabolism of hemoglobin and other iron-bearing proteins. This is important to restrict the loss of iron from the body, and the body carefully guards its content of iron. About 200 billion red cells are broken down per day under normal circumstances, representing the release of about 25 mg of iron. It sounds like a lot, but, in fact, this represents about 20 mL of red cells. Binding to transferrin also prevents the toxicity associated with free iron in the body. A potential danger coming from the free iron stems from infections with bacteria that are supported by free iron; these can occur with the ingestion of certain shellfish that contain such bacteria. Transferrin does not usually carry a full iron load; rather, about 33% of the sites on transferrin are saturated with iron.

Transferrin is a transport vehicle for iron, and thus, transferrin is also involved in an iron delivery mechanism. This involves the binding of transferrin to a transferrin receptor located on the surface of cells, such as hepatocytes (Figure 2–7). The receptor is a protein that spans the plasma membrane. Low concentrations of iron within cells will initiate the synthesis of more of the transferrin receptor to improve the binding of transferrin at the cell surface. Once transferrin is bound, a process called **receptor-mediated endocytosis** is initiated. The transferrin receptor with bound transferrin is localized to areas of the plasma membrane called **coated pits**. Here, the transferrin receptor and bound transferrin are internalized as coated vesicles that enter the cell. These vesicles undergo fusion events with other intracellular vesicles called **endosomes**. The iron subsequently dissociates from

Table 2–2
Iron in the Body

	Adult Male (70 kg)
Transferrin	0.003 g
Hemoglobin	2.5 g
Myoglobin, Enzymes, Cytochromes	0.30 g
Ferritin, tissue	1.0 g
plasma	0.0001 g

transferrin because of the low pH within the endosomes. While the iron is retained by the cell and either stored or used in the synthesis of iron-containing compounds, the apotransferrin–transferrin receptor complex returns to the cell surface, where the apotransferrin is released back into the extracellular fluid. Thus, the transport protein can be reutilized within the plasma. Note the prefix "apo" in this context. When a protein carries or is associated with a metal ion, the removal of such ions produces an apoprotein. Thus, apotransferrin simply has both its iron-binding sites free so that it can function as a transport protein for iron atoms.

Ferritin is the principal intracellular protein associated with iron (Fe^{3+}) storage, and its synthesis is elevated when levels of iron increase. It is considerably more complex than transferrin because it consists of 24 subunits (single polypeptide chains) and has a molecular weight of 440 kDa. Thus, ferritin is really a complex of subunits that creates a shell that surrounds a

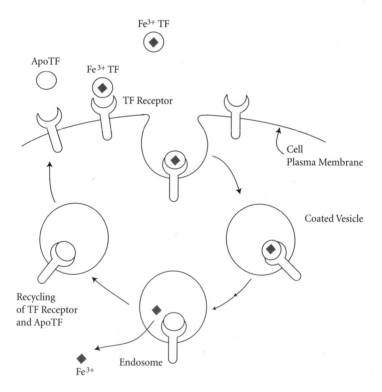

Figure 2–7 Receptor-mediated endocytosis of transferrin. Transferrin (TF) carrying iron can bind to a transferrin receptor located at the plasma membrane of cells, such as hepatocytes. Once bound, the transferrin is internalized with its receptor by endocytosis and by the formation of coated vesicles. These vesicles can fuse with endosomes, where the low internal pH facilitates the removal of iron from transferrin. The apotransferrin (ApoTF) and its receptor are returned to the cell surface, where apotransferrin is released.

core in which iron can be stored. Each ferritin complex has the potential to store 4,500 iron ions, although, on average, ferritin usually carries close to 3,000. There are channels that allow iron to enter and leave the complex. About 23% of the weight of the ferritin complex is iron. Apoferritin has no iron (following our terminology discussed for transferrin). Hemosiderin refers to iron deposits that are found close to ferritin when there is excess iron available. It is also considered that hemosiderin may represent a form of partly degraded ferritin. Usually, ferritin is found within cells and tissues, and there is very little ferritin found in plasma. Plasma ferritin is useful because it can serve as a measure of iron levels within the body. For example, in iron deficiency anemias, levels of plasma ferritin are depressed.

These levels can be measured using a radioimmunoassay (RIA). A radioimmunoassay of ferritin (Figure 2–8) employs a complex of commercial radioactive ferritin with a specific antibody to ferritin. Antibodies are proteins that are produced by the body's immune system in response to exposure to bacteria, virus, or foreign compounds. Specific antibodies can recognize specific foreign proteins and bind to them noncovalently in an effort to neutralize the function of the foreign protein. This is another function of proteins. The injection of human ferritin into animals will stimulate the production of antibodies to human ferritin, and these can be isolated. In the RIA for ferritin, the addition of an unknown quantity of ferritin (supplied in a human tissue or plasma sample) will displace a certain quantity of radioactivity from the radioactive ferritin–antibody complex. The percentage loss of radioactivity from the complex can be measured and used as an index of the quantity of unlabelled ferritin in the sample.

Primary hemochromatosis is a relatively common genetic disorder. It is more common in men and is caused by excessive iron absorption at the intestine. Liver, pancreas, heart, skin, and other tissues can be affected by the disease. Body levels of iron can be raised as high as 100 g. The high levels of iron will lead to cirrhosis of the liver, diabetes mellitus (with pancreatic damage), heart failure, and a bronzing of the skin because of increased pigmentation. Primary hemochromatosis is also referred to as bronze diabetes. Treatment of the disease consists of blood withdrawal (phlebotomy). Women are less likely to manifest the disease because of loss of iron in menstruation.

Specific genetic changes are associated with hemochromatosis. The *HFE* gene has been identified as a candidate gene for primary hemochromatosis. The HFE protein, whose synthesis is effectively directed by the genetic sequence within the *HFE* gene, is found at the surface of intestinal mucosal cells and can show several distinct changes in amino acid sequence. In many cases, a cysteine residue (remember, it has the distinctive -SH side chain) at position 282 in the normal protein is replaced by the amino acid tyrosine. This will happen because of a specific change (mutation) in the corresponding genetic sequence. We will go into the nature of mutations, disease, and genes in more depth in Chapter 8, but this specific change in

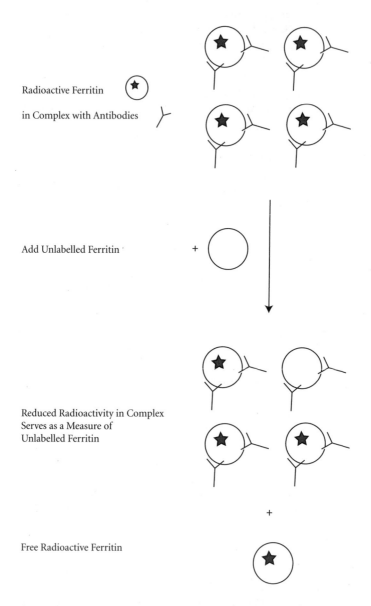

Figure 2–8 Radioimmunoassay (RIA) for ferritin. Very small quantities of ferritin can be measured in plasma samples using commercial radioactive ferritin, complexed with antibody for ferritin. The addition of a small quantity of unlabelled ferritin (in the serum or plasma sample) will liberate radioactive ferritin from the complex. Free radioactive ferritin can be separated from the complex. The loss of radioactivity from the complex will be proportional to the ferritin in the serum or plasma sample, which was initially added to the complex, and allow a quantitation of the unknown ferritin sample.

an amino acid occurs when a specific guanine base (G) in the genetic sequence is simply replaced by adenine (A). The resulting change in the protein structure is associated with higher levels of iron uptake from the intestine. One lab test for the disease is elevated levels of iron saturation of plasma transferrin. Another is increased levels of plasma ferritin as shown by RIA. Mutations associated with hemochromatosis can be shown by the use of appropriate DNA probes.

Secondary hemochromatosis is not a genetic disease but can have other causes, such as excess blood transfusions.

Ceruloplasmin and Copper Transport

Copper ions are transported by the plasma protein ceruloplasmin (160 kDa), which has a blue color because of its copper content. Most of the circulating copper (90%) is carried by ceruloplasmin (six copper ions per molecule of protein). However, the binding of copper to this protein is very tight, and the copper ions cannot be easily exchanged. Albumin can carry the remainder of the circulating copper, and this represents a more easily exchanged pool of soluble copper ions. Liver disease will reduce levels of ceruloplasmin, and Wilson's disease, which we will discuss later, is marked by low levels of this plasma protein.

Copper is an important mineral micronutrient that is required for the activities of a number of enzymes in the body. Two examples are copper-dependent superoxide dismutase (SOD) and cytochrome oxidase. SOD catalyzes a reaction that removes superoxide radicals and generates hydrogen peroxide.

$$O_2^- + O_2^- + 2H^+ \rightarrow H_2O_2 + O_2$$

The oxygen radicals, indicated as O_2^-, are made as a consequence of oxidation reactions and are remarkably reactive and toxic. Thus, SOD is part of a defense mechanism to disarm these oxygen radicals before damage is done to the other molecular components of cells. Admittedly, the product of the enzyme is hydrogen peroxide (H_2O_2), hardly an innocuous molecule (as you can tell by its effects on human hair). However, the enzyme catalase readily transforms hydrogen peroxide into water and oxygen. Cytochrome oxidase is an enzyme component of the electron transport chain in mitochondria, which is essential in the generation of ATP. We will discuss energy production in more detail in Chapter 7. We need far less copper than iron; therefore, dietary deficiency of copper is rather rare. Conceivably, some of the copper ingested can be attributed to the prevalence of copper plumbing in certain parts of the world. You should know that there are other dietary sources of copper ions, if you now use filtration at home to remove a variety of metal ions from the water source.

An adult has about 100 mg of copper, found in bone, liver, kidney, and muscle. Copper (2 to 4 mg) is ingested daily, and about half of this is taken up by the stomach and small intestine. In the liver, copper ions bind to ceruloplasmin, which then enters the blood. Albumin also serves as a transporter of copper ions. Like iron, free copper can have toxic effects, including oxidation of cellular components. After cellular entry, copper ions can bind to a class of proteins called **metallothioneins** (6.5 kDa). These proteins bind a variety of metal ions, including copper, cadmium, mercury, and zinc. The metallothioneins contain cysteine residues that participate in the binding of the metal ions, effectively blocking the potentially harmful effects of the free ions. When elevated levels of these ions are present, the levels of these proteins increase.

Menkes' Disease

This disorder involves a defect in copper handling. It is a genetic defect, and as it is X-linked, only males are affected. We talked briefly in Chapter 1 about hemophilia as an X-linked defect that affected certain males descended from Queen Victoria. The problem with males (among others, we can hear our women readers saying) is the XY pairing of the sex chromosomes. As there is no second X chromosome, a genetic defect in the single X-chromosome inherited from one parent will manifest itself in male children.

Menkes' disease principally affects the nervous system, connective tissue, and vascular system; infants with the disease do not usually survive. The genetic flaw has been traced to a defective form of ATPase that binds copper and is involved in the removal of copper ions from cells. Remember, in Chapter 1, we described the Na^+, K^+-ATPase responsible for pumping Na^+ ions out and K^+ ions into the cell across the plasma membrane. The use of ATP by the pump indicates a form of active transport. There are also ATPase activities associated with the pumping of copper ions out of cells. In Menkes' disease, a defective copper-binding ATPase leads to an accumulation of copper in the intestine and other tissues (with the exception of liver) and is shown by low levels of serum copper and ceruloplasmin and low copper in the liver. While you might consider that this type of defect could be treated by chelation therapy to assist in the depletion of cellular copper outside the liver, unfortunately, there is another aspect to the disease. In Menkes' disease, the activities of copper-dependent enzymes (e.g., SOD and cytochrome oxidase) are low, suggesting a problem with incorporation of copper ions into proteins in spite of the accumulation of copper. Thus, these patients will show predominantly apoenzyme forms of copper-dependent enzyme activities. Interestingly, the liver is not affected by the defect as the copper-binding ATPase in the liver appears to be the product of a different gene that is not defective in Menkes' disease. There is as yet no treatment for the disease.

Wilson's Disease

This is a second genetic disease affecting copper and has a later onset than Menkes' disease. The two diseases are compared in Table 2–3. Wilson's disease is not X-linked and is autosomal recessive. The latter term indicates that in this disease there are defective genes on both chromosomes so that the two parents may be carriers of the gene defect; that is, each has one chromosome with a mutation in the affected gene. Again, a copper-binding ATPase is affected, but in this case, it is the enzyme found in the liver that is defective. It operates in the removal of copper ions from the liver into the bile, and the defective liver ATPase prompts a rise in levels of copper in the liver. These can be toxic and lead to a lowering of the liver's output of ceruloplasmin and poor incorporation of copper ions into ceruloplasmin. Liver disease can result. The defective copper pump in the liver leads to a build-up of copper in other tissues. An accumulation of copper ions in the basal ganglia of the nervous system causes neurologic degeneration. Copper can also accumulate in the red blood cells (where it is associated with hemolytic anemia) and in the kidney. A green or golden ring (the Kayser-Fleischer ring) can be seen around the cornea as a result of copper deposits. As the problems can be traced to levels of excess copper within cells, chelation therapy can be used. The drug penicillamine will chelate copper ions, and the complex is excreted in urine.

LIPOPROTEINS, LIPID TRANSPORT, AND ATHEROSCLEROSIS

While our previous examples of plasma proteins involved the transport of discrete numbers of molecules or ions around the body in association with transferrin, albumin, haptoglobin, or ceruloplasmin, lipoproteins are plasma proteins that work in a rather different way. As the prefix "lipo" suggests, these proteins are associated with lipids. Lipids are a rather diverse group of compounds that are hydrophobic and include triglycerides (or triacylglycerols), phospholipids, and cholesterol. Triglycerides are made up of glycerol and three fatty acids in ester linkage (Figure 2–9A) and are found as the principal stored fat component of fat cells or adipocytes. Phospholipids are somewhat similar, usually consisting of two fatty acids and glycerol, but they also possess a polar group, as they contain phosphate that is linked to another water-soluble molecule. Phospholipids are the principal lipid structural elements in cell membranes. Cholesterol is a steroid composed of several characteristic interlocking rings and has one -OH functional group that can be esterified to fatty acids. Cholesterol is also a component of membranes and is particularly abundant in the plasma membrane that surrounds a cell.

Lipoproteins are large multimolecular particles that consist of a central lipid core made up of triacylglycerols and fatty acid esters of cholesterol and surrounded by a thin outer shell composed of phospholipid, cholesterol, and proteins (Figure 2–9B). While a plasma protein, such as albumin,

Table 2–3
Menkes' and Wilson's Diseases

	Menkes'	**Wilson's**
Genotype	X-linked	Autosomal recessive
Defective protein	Cu^{2+}-ATPase	Cu^{2+}-ATPase
Location	All tissues but liver	Liver
Copper levels	Low in serum Low in liver Elevated in other tissues Low ceruloplasmin Poor production of copper-dependent proteins	Low in serum High in liver Elevated in other tissues Low ceruloplasmin Impaired copper loss in bile
Pathology	Cerebral degeneration Early death	Neuronal degeneration Hemolytic anemia Liver disease Survival into late adulthood
Treatment	None	Chelation of Cu^{2+} by penicillamine

functions like a bus with a certain number of seats or binding sites for smaller molecules or ions, lipoproteins, in contrast, are almost like small oil tankers, traveling within the blood.

When you eat a meal rich in fat, be it meat (the inevitable hamburger or hot dog) or vegetable (your favorite avocado dip prepared with soybean or canola oil), the dietary fat, which is largely triglycerides, is hydrolyzed in your intestine by pancreatic enzymes called **lipases**. The breakdown products can be absorbed by the intestinal mucosal cells, which, in turn, use energy in the form of ATP to reassemble these products into triglycerides (Figure 2–10). Cholesterol from ingested animal fat can also be absorbed and metabolized into cholesterol ester. The mucosal cell will synthesize certain proteins at the same time and will take both the lipid and protein components to assemble large lipoprotein particles called **chylomicrons**. These are secreted by the mucosal cell and eventually enter the blood. After a fat-rich meal, your plasma can look rather like a miniature snowstorm (albeit somewhat yellow), created by the lipoproteins in the blood. Another lipoprotein, VLDL, is assembled from lipid and proteins in the liver and released into the blood. VLDLs are smaller particles than chylomicrons (Table 2–4). Liver can make its own lipids, such as triglycerides. Carbohydrates (e.g., sugars and starches), broken down in the gastrointestinal tract

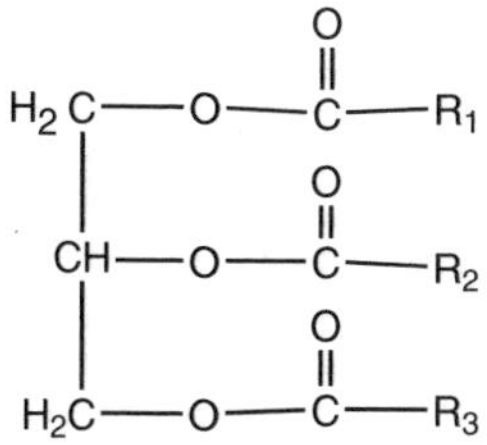

Triglyceride

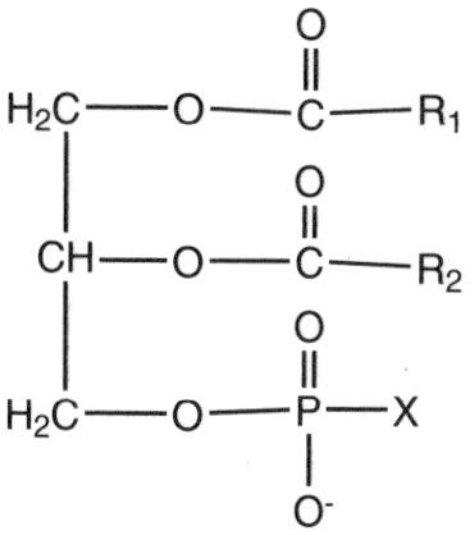

Phospholipid

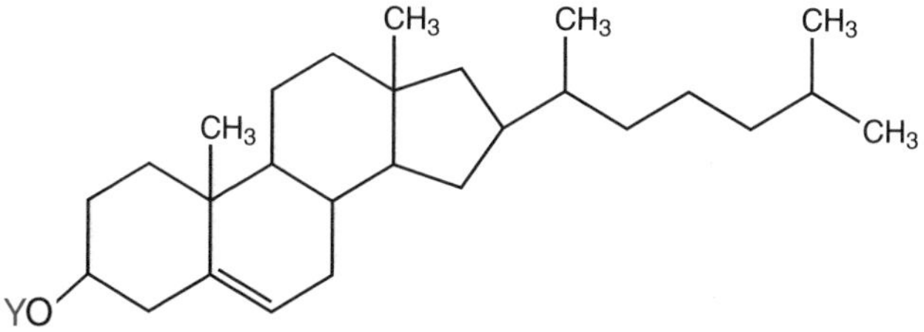

Cholesterol (Y = H)
Cholesterol Ester
(Y = R — C —)
‖
O

Figure 2–9 *A,* Structures of triglyceride, phospholipid, cholesterol, and cholesterol ester. "X" is a water-soluble compound, such as choline, "R-C-O-" is a fatty acid in ester linkage.

to simple sugars, can enter the bloodstream and be used by the liver to make lipids. As you know, eating carbohydrate instead of fat certainly does not prevent you from gaining weight.

One point of information: many of your patients may be aware of digestion and certainly of the dramatic consequences of gastrointestinal upsets, but there is a critical and often widespread misconception that whatever is eaten will arrive unaltered in the bloodstream or in the tissues of the body. For example, an individual may buy chondroitin sulfate in a health food store and consume this in the belief that this macromolecule is entering the bloodstream and is being used to repair cartilage in joints, if he or she happens to suffer from osteoarthritis. Now, chondroitin sulfate is found in cartilage, but it is a macromolecule composed of long chains of sugars, half of which are sulfated. To be absorbed, these sugar chains must be broken down to simple sugars. It is, indeed, possible that such simple sugars, once in the body, could be used to promote reconstruction of connective tissue and thus be of benefit, but the original macromolecule will not pass intact into the mucosal cells of the intestine. Rather, for large molecules with bonds that can be broken by hydrolytic digestive enzymes, there is a cycle of disas-

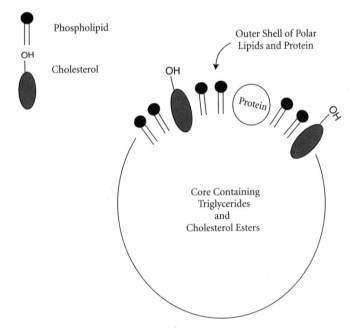

Figure 2–9 *B,* General lipoprotein structure. Lipoproteins are composed of a core containing triglycerides and fatty acid esters of cholesterol and a thin shell consisting of a monolayer of phospholipids, cholesterol, and specific proteins.

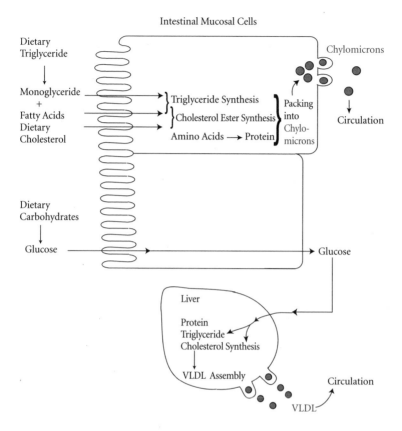

Figure 2–10 Lipoprotein synthesis. The intestinal digestion of dietary triglycerides yields fatty acids and monoglycerides that can be absorbed by the intestine and used in the synthesis of triglycerides within the mucosal cells. Dietary cholesterol is also taken up and used to form fatty acid esters of cholesterol. The intestinal cell uses these lipid components and proteins to assemble lipoproteins called chylomicrons, which are released and eventually enter the circulation. Dietary carbohydrate provides glucose that can enter the circulation from the intestine. Circulating glucose can be metabolized by the liver to make lipids that can be packaged and released as the lipoprotein VLDL (very-low-density lipoprotein).

sembly to simpler subunits in the gastrointestinal tract and assembly of absorbed simple molecules in the body's cells and tissues to more complex molecules. This disassembly–reassembly principle also applies to dietary fats and the assembly of lipoproteins.

Both VLDLs and chylomicrons function to transport lipids so that other cells in the body will be provided with fuel molecules for metabolism (e.g., muscle cells) or simply be able to store the fat against future needs (e.g., in fat cells or adipocytes). As you might expect, lipoproteins cannot simply unload triglycerides into cells. Rather, the lipoproteins are actually broken

Table 2–4
Characteristics of Lipoproteins

	Chylomicrons	VLDLs	LDLs	HDLs
Density (g/mL)	<0.95	0.95–1.006	1.019–1.063	1.063–1.21
Diameter (nm)	100–1200	25–80	20–25	7–12
Components (% of dry weight)				
Protein	2	8	23	32
Triglycerides	85	55	10	7
Cholesterol (+ esters)	6	20	47	32
Phospholipid	8	17	18	29

down by an enzyme called **lipoprotein lipase** that acts on the VLDLs and chylomicrons in the blood to generate smaller breakdown products, such as fatty acids (Figure 2–11). Fatty acids can be taken up by cells, such as adipocytes, in the vicinity of this attack. Naturally, the lipoproteins will decrease dramatically in size as a result of hydrolysis by lipoprotein lipase. Smaller lipoproteins called low-density lipoproteins (LDLs) are created from the digestion of VLDLs. The terminology for lipoproteins is based on density, simply because the more fat there is in a lipoprotein, generally the lighter the particle is. Thus, LDL is a heavier particle than VLDL, and LDL contains a higher percentage of protein and cholesterol and a much lower percentage of triglyceride than does VLDL (see Table 2–4). The lipoproteins can be separated from one another on the basis of density.

You have probably heard of LDL because of its important role in the development of cardiovascular disease. After the digestion of VLDL by lipoprotein lipase, LDL particles do not simply circulate in the blood like so many abandoned rockets in space. Rather, they are taken up by a process known as **receptor-mediated endocytosis**. This process was described earlier in this chapter for the delivery by transferrin of iron to cells. LDL receptors are located on the surface of the liver and adrenal and adipose cells and bind a protein component found in LDL. This is the protein apo-B100, which is also found on the surface of the parent VLDL. (Again, note the "apo" prefix used for the protein when considered as a single element away from the lipoprotein particle.) The LDL–LDL receptor complex is taken into the cell within the coated vesicles formed during endocytosis in a manner very similar to that shown for transferrin in Figure 2–7. The coated vesicles fuse with other cellular vesicles, and the lipid and protein components of LDL are degraded within the lysosomal system, yielding amino acids, fatty acids, and cholesterol. The LDL receptor returns to the plasma membrane, where it can bind more LDL particles. The cellular content of cholesterol can rise, and this can suppress the synthesis of the LDL receptor by the cell.

The problem associated with LDL arises when the particles are not cleared quickly enough from the circulation, and levels of plasma choles-

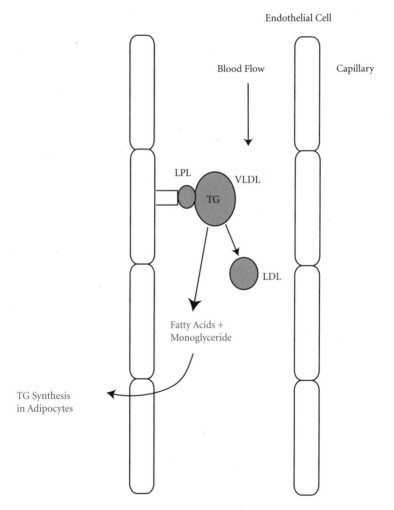

Figure 2–11 Hydrolysis of circulating VLDL by lipoprotein lipase (LPL). LPL is located within capillaries and can bind to and hydrolyze triglycerides of lipoproteins. The products, fatty acids and monoglycerides, move out of the capillary and can be used by nearby fat cells (adipocytes) in the synthesis of triglycerides for storage. LDL (low-density lipoprotein) is also a product of the LPL attack on VLDL. LDL can be taken up by the liver and other cells in receptor-mediated endocytosis. Inefficient uptake of LDL can lead to increased levels of circulating cholesterol, which are associated with cardiovascular disease.

terol rise with increasing concentration of LDL. The underlying problem is a defective LDL receptor, and this has a genetic basis. The resulting disease is referred to as **familial hypercholesterolemia** and is a very common inherited metabolic disorder. If both genes for the LDL receptor are defective (homozygous form of the disease), patients will usually die before the age of 20 years. Cardiovascular disease is a common cause of death. If they have one defective gene (heterozygous form), the individuals will have a longer lifespan and manifest lower levels of serum cholesterol than do homozygotes, although these levels will still be elevated in comparison with normals. Generally, levels of plasma cholesterol ≤5.2 mMol/L or 200 mg/dL are desirable. Be aware that elevated serum cholesterol in one individual, if it has a genetic basis, will have implications for other family members. Patients with elevated levels of serum cholesterol are usually first placed on diets with restrictions on meat and dairy products, which are rich sources of cholesterol. In contrast, plant and fish oils tend to reduce the incidence of cardiovascular disease, as does exercise. Generally, it is recommended that fat intake be reduced from 40 to 30% of calories ingested, with increased ingestion of vegetables and fish. Such approaches may lead to weight loss, which can, for some, be a desirable end result.

On the basis of serum cholesterol values, these dietary approaches may not be sufficient, as you may certainly see patients who conscientiously remove dairy and meat from their diets, yet their levels of serum cholesterol remain high. You will also see patients who say they are following a diet but, in fact, are not complying very well with your advice. This is all part of the real-world experience, as you cannot literally "spoon feed" your patients. When diet does not succeed, the use of drugs (such as lovastatin; related medications also have the -statin suffix) to inhibit the synthesis of cholesterol may be desirable. This therapy can be combined with the ingestion of certain resins that complex with bile salts in the intestine. Bile salts are synthesized from cholesterol and represent an important product of this molecule. They enter the intestine where they function as detergents to break up lipid droplets to promote their enzymatic hydrolysis. Bile salts can be resorbed from the intestine, and their loss in resin complexes from the intestine may promote the conversion of cholesterol in the liver into these derivatives. This conversion of cholesterol to bile salts is one way of reducing body levels of cholesterol.

You likely have heard, through the mass media, that cholesterol exists in two forms: "bad" and "good" cholesterol. "Bad" cholesterol is associated with LDL, while "good" cholesterol resides in high-density lipoprotein (HDL), a lipoprotein particle we have yet to describe (see Table 2–4). HDL is the smallest of the lipoproteins and is made by the liver but is initially rich in protein, with very little cholesterol ester. HDL functions to pick up cholesterol from cells and to convert this to cholesterol esters, which can then be transferred from HDL to LDL or VLDL (Figure 2–12). It is known that elevated levels of HDL in plasma correlate with reduced risk of cardiovascular disease. It is believed that HDL participates in reverse cholesterol transport, promoting the transport of cholesterol to the liver from nonhepatic tissues.

The pathology associated with elevated levels of LDL is related to atherosclerosis (see Figure 2–12). Over long periods of time, high levels of circulating LDL may promote the infiltration of these particles into the walls of arteries. This process can be accelerated by damage to the endothelial layer of the wall, such as that found with high blood pressure, diabetes, and smoking. The atherosclerotic process can be accelerated if the LDL particles are oxidized. Certain oxidized lipids can actually stimulate other cells, such as macrophages and monocytes. The LDL particles within the wall can provoke the entry of monocytes (leukocytes) from blood, which develop into macrophages that phagocytose the lipoproteins. These macrophages develop into foam cells, which have large fat deposits principally containing cholesterol. It is also possible that the infiltrating LDL particles aggregate and form larger particles in the vessel wall. Because of the cellular differentiation events in the arterial wall provoked by the invading macrophages, LDL particles, and damaged endothelial cells, there can be remarkable morphologic changes to the wall. Eventually, it accumulates an extracellular pool of lipid (that is largely cholesterol) as well as connective tissue proteins and bulges into the lumen, altering the blood flow dynamics in the artery. This bulge of material constitutes the atherosclerotic plaque that can be found in the coronary, carotid, and other arteries. Should the plaque fragment, complete arterial blockage and death can ensue. More often, the surface of the plaque is a site for the aggregation of platelets of the blood, forming what are called **thrombi**. These particles can dislodge from the plaque as **emboli** and flow with arterial blood, until they block a small blood vessel and provoke an ischemic event in the nearby tissue. Transient ischemic attacks (TIAs) are produced, for example, when there is a shut-down in the blood flow in a discrete area of the brain. This can come from a thrombus originating from a plaque in the carotid or vertebrobasilar artery and results in an episode of specific neurologic malfunction for a short time period. For example, a friend of your father, in his 50s, may rise at a wedding to give a toast to the bride and be quite unable to speak, although he can hear, see, and move. In another instance, a patient with a TIA may show temporary blindness in one eye or an episode of dizziness or blackout (e.g., a fall down a flight of stairs). TIAs can be events that are preliminary markers for stroke, and it is critical that such patients be examined thoroughly and receive treatment to prevent death or debilitating disease.

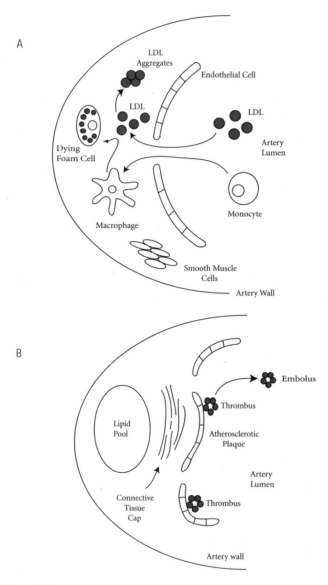

Figure 2–12 Atherosclerosis. *A*, Damage to the arterial endothelial cell layer can lead to infiltration of the lipoprotein LDL (rich in cholesterol) into the artery wall. The LDL may be followed by monocytes of the blood, which differentiate into macrophages inside the wall. LDL may aggregate within the arterial wall or be phagocytosed by macrophages. The macrophages can turn into foam cells with lipid deposits consisting largely of cholesterol. *B*, Infiltration by macrophages and damage to endothelial cells can promote cellular proliferation and differentiation events. A build-up of connective tissue proteins and a pool of lipid left behind after the death of the foam cells can contribute to an arterial atherosclerotic plaque that hinders blood flow and serves as a site for the formation of thrombi.

3

Enzymes

In Chapter 1, we introduced enzymes as proteins that catalyze specific reactions in the context of muscle and membrane functions. These included the action of Ca^{2+} ATPase in muscle contraction, Na^+, K^+-ATPase in active transport, kinases that phosphorylate proteins, and nitric oxide synthase (NOS), an enzyme that produces NO from the amino acid arginine. In this chapter, we wish to describe enzymes in more detail so that you can visualize how these very dynamic proteins work. As well, we will outline the variety of different reactions enzymes catalyze, how enzyme activities can be controlled and also altered by the administration of drugs, how enzymes can be used in diagnosis (following tissue injury), and how enzymes can be used to treat disease.

An enzyme (E) can take a molecule called the substrate (S) and convert this into a product molecule (P). An enzyme reaction may use two (or more) substrates and may lead to the formation of more than one product, as shown in the examples below:

$$\overset{E}{S \rightarrow P} \qquad \overset{E}{S_1 + S_2 \rightarrow P_1 + P_2} \qquad \overset{E}{S \rightarrow P_1 + P_2}$$

Enzymes often work in series, in pathways or cycles, so that the product of one enzyme is used as substrate by the next enzyme to produce a new product. In turn, this new compound can be used by a third enzyme to yield a third product. This occurs because each enzyme can catalyze a specific reaction, and usually a string of different reactions is required to generate a desired end product (F in our example below).

$$\overset{E_1 \quad E_2 \quad E_3 \quad E_4 \quad E_5}{A \rightarrow B \rightarrow C \rightarrow D \rightarrow E \rightarrow F}$$

This is similar to the assembly of a car by a number of workers or machines employed on an assembly line. Each has a specific task performed as part of a sequence, for example, installing the engine, wheels, seats, electronic equipment, and so on, that contributes to the final product emerging at the end of the line. When your cells or tissues construct a new molecule in such a manner, this molecule is usually more complex than the initial substrate molecule that entered the chain of reactions (rather like the bare metal chassis of a car entering our assembly line), and accordingly, this sequence of enzyme events is termed **anabolic** (Figure 3–1). One example of anabolism is the conversion of glucose molecules (monosaccharides called **hexoses**) into a long-branched polymer called **glycogen** (a polysaccharide) that has glucose as its subunit. Glycogen is somewhat like starch and represents a convenient storage form of glucose. Such anabolic reactions (including the assembly of proteins from amino acids, nucleic acids from nucleotides, and the synthesis of lipids from fatty acids and glycerol) require energy that is provided by the molecule adenosine triphosphate (ATP).

In a similar manner, molecules can be taken apart by a sequence of specific enzyme actions to produce smaller, simpler molecules. Often, these pathways are associated with the production of energy for your cells and are very important in the generation of the energy molecule ATP, which we mentioned in Chapter 1. Such sequences of enzymes involved in the breakdown of substrates are called **catabolic**. An example of catabolism is the breakdown of the simple hexose sugar glucose (a fuel substrate) to form the smaller compound pyruvate. Pyruvate is then converted to the central molecule acetyl-CoA, which, as you can see, may also be formed during the catabolism of amino acids derived from protein breakdown, from nucleotides coming from the disassembly of nucleic acids, or from the breakdown of fatty acids derived from lipids (see Figure 3–1). All these catabolic paths can contribute to the formation of acetyl-CoA, and acetyl-CoA can be used in a further catabolic sequence in the Krebs cycle, in which carbon dioxide is released. This cycle is associated with processes known as **electron transport** (which produces water) and **oxidative phosphorylation** (which drives the formation of ATP using power supplied by electron transport). ATP is a very important product formed by these catabolic paths.

Metabolism is really the sum total of all the enzyme reactions in your body, including both anabolic and catabolic sequences. We will discuss anabolism and catabolism (with ATP generation) in greater detail in Chapter 7.

PROPERTIES OF ENZYMES

Now that you have the "big picture," let's investigate individual enzymes and what they can do. The first important observation is that there are relatively few molecules of enzyme, compared with the substrate molecules that they handle. One analogy that can be used is the turnstile. You quite likely inter-

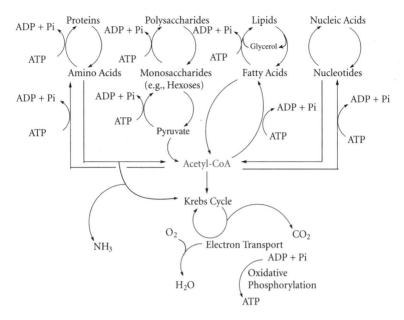

Figure 3–1 An overview of catabolic and anabolic paths in metabolism. Note that anabolic paths usually form more complex molecules (proteins, polysaccharides, lipids, nucleic acids) from simpler building blocks and require energy supplied by ATP. Catabolic paths are separate from anabolic ones and involve the breakdown of the more complex to the simpler molecules. Of these, acetyl-CoA is a central molecule both in catabolism and anabolism. Note the importance of the Krebs cycle in the generation of ATP by associated processes known as electron transport and oxidative phosphorylation.

face with this piece of transit machinery as you enter the subway, metro, or underground on your trip to your university or college in the morning. The turnstiles can represent the few molecules of enzyme that can handle an enormous number of commuters passing through them. Thus, the commuters are molecules of substrate that are converted into molecules of product by passing through the turnstiles. The token or cash surrendered or the ticket punched during the process may represent the change effected in your turnstile-mediated conversion from S to P.

Enzymes are also rather specific for the substrates that they handle because substrates actually bind to specific sites on the enzyme before the chemical change will take place. Continuing with our analogy, you initially enter the turnstile before you deposit your cash, token, or ticket and then push through the turnstile. Obviously, a horse, a cow, or even a student couple holding hands could not be accommodated within the turnstile (and thus not converted to the product). Often, a lock-and-key model of enzyme–substrate interaction is used to show the precision of the fit (Figure 3–2). Thus, an enzyme that handles glucose may not be able to handle another sugar, such as sucrose (table sugar), that is larger and has a different overall configuration.

This brings us to the remarkable speed or velocity of an enzyme-catalyzed reaction. Why is it that enzymes are so efficient? One reason is simply that enzymes do have specific binding sites for substrates. Thus, if a reaction requires the union of two molecules, a suitable enzyme allows both molecules to be bound close to each other within the enzyme. This binding feature is considerably superior to the corresponding nonenzymatic

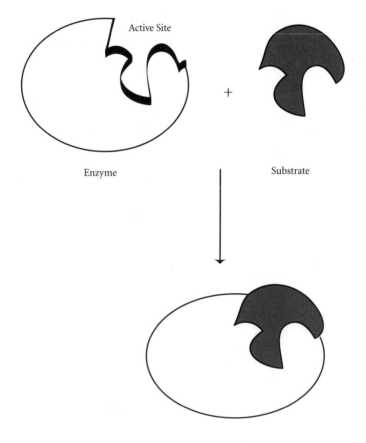

Figure 3–2 A lock-and-key model for enzyme–substrate binding. The substrate usually has a three-dimensional shape that allows it to fit rather specifically within the active site of the enzyme.

reaction, in which, for example, two molecules (likely in dilute solution) meet each other by chance and react chemically. The enzyme in this case is somewhat like a dating service. You may have little chance of finding your true match simply by circulating through your classes, your neighborhood, or shopping malls (not to mention the potential dangers in attracting the attention of law-enforcement personnel by your activities!). But submit your name and video bio to a dating service (the enzyme-binding site), and the chances of finding that suitable someone are definitely increased. There are other advantages to enzyme binding. The binding event actually promotes the reaction by increasing the probability of interaction. As per our dating service analogy, two singles, by joining such a service, are indeed much more likely to interact. You are at the service because you wish to find a match, and you have paid money to do this. You are serious about the process; another individual also at the service has similar objectives, and an interaction is that much more likely to occur. (Unlike the desirable individual you see in class, who may be more interested in someone else, or perhaps even more interested in pizza than in you!) The increased probability of the interaction between the two substrates at the enzyme-binding sites is explained chemically by the decreased entropy that each molecule has following binding. Entropy (although you may have rather painful memories associated with this term, depending on your experiences in the often medicine-unfriendly spheres of physical chemistry) is simply a measure of disorder, and a substrate binding to an enzyme tends to decrease entropy and promote a chemical reaction.

Another important reason for the efficiency of enzyme reactions is that the substrate molecules, when held at binding site(s), are usually placed in close proximity and favorable orientation to the R-groups of other amino acids of the enzyme that can carry out the reaction. In Chapter 1, we noted some of the different R-groups of the common amino acids. We also discussed the dissection of the muscle protein myosin by the enzyme trypsin. Trypsin hydrolyzes specific peptide bonds in protein substrates, and trypsin has a binding site for the side chains of arginine or lysine, two amino acids with long, positively charged R-groups in the protein substrate (see Figure 1–3). Once the side chain of the protein substrate is held at this binding site, the peptide bond linking arginine or lysine to the next amino acid in the substrate is held in favorable orientation to the serine, histidine, and aspartate amino acid side chains in trypsin that carry out the enzyme reaction (Figure 3–3). These amino acids in trypsin participate in a catalytic mechanism that breaks the peptide bond on the carboxyl side of arginine or lysine within the substrate and then releases the two pieces derived from the original protein. It is of interest that there is a family of proteases (the serine proteases), including trypsin, that have virtually identical catalytic mechanisms but differ in their binding sites for certain amino acid side chains found in

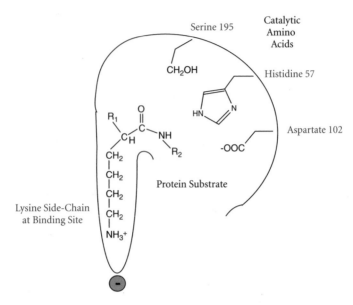

Figure 3–3 The interaction of the proteolytic enzyme trypsin with a protein substrate. Trypsin has a binding pocket within the active site that specifically accommodates the long positively charged side chains of lysine and arginine in the substrate protein. Following this binding, the peptide bond linking lysine or arginine to the next amino acid (toward the carboxyl terminus) is hydrolyzed by the catalytic mechanism of the enzyme.

protein substrates. And it is the binding site that determines what peptide bonds can be hydrolyzed by a specific protease in this family.

Thus, you can see the sequence of enzyme events: specific binding of substrate(s) to the binding site(s), optimized chemical reaction via the catalytic amino acid residues, and release of products. The binding site(s) and catalytic amino acids within the enzyme constitute what is called the **active site** of the enzyme. The active site usually takes up a rather small percentage of the total enzyme volume and has a particular three-dimensional structure, depending on the nature of the substrates, binding site(s), and catalytic amino acids. The active site is formed during the folding of the enzyme, as it comes to assume its mature three-dimensional structure. The active site can be made up of amino acid residues brought from many different locations in the linear structure. Thus, in the enzyme lysozyme (a small protein found in tears), which can hydrolyze components of bacterial cell walls (and serves as an antibiotic), the amino acids numbered 35, 52, 62, 63, 101, and 108 in the linear sequence of amino acids come together during folding and contribute to the geography of the active site (Figure 3–4). Denaturation of an enzyme (e.g., when the enzyme is exposed to ethanol or detergent) involves unfolding and, thus, loss in activity.

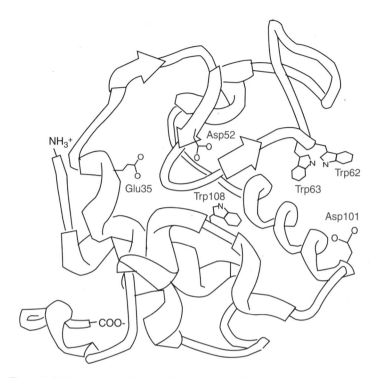

Figure 3–4 The active site of lysozyme. Lysozyme is a small enzyme (129 amino acids) found in tears that can hydrolyze bacterial cell walls. When it folds, different parts of the linear sequence of amino acids in lysozyme are brought together. The active site is made up of amino acids numbered 35, 52, 62, 63, 101, and 108. Thus, contributions to the active site can be made from throughout the linear amino acid sequence. Adapted from Voet D, Voet JG. Biochemistry. 2nd ed. New York: Wiley and Sons; 1995.

You might wonder about the function of the rest of the enzyme situated outside the active site. This bulk of the protein, of course, contributes to the conformation of the enzyme and of the active site, and it may contain other binding sites for nonsubstrate molecules that can regulate the enzyme activity. An enzyme is, after all, a powerful catalytic activity that can participate in the rapid depletion of a specific molecule or molecules. Naturally, an override mechanism is needed to slow down an enzyme pathway at a control point should there be an accumulation of the end product made by the path. Thus, an end product may interact with a control enzyme in the path by binding at a site outside the active site (Figure 3–5). This binding may lead to a conformational change that slows this key enzyme reaction. The control of enzyme activity is a very important feature within the regulation of metabolism that we will discuss in Chapter 7.

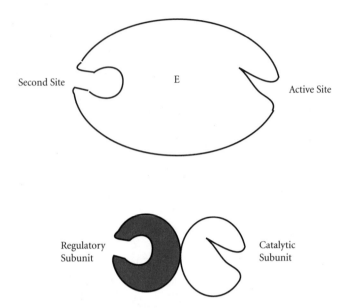

Figure 3–5 Second sites on enzymes. Besides the active site, which binds substrates and carries out the enzyme reaction, there can be other binding sites on the enzyme. These are referred to as regulatory sites. It is possible for a molecule (which is not the substrate) to bind at a second site and to influence the activity of the enzyme by promoting a conformational change in the enzyme. This is called allosteric regulation. Regulatory enzymes are often made up of different polypeptide subunits, and regulatory sites are more commonly found on regulatory subunits that are distinct from subunits that carry out the reaction (catalytic subunits).

Specificity

By utilizing a relatively large macromolecule, a protein, as the site for a reaction, one advantage over a purely chemical reaction in solution is considerable control over the compounds that can be used as substrates. We briefly noted this in our turnstile analogy, with images of cows and horses as ineffective substrates for the turnstile enzyme. This selection of substrates is referred to as **enzyme specificity**. Specificity can be absolute for one molecule. For example, the enzyme urease, the first protein to be crystallized, handles only urea as its substrate. Urease is a bacterial enzyme (whose abundance is particularly noticeable at campsite outhouses, as this enzyme converts urea into water and ammonia). Other enzymes may not be specific for a single molecule but rather for a particular functional group within that molecule. For example, the enzyme alcohol dehydrogenase can utilize a number of alcohols as substrates, converting the alcohol function to that of an aldehyde. Parenthetically, aldehydes are very reactive and can be used as the basis for blood alcohol determinations using breathalyzers at police check-points on New Year's Eve (and other festive occasions). There are also enzymes that can hydrolyze chemical bonds that are related to one another. For example, trypsin, as we have noted, can hydrolyze peptide bonds at lysine and arginine amino acid residues but can hydrolyze certain ester bonds as well. One further feature of the active site and substrate specificity is the recognition of stereoisomerism. Stereoisomers are molecules that are almost completely identical, with the same numbers and types of functional groups at each carbon atom, but differ in the orientation of these chemical groups. Your two hands are a good analogy. Each has the same number of fingers and thumb (hopefully), but the orientation is different. Essentially your two hands are mirror-images of one another and are, thus, not identical and cannot be superimposed one upon the other. In a similar manner D-glucose and L-glucose are mirror images (Figure 3–6), but it is only D-glucose that can be used by your cells in their metabolic processes.

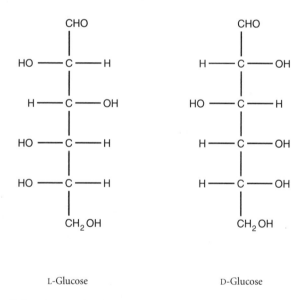

L-Glucose   D-Glucose

Figure 3–6 D-glucose and L-glucose as stereoisomers. These two forms of glucose are mirror images of each other and are very distinct molecules, even though they have the same number of carbons and the same number of functional groups. Enzymes can discriminate between these two stereoisomers so that only D-glucose is used in metabolism.

Velocity

Of course, it is the actual rate or velocity of reaction catalyzed by an enzyme that is the most prominent feature of enzyme function. And these reaction rates can be very impressive, indeed. Without unduly knocking organic chemistry, comparing rates in standard organic reactions in solution with enzyme-based reactions is like comparing a World War I biplane (Sopwith Camel) with an F-18 or, perhaps more accurately, with the USS Enterprise, if you happen to be a Star Trek fan. Enzymes usually increase reaction rates (conversion of substrates to products) by at least a factor of one million. For urease, the enzyme that renders the contents of outhouses alkaline by the production of ammonia from urea, this factor is closer to 10^{14}.

Turnover number is a measure of enzyme efficiency and gives the number of substrate molecules converted into product per molecule of enzyme within a unit of time. This is determined when the enzyme is operating at optimal efficiency, when there is a relatively high concentration of substrate for the enzyme. Thus, substrate availability does not limit the enzyme reaction rate. In our turnstile analogy, there is a steady and rapid rush hour flow of commuters into the turnstiles. The turnover number can also be referred to as the catalytic constant (kcat) for an enzyme. For the enzyme urease, the turnover number is 30,000/sec. For the enzyme carbonic anhydrase, which converts carbon dioxide and water into carbonic acid, the turnover number is 1 million/sec. Using the turnstile image, the rate of rotation would be quite frightening if it were to approach that of an enzyme in velocity. Under such conditions, entering the subway or metro would be like walking into a rather blunt food processor. Perhaps such an image should be left for the next "slice-and-dice" or, perhaps more accurately, blunt-trauma movie.

Activation

Enzymes are efficient catalysts, largely because they reduce the so-called free energy of activation associated with a reaction (Figure 3–7). This is because a substrate or substrates have to pass through a transition state before the formation of product. In the transition state, molecules are considered to be most reactive. And this transition state has an elevated free energy associated with it. Because of the binding of substrates, the reduction in entropy, and the proximity of catalytic groups, enzymes reduce the energy of this transition state quite sizably, thus accelerating the reaction. This is necessary for the enzyme reaction to take place within the bounds of body temperature. One advantage for organic nonenzyme reactions is that a greater efficiency can be achieved by simply increasing the heat of the reaction vessel. For living systems, this is not an option. You should also note that enzymes, like other inorganic catalysts, do not change the equilibrium constant for a reaction (the inherent balance between numbers of substrates and product molecules based on the free energies of these compounds); rather, enzymes accelerate the speed at which equilibrium is attained.

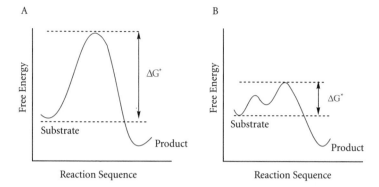

Figure 3–7 Free energy changes associated with non-enzyme (*A*) and enzymatically catalyzed (*B*) reactions. The conversion of substrate to product involves a free energy of activation as the substrate passes through a transition state. In the transition state, molecules are most reactive, and an elevated free energy is associated with it. Enzyme-catalyzed reactions (*B*) occur more readily, as the free energy of the transition state is considerably lower for the enzyme reaction.

Cofactors

Often, enzymes make use of not only substrates but also molecules or inorganic ions called **cofactors**. These participate in a variety of enzyme reactions and are present in the cytoplasm of cells or in organelles. Cofactors are often divided into two classes: the inorganic ions and the small organic molecules, which are called **coenzymes**. The inorganic ions include some that we have already discussed: iron (Fe), zinc (Zn), cobalt (Co), calcium (Ca), magnesium (Mg), and copper (Cu). Coenzymes, on the other hand, are usually derived from the vitamins within the diet, and much of the early biochemistry of nutrition was devoted to identifying vitamins as well as the diseases associated with vitamin deficiencies. One well-known vitamin is vitamin C (ascorbic acid), which is needed in the synthesis of connective tissue. In the early exploration of North America, it was quite common for European sailors on long ocean voyages or enduring the long winter in the Northern United States or Canada (areas not particularly well known as producers of citrus fruits) to become deficient in vitamin C and develop symptoms of scurvy. In the 18th century, Captain Cook had an interest in this disease, and he attempted to identify the fruit or vegetable that would cure his sailors of this disease. Once citrus fruits were identified as curatives/preventives for scurvy (by Captain James Lind, a naval physician), British sailors, and ultimately the English population, became known as "limeys." If you are an old-film buff, you may recall Gregory Peck as Captain Horatio Hornblower striding on his quarterdeck ordering the juice of 10,000 limes for his crew before they set off in pursuit of the Napoleonic fleet. You may think that this nutritional-deficiency disease was eradicated by the 19th century; however, it was quite likely that explorers traveling to the South Pole within the 20th century suffered from scurvy. It is conceivable that the members of the ill-fated Scott expedition to the South Pole (1910 to 1911) perished because of vitamin C (and other) deficiencies, even though the dietary basis of this disease was well known. Even today, you will likely encounter vitamin C deficiency among the elderly, particularly those who exist largely on a diet of tea and toast. Vitamins and their derivative coenzymes are vitally important for enzyme activity and good health, and it is critical in this fast food era that you be very aware of the potential dangers of this form of malnutrition.

Some enzymes rely on cofactors; in the absence of these cofactors, they are called **apoenzymes**, and in their presence, they are called **holoenzymes**.

$$\text{apoenzyme} + \text{cofactor} \Leftrightarrow \text{holoenzyme}$$
$$\text{(nonfunctional)} \qquad \text{(functional)}$$

Inorganic ions can participate in oxidation–reduction reactions catalyzed by enzymes and assist in the binding of organic substrates at the active site. ATP, the energy molecule, can be used in a variety of reactions but is usually active as its Mg^{2+} salt. Likely, this divalent cation helps to neutralize the negative charges associated with the phosphate groups in ATP. Metal ions can also be bound tightly to proteins to assist in reactions. Coenzymes (the organic cofactors) also play essential roles in enzyme-catalyzed reactions. Coenzymes can exist as free molecules that associate with the active site of enzymes, or they can be bound tightly to the active site. These latter coenzymes are often called **prosthetic groups**. Thiamine pyrophosphate (Table 3–1) is formed from the vitamin thiamine and acts as a coenzyme for the enzyme pyruvate dehydrogenase, a key enzyme that produces acetyl-CoA using pyruvate as substrate. The flavin nucleotides FAD (flavin adenine dinucleotide) and FMN (flavin mononucleotide), which participate in oxidation–reduction reactions, are derived from the vitamin riboflavin. The nicotinamide-containing coenzymes NAD^+ (nicotinamide adenine dinucleotide) and $NADP^+$ (nicotinamide adenine dinucleotide phosphate) also play roles in enzyme-catalyzed oxidation–reduction reactions and are derived from the vitamin niacin. The structures of NAD^+ and $NADP^+$ are shown in Figure 3–8. Parenthetically, these two coenzymes are <u>not</u> derived from nicotine. The deficiency disease pellagra is caused by lack of dietary niacin, while a deficiency of thiamine causes beriberi. Thiamine, niacin, and riboflavin are B vitamins and are water-soluble. We will talk about other water soluble vitamins, vitamins B_6 and B_{12} and folic acid, in Chapters 6 and 7. One important note: deficiencies of folic acid are associated with fetal neural tube defects (resulting in spina bifida), and it is very important that women even contemplating pregnancy should be taking this vitamin, as these defects can be initiated very early in fetal development. Multivitamins (and multiminerals) are available and

Table 3–1
Vitamins and Their Coenzyme Derivatives

Coenzyme	Vitamin
NAD$^+$, NADP$^+$	Niacin (vitamin B$_3$)
FAD, FMN	Riboflavin (vitamin B$_2$)
Thiamine pyrophosphate	Thiamine (vitamin B$_1$)
Pyridoxal phosphate	Pyridoxine, pyridoxal, pyridoxamine (vitamin B$_6$)
Coenzyme A (CoA)	Pantothenic acid*
Biotin (covalently linked)	Biotin*
Tetrahydrofolate	Folic acid*
Cobalamin derivatives	Cobalamin (vitamin B$_{12}$)

*These vitamins are also, historically, considered to be part of the vitamin B complex, which was a crude, water-soluble fraction isolated from yeast and liver and found to be essential for life.

should be taken during pregnancy. Fat-soluble vitamins include vitamin A (needed for the formation of retinal, a molecule bound to the protein rhodopsin, which is involved in vision), vitamin D (involved in Ca^{2+} absorption), vitamin E (an antioxidant of particular potency), and vitamin K (necessary for blood coagulation, and noted in Chapter 4). Not all fat-soluble vitamins fill cofactor roles in enzyme reactions.

ENZYME CLASSIFICATION AND NOMENCLATURE

It is estimated that there are about 10,000 enzymes in the human body. As we have noted earlier, one common suffix used to denote an enzyme is -ase (e.g., phosphatase, lipase, protease, nuclease). However, some enzymes do not have this useful ending (e.g., trypsin, papain). As more and more enzymes were described and purified, it became very important to adopt a classification system, somewhat like Linnaeus systematically classifying plants and animals. One logical approach to enzyme classification is based on the nature of the reaction catalyzed. Thus, there are six main classes of enzymes (Figure 3–9) that include the following:

1. Oxidoreductases catalyze oxidation–reduction reactions. These enzymes may also be called dehydrogenases or reductases. Usually, coenzymes, such as NAD$^+$, NADP$^+$, FAD, or FMN, are involved in these enzyme-catalyzed reactions. You may remember from school the chemical rubric LEO GER: loss of electrons is oxidation, gain of electrons is reduction. In these oxidation–reduction reactions, electrons can travel from a substrate to a coenzyme (thus oxidizing the substrate and reduc-

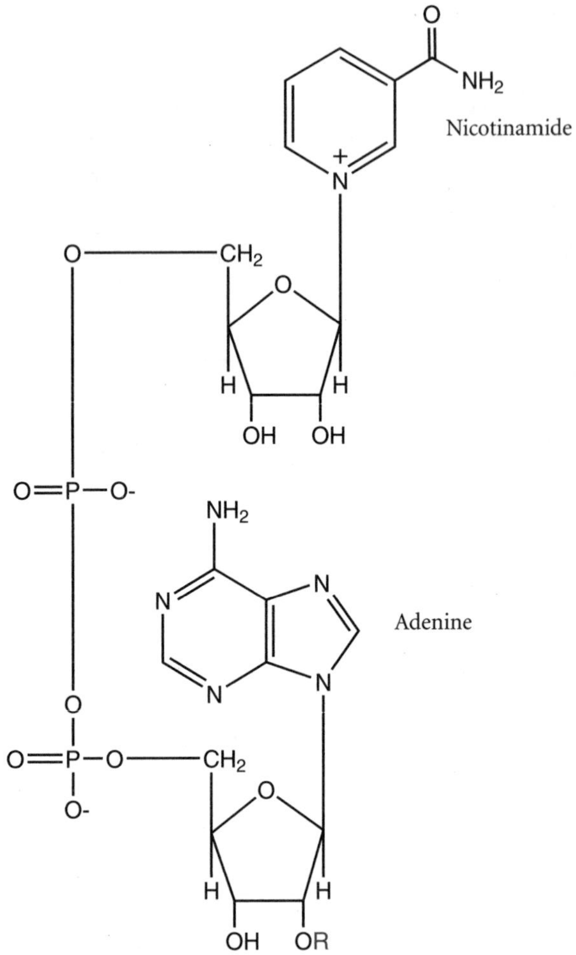

Figure 3–8 The structure of the related coenzymes NAD⁺ and NADP⁺. These two coenzymes are derived from the vitamin niacin, a B vitamin found in the diet. The one difference between these two nicotinamide coenzymes is the presence of a phosphate monoester (designated R) linked to the hydroxyl group of C2 of ribose. Adapted from Murray RK, Granner DK, Mayes PA, Rodwell VW. Harper's biochemistry. 25th ed. Stamford (CT): Appleton and Lange; 2000.

ing the coenzyme), or the flow of electrons can be in the opposite direction (oxidizing the coenzyme and reducing the substrate). Often, oxidation–reduction reactions are reversible. One such reaction is catalyzed by the enzyme alcohol dehydrogenase (see Figure 3–9). The enzyme can oxidize ethanol to acetaldehyde, with the concomitant acceptance of electrons by the cofactor NAD⁺ to give its reduced form: NADH. In this case, and in many examples of oxidation–reduction, the electron pair

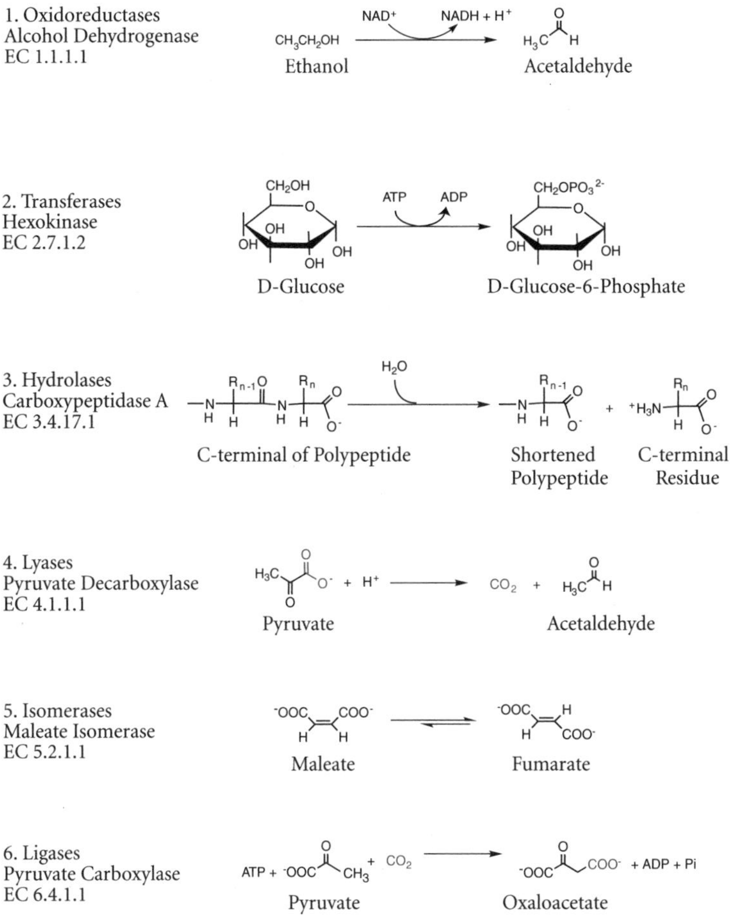

1. Oxidoreductases
Alcohol Dehydrogenase
EC 1.1.1.1

$$CH_3CH_2OH \xrightarrow{\quad NAD^+ \quad NADH + H^+ \quad} H_3C \overset{O}{\underset{}{\diagdown}} H$$

Ethanol   Acetaldehyde

2. Transferases
Hexokinase
EC 2.7.1.2

D-Glucose $\xrightarrow{\quad ATP \quad ADP \quad}$ D-Glucose-6-Phosphate

3. Hydrolases
Carboxypeptidase A
EC 3.4.17.1

$$\xrightarrow{\quad H_2O \quad}$$

C-terminal of Polypeptide → Shortened Polypeptide + C-terminal Residue

4. Lyases
Pyruvate Decarboxylase
EC 4.1.1.1

$$H_3C \overset{O}{\underset{O}{\diagdown}} O^- + H^+ \longrightarrow CO_2 + H_3C \overset{O}{\underset{}{\diagdown}} H$$

Pyruvate   Acetaldehyde

5. Isomerases
Maleate Isomerase
EC 5.2.1.1

Maleate ⇌ Fumarate

6. Ligases
Pyruvate Carboxylase
EC 6.4.1.1

$$ATP + {}^-OOC \overset{O}{\underset{}{\diagdown}} CH_3 + CO_2 \longrightarrow {}^-OOC \overset{O}{\underset{}{\diagdown}} COO^- + ADP + Pi$$

Pyruvate   Oxaloacetate

Figure 3–9 Enzyme classification. Enzymes are divided into six classes, depending on the reaction they catalyze. Each enzyme also receives a four-digit EC (Enzyme Commission) or classification number, the first digit representing the class to which the enzyme belongs. Adapted from Mathews CK, van Holde KE, Ahern KG. Biochemistry. 3rd ed. San Francisco (CA): Addison Wesley Longman; 2000.

travels as a hydride ion, H$^-$, that is a hydrogen atom with an extra electron. You will note that each enzyme in this classification is assigned a four-digit EC (Enzyme Commission) number that is a specific catalogue number. The first digit specifies which of the six main classes the enzyme belongs to. Alcohol dehydrogenase has the number EC 1.1.1.1.

2. The transferases are the second class of enzymes, which catalyze the transfer of specific groups to substrates during these reactions. The example given is hexokinase, an enzyme that transfers a phosphate group from ATP to the C6 position of D-glucose, forming D-glucose-6-

phosphate. You should know that kinases either utilize ATP (we noted protein kinases in Chapter 1) or generate ATP.

3. Hydrolases make up the third class of enzymes. As the name suggests, these enzymes catalyze hydrolytic reactions, using water molecules to break chemical bonds. The example given is carboxypeptidase A, which liberates the C-terminal amino acid of a polypeptide by hydrolyzing the C-terminal peptide bond.

4. Lyases constitute the fourth class, possibly the category whose actions are most difficult to remember. A lyase will catalyze a reaction that generates a double bond or the addition of one substrate to the double bond of a second substrate molecule. The example is perhaps more illuminating. Here, pyruvate decarboxylase effectively removes a carboxyl group from pyruvate, thus liberating carbon dioxide (creating a new double bond as seen in CO_2) and producing acetaldehyde.

5. The fifth class comprises the isomerases, which convert one isomeric form into another. The example shows how maleate isomerase converts maleate into fumarate by changing a cis isomer (both large groups on the same side of the double bond) to a trans isomer.

6. Ligases make up category six, and these enzymes effectively join two molecules. Pyruvate carboxylase is a ligase that catalyzes the addition of carbon dioxide to pyruvate in the formation of oxaloacetate. Reactions employing ligases require the participation of ATP or another nucleotide that can provide energy to drive such anabolic reactions. DNA ligases can join two nucleotides in DNA strands at a break in DNA structure.

MEASUREMENT OF ENZYME ACTIVITY (ENZYME ASSAYS)

Within medicine and the health sciences, your grasp of enzymes must extend from the theoretical to the practical. You may be using enzymes therapeutically or, more often, using measurements of enzyme activities as a diagnostic tool. Others will carry out these clinical assays for you, but it is imperative that you understand the process. Remember that enzymes are dynamic molecules, converting substrates to products at considerable speed and efficiency. While the actual quantity of an enzyme may be measured, the relatively small number of enzyme molecules makes this a rather costly procedure, if done routinely. The easier way to measure enzymes is by their activity. By our earlier analogy of the transit turnstiles, the clinician does not measure the number of turnstiles but takes the easier course in measuring the number of commuters who have passed through the turnstiles on their way to the subway or metro. The large numbers of commuters (product molecules) make this measurement both sensitive and accurate. Remember that five turnstiles could effectively handle some 300 or more commuters per minute.

The measurement of an enzyme in a clinical lab means a measurement of rate, that is, so many molecules of product formed or substrates utilized per minute. Usually, one wishes to measure a maximal rate to quantitate enzyme performance, and thus a relatively high concentration of substrate(s) is used in the reaction. Enzyme measurements or assays are usually carried out using automated equipment that sets up, within test tubes, a mixture of components that include both the substrate and the sample to be measured for enzyme activity (e.g., plasma or serum). There are a number of variables in an enzyme assay. One is the pH of the medium for the assay. An enzyme will show an optimal pH (Figure 3–10); thus, it is important to maintain the pH of an enzyme reaction. This is normally done by the inclusion of a buffer, a weak acid or base that will hold the pH of the reaction during the addition of assay components (e.g., a substrate that is acidic). For example, a phosphate, Tris or Hepes buffer can be used to maintain a reaction at pH 7.4. Another variable is the temperature of the reaction, and a temperature optimum can be determined for an enzyme (Figure 3–11). An enzyme assay can

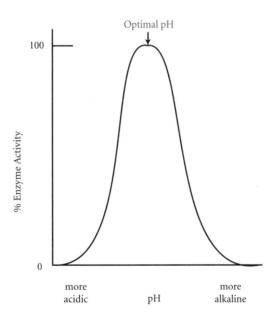

Figure 3–10 The effect of pH on enzyme activity. Enzymes usually have characteristic optimal pH values for the reactions they catalyze. These pH optima may reflect the nature of the reaction and also the location for the reaction within the cell. For example, many anabolic reactions take place in the cytoplasm or on the membrane of the endoplasmic reticulum, optimally at a pH of 7.4. In contrast, the actions of lysosomal acid hydrolases have optima in the acidic range, reflecting the acidic environment of the lysosome.

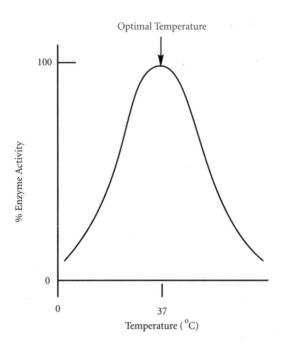

Figure 3–11 The effect of temperature on enzyme activity. Enzymes show optimal temperatures for their reactions. These may be close to body temperature. Raising the temperature of the environment of the enzyme above the optimal temperature can lead to denaturation of the enzyme as it loses its conformation.

be run at room temperature, as long as this value is fairly constant from day to day or season to season. Be careful during fall or spring, when room temperature may vary significantly depending on the switchover between heating and air conditioning. Another variable is the presence of drugs that may function to inhibit the enzyme of interest. It can be quite enlightening to see exactly what medications and other compounds an individual is taking, particularly if she or he is under the care of a number of health-care practitioners (chiropractor, naturopath, practitioner of Chinese medicine) who are functioning independently of each other. Other sources of less legal forms of medication should also be of interest, although such information will likely be less readily accessible for you.

An example of an enzyme assay is the measurement of alcohol dehydrogenase (an oxidoreductase).

$$\text{ethanol} + NAD^+ \rightarrow \text{acetaldehyde} + NADH + H^+$$

The enzyme reaction mixture will contain a buffer that holds the pH at 7.4, ethanol (at a concentration that will maximize enzyme activity without denaturing the enzyme itself), the coenzyme NAD⁺, and a sample of enzyme. The enzyme sample can be taken, for example, from a liver biopsy, which is homogenized in buffer (i.e., all the cells are broken to free the soluble enzymes inside). Thus, the enzyme source is a liver homogenate. These components are mixed within a test tube or a cuvette (a square glass or plastic container that usually measures 1 cm × 1 cm and is 4 to 5 cm tall). The volume of the assay is usually adjusted by the addition of water to give a standard final volume (e.g., 1 mL) so that concentrations of buffer, ethanol, NAD⁺, and enzyme will be standardized over a series of assays. Often, the enzyme is added last, and its addition to the assay initiates the enzyme reaction. With time, the enzyme will convert the ethanol to acetaldehyde and simultaneously will convert NAD⁺ to NADH. Not only does the cofactor serve as an electron acceptor in this reaction, the reduced NADH product also absorbs ultraviolet light at a characteristic wavelength. In Figure 3–12, the absorption spectra of NAD⁺ and NADH are shown. A compound may absorb either visible or ultraviolet light. For example,

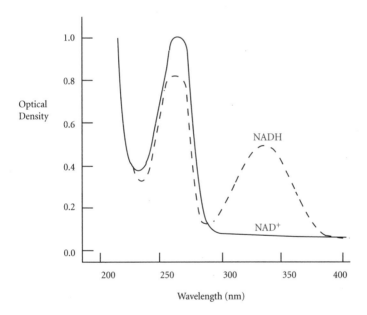

Figure 3–12 The absorption spectra of the coenzymes NADH and NAD⁺. Absorption spectra are recorded by shining light of different wavelengths through solutions containing the two coenzymes. When there is absorption at a particular wavelength, this is registered as an increased optical density or absorbance. Both NADH and NAD⁺ have an absorbance peak near 260 nm, but only NADH shows an absorption peak at 340 nm. This is an extremely useful distinction, as the formation of NADH or the loss of NADH in a reaction can be followed specifically by monitoring light absorbance at 340 nm. Similar principles apply to NADP⁺ and NADPH. Adapted from Murray RK, Granner DK, Mayes PA, Rodwell VW. Harper's biochemistry. 25th ed. Stamford (CT): Appleton and Lange; 2000.

hemoglobin is red because it can absorb blue light from the visible spectrum of light (made up of all the colors of the rainbow). The absorption of blue light by hemoglobin in solution will make the hemoglobin solution appear red in color.

So, too, molecules with unsaturated ring structures, as found in NAD$^+$ or NADH (see Figure 3–8), can absorb ultraviolet light. However, NADH, the reduced form of this coenzyme, shows a characteristic peak of absorbance of ultraviolet light at 340 nm that is not found for NAD$^+$. This is very useful, as the reaction can be monitored by passing ultraviolet light at a 340-nm wavelength through the reaction cuvette. The cuvette is held in a spectrophotometer, which can direct the light of an individual wavelength through the cuvette and also measure the intensity of light emerging from the cuvette. A spectrophotometer will measure light absorption by solutions in terms of absorbance (also known as optical density). Thus, a high absorbance at 340 nm would indicate a relatively high concentration of NADH in the reaction cuvette. If you mix the assay components for alcohol dehydrogenase together within the cuvette (as noted above), the absorbance at 340 nm will increase. As the enzyme converts more ethanol to acetaldehyde, there is an equivalent conversion of NAD$^+$ to NADH. Thus, as the enzyme reaction progresses, there is a rising concentration of NADH in the reaction cuvette. The spectrophotometer can plot absorbance on a graph with time to give a progress curve (Figure 3–13). As the absorbance is a direct indication of the concentration of NADH, the enzyme rate can be calculated as the initial slope of the line (i.e., change of optical density per minute). This slope is also known as the initial velocity (v_o), as the slope can fall off with time. This fall away from linearity may come from the loss of substrate concentration (as the enzyme rate will slow down if the substrate concentration falls significantly) or the possibility that rising concentration of product may inhibit the enzyme reaction. It is also possible that the enzyme is not stable under the assay conditions, for example, the enzyme may denature or be destroyed, possibly by a protease activity that is also present in the enzyme sample.

There is a direct correlation between the concentration of NADH and absorbance at 340 nm (usually referred to as a molar extinction coefficient for NADH). Thus, an absorbance reading can be readily converted into a concentration of NADH, and a change in absorbance with time can be converted into a rate based on millimoles of NADH formed per minute.

Two guiding principles for clinical enzyme assays are simplicity and cost. Thus, reactions that can be monitored using a spectrophotometer are preferred to assays using radioactive substrates and the need to separate radioactive products for measurements of enzyme activity. Clinical enzyme assays can also utilize artificial substrates that are colorless themselves but release colored products or products that absorb ultraviolet light. An

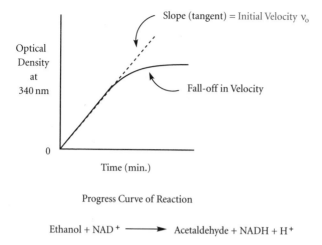

Progress Curve of Reaction

$$Ethanol + NAD^+ \longrightarrow Acetaldehyde + NADH + H^+$$

Figure 3–13 The time course of an enzyme reaction. In this example, the production of NADH is being monitored at 340 nm. As more NADH is produced in the reaction cuvette, the optical density or absorbance increases. Thus, the rate of change of optical density (the slope to the initial part of the progress curve) can be used to calculate the initial velocity of the enzyme (v_o). As there is a direct relation between the optical density and concentration of NADH, a rate can be calculated on the basis of the number of millimoles of NADH produced per minute.

enzyme reaction may also be monitored by the loss of a substrate that absorbs light. A reaction that utilizes NADH in the formation of NAD^+ may be monitored by a decline of absorbance at 340 nm in an enzyme catalyzed reaction. For example, the enzyme lactate dehydrogenase can be monitored by the conversion of NADH to NAD^+, as pyruvate is reduced to lactate.

$$CH_3\text{-}CO\text{-}COO^- + NADH + H^+ \leftrightarrow CH_3\text{-}CHOH\text{-}COO^- + NAD^+$$
$$\text{pyruvate} \text{lactate}$$

Spectrophotometers can be automated so that hundreds of enzyme samples and their reactions can be measured within a day, as is done in a busy hospital laboratory.

As you might imagine, not all enzyme reactions can be measured as conveniently as described above. Some reactions do not produce products that absorb light, either in the ultraviolet or visible range. For example, hexokinase converts glucose to glucose-6-phosphate with the parallel conversion of ATP to adenosine diphosphate (ADP), as a phosphate group leaves ATP and is transferred to the carbon 6 position of glucose (Figure 3–14). None of the substrates or products has a unique light absorbance property that can be used to follow the reaction directly. In this circumstance, a coupled assay may be used. The hexokinase reaction is set up (glucose, ATP, source of enzyme, buffer at pH 7.4), but a further addition of the purified enzyme

Coupled Assay:

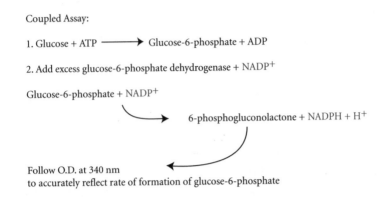

1. Glucose + ATP $\longrightarrow$ Glucose-6-phosphate + ADP

2. Add excess glucose-6-phosphate dehydrogenase + NADP$^+$

Glucose-6-phosphate + NADP$^+$

$\searrow$ 6-phosphogluconolactone + NADPH + H$^+$

Follow O.D. at 340 nm
to accurately reflect rate of formation of glucose-6-phosphate

Figure 3–14 The coupled enzyme assay. It is highly practical for an enzyme used clinically to be determined by a spectrophotometric change (i.e., a change in optical density or absorbance). For a reaction such as that catalyzed by hexokinase (the conversion of glucose to glucose-6-phosphate), it is not possible to monitor this reaction directly in this way. What can be done is to couple a second reaction to hexokinase. In this case, an excess of the enzyme glucose-6-phosphate dehydrogenase is added to the reaction as well as an excess of NADP$^+$. This dehydrogenase rapidly converts glucose-6-phosphate to the phosphogluconolactone, with the accompanying production of NADPH. This second reaction can be monitored at 340 nm and reflects the rate of the first enzyme (hexokinase).

glucose-6-phosphate dehydrogenase is made, along with its coenzyme NADP$^+$. This second enzyme is present in excess concentration, very efficiently takes the glucose-6-phosphate product of the hexokinase reaction, and rapidly oxidizes it to 6-phosphogluconolactone, while reducing NADP$^+$ to NADPH + H$^+$. NADPH, like NADH, has the characteristic absorbance at 340 nm. Thus, the hexokinase reaction can be followed in this coupled assay, as a second enzyme reaction is coupled to the first. The production of NADPH will accurately reflect the rate of production of glucose-6-phosphate. As glucose-6-phosphate dehydrogenase is present in excess, compared with hexokinase, the rate of production of glucose-6-phosphate will determine the rate of the dehydrogenase.

Remember, the initial velocity measured in an enzyme assay will depend on a variety of factors. Usually, substrate concentration is high so that substrate availability will not limit the enzyme. The pH is optimized for the reaction. There may also be an optimal temperature for the reaction that is above room temperature, but it may be more convenient (if the enzyme is sufficiently active) simply to perform the assays at room temperature. If the patient has taken medication, this may influence the enzyme velocities. As well, if the concentration of enzyme is increased, there will be a proportional increase in initial velocity. For example, in the assay of alcohol dehydrogenase outlined earlier, if the volume of liver homogenate added to the reaction cuvette (in a fixed final volume) is doubled, you would expect to see a doubling in the initial velocity. This linear relationship between enzyme concentration and initial velocity is shown in Figure 3–15.

If the substrate concentration is lowered below the high value that is standard for clinical enzyme assays, you will find that the initial velocity will eventually decline. A plot of enzyme velocity versus substrate concentration is shown in Figure 3–16. As the substrate concentration is increased, the initial velocity will also increase, but this curve will have the form of a rectangular hyperbola as the substrate concentration gets higher and higher. You must realize that each point on this curve is an initial velocity determined from the progress curve shown for one enzyme assay at one substrate concentration. Essentially, as the concentration of substrates increases, the enzyme approaches a rate that is called the **maximum velocity** (Vmax). Returning to our turnstile analogy, you can appreciate that there is indeed a maximum speed at which each turnstile can handle commuters (perhaps 120/min, if the commuters are lined up in front of the turnstiles and if they all have their tickets/tokens ready). This Vmax value is an asymptote to the hyperbolic curve and can be approached closely with high substrate con-

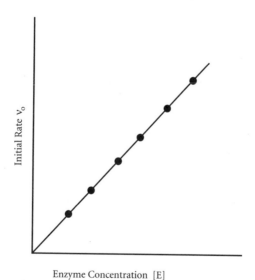

Enzyme Concentration [E]

Figure 3–15 Enzyme concentration in enzyme assays and enzyme velocity (v_o). There is a linear relationship between enzyme concentration and enzyme velocity. Thus, doubling the enzyme concentration doubles the concentration of enzyme molecules in the assay, and this is shown by a doubling of enzyme rate. It is possible at high enzyme concentration that there may be a deviation from linearity if it is difficult to calculate an accurate initial velocity in the face of rapid substrate depletion. Each point on this plot is an initial velocity taken from a separate enzyme assay with a specific enzyme concentration.

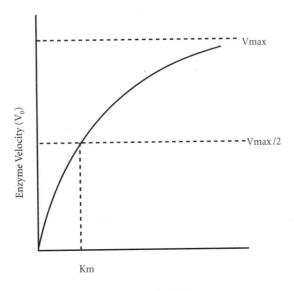

Figure 3–16 Substrate concentration and enzyme velocity. As substrate concentration increases, so too does enzyme velocity up to a maximum velocity (Vmax). The curve is a rectangular hyperbola; thus, increasing substrate concentration from a relatively low value will result in a relatively rapid increase in enzyme rate. Increasing substrate concentration at relatively high values will have less effect on enzyme rate. The substrate concentration that gives a rate equivalent to Vmax/2 is known as the Michaelis constant (Km) for the enzyme. Usually, a low value for Km indicates a high efficiency in enzyme-substrate binding.

centration. The Vmax can be given as millimoles of product per minute per enzyme sample (e.g., per millilter of plasma). There is a second parameter that can be gained from this curve, and that is the Km value. Km is the Michaelis constant and is derived from the Michaelis-Menten equation, which was formulated by Leonor Michaelis and Maud Menten in the early part of the 20th century. Maud Menten is notable for a number of things: she was a productive woman scientist during this male-dominated time period, she was Canadian, she was remarkably talented, and she was very attractive (a feature, most students will agree, that is not common among their various male and female professors today). The Michaelis constant (if you would like to call it the Menten constant we would have no philosophical or national objection) is expressed in terms of molarity, and it is the substrate concentration at which the initial velocity is half the Vmax value. You can see that an enzyme that very rapidly attains its Vmax with increasing substrate concentration will have a relatively small Km. The Km is often taken as an indication of the efficiency of substrate binding by the enzyme, with lower Km values indicating better efficiency.

ENZYME RATE AND END-POINT ANALYSIS

An enzyme rate or initial velocity (the two terms are often used interchangeably) will indicate the activity of an enzyme in a particular sample. This activity may reflect the actual numbers of enzyme molecules available, although enzymes can be activated or deactivated by chemical modification. Remember, in Chapter 1, we noted the lowered affinity of myosin light chain kinase for Ca^{2+}–calmodulin, when the kinase is phosphorylated. Enzyme rates can also be lowered or eliminated by the action of drugs on the enzyme. One important clinical use of the enzyme rate is to determine tissue damage. For example, there is not usually much of the enzyme lactate dehydrogenase (LDH) present in serum or plasma. This enzyme is found within cells and can reversibly convert pyruvate to lactate. In a heart attack (myocardial infarction [MI]), muscle cells are damaged, and LDH leaks into the blood. Thus, elevated levels of serum or plasma LDH can be indicative of MI. Enzyme activities are often given in International Units (IU), where one unit is defined as the amount of enzyme catalyzing the conversion of a certain quantity of substrate (often 1 millimole) per unit of time (often 1 minute). Be very aware that different tables of enzyme values or different commercial sources of enzyme may use the term enzyme "unit," but this may be based on different substrate (millimole, micromole) or time (minute, hour) units. As we will discuss shortly, a variety of different enzymes can be released from different tissues and can be used diagnostically for a variety of diseases.

Another principle is used when the amounts of various compounds (e.g., ethanol or glucose) are measured using enzymes. This method is called **end-point analysis** (Figure 3–17). In this procedure, enzymes are purchased commercially and are used to convert a substrate quantitatively to a product. For example, a sample of serum or plasma containing ethanol is usually treated to remove protein (deproteinization) and then added to a solution of NAD^+. An excess of pure alcohol dehydrogenase is next added; there is a rapid increase in absorbance at 340 nm, and a plateau or maximum absorbance is reached. The increase in absorbance represents the concentration of NADH formed, as ethanol is quantitatively oxidized to acetaldehyde. The difference between the absorbance reading before enzyme addition and the maximal absorbance plateau at the end of the reaction can be used to calculate the concentration of NADH at the end point. As there is one molecule of NADH generated per molecule of ethanol used by the enzyme, the concentration of NADH will be equivalent to the initial concentration of ethanol in the sample. For example, the absorbance change may indicate a concentration of 1 mM NADH at the end point. As your reaction cuvette contains 1 mL, you can calculate the quantity of NADH in 1 mL to be 1 micromole. Thus, your sample of serum or plasma contained

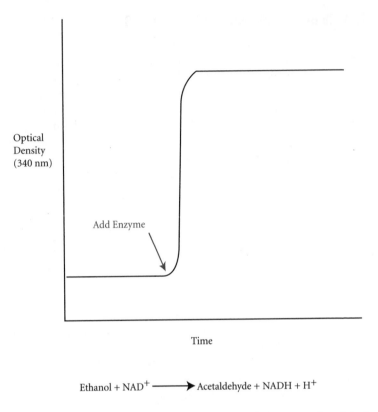

Ethanol + NAD$^+$ $\longrightarrow$ Acetaldehyde + NADH + H$^+$

Figure 3–17 End-point assays. Enzymes may be used to quantitate concentrations of simpler molecules within biological fluids, for example, ethanol or glucose in plasma. In this assay, an excess of purified enzyme (commercially available) is added to a reaction with a small quantity of substrate. In the example given, alcohol dehydrogenase is added to a reaction mixture containing an unknown quantity of ethanol (supplied in a plasma or serum sample) and an excess of the coenzyme NAD$^+$. The enzyme rapidly converts ethanol to acetaldehyde, with a matching conversion of NAD$^+$ to NADH + H$^+$. The formation of NADH is measured by the increase in absorbance (optical density) at 340 nm. From this increase in absorbance, the concentration of NADH can be calculated, and from this value the concentration of ethanol can be determined. By considering the volume of plasma or serum initially used in the end-point assay, the concentration of ethanol within the biological sample can be determined.

1 micromole of ethanol in the volume of plasma or serum used. If this was 0.1 mL of plasma, the plasma concentration of ethanol would be 10 mM. End-point analyses using enzymes can be used to calculate concentrations of a variety of substrates in biological fluids or tissues. You can also see from Figure 3–14 that a coupled assay could be used in end-point analysis by using an excess of both hexokinase and glucose-6-phosphate dehydrogenase to determine an unknown concentration of glucose in plasma.

MODULATION OF ENZYME ACTIVITY BY DRUGS

In Chapter 7, we will discuss in more detail how enzymes can be regulated within metabolism, and how various types of inhibitors have their effects on enzymes. You should know that drugs can modify enzyme activities in several ways. For example, aspirin (acetylsalicylic acid [ASA]) was known for years as a pain killer and an anti-inflammatory drug. It was only in the 1970s that the action of ASA was elucidated. ASA can acetylate the enzyme cyclooxygenase (COX) at an active site serine, thus killing the enzyme activity. COX is an enzyme that generates a parent compound for the production of a variety of compounds known as **eicosanoids**. We shall discuss these in greater detail in Chapter 4, but certain of the eicosanoids are associated with pain, fever, and inflammation. Thus, ASA, by inhibiting COX, is an analgesic, anti-inflammatory, and antipyretic (reduces fever) agent. Corticosteroids (e.g., budesonide) can also be used as anti-inflammatory agents, and these drugs prevent the elevation in COX activity by actually blocking the passage of the DNA code for the enzyme into its messenger RNA (a process called **transcription**, which we shall discuss in Chapter 8). Corticosteroids can also promote the synthesis of other proteins that can function to alleviate inflammation by preventing the generation of the substrate for COX. These are only a few examples of drug-based interventions and emphasize the need to determine what medications an individual is taking before efforts are made to measure his or her enzyme activities for diagnostic purposes.

DIAGNOSTIC ENZYMOLOGY

This is a very important area for the use of enzymes within medicine. As we briefly noted before, diagnostic enzymology is used in the detection of a particular disease or pathologic condition. Most cells will go through a normal cycle of cell division and cell death, releasing intracellular enzymes into extracellular fluids and blood. However, in certain pathologic states, there is an accelerated rate of cell death and, thus, an increase in the loss of intracellular enzymes. This could occur in heart muscle, following a blockage in coronary artery blood flow to the heart (MI). About 12 enzymes are commonly used in diagnosis, and these are noted in Table 3–2. We discuss a few of the more prominent diagnostic enzymes below.

Creatine Kinase

We drew attention to this enzyme in Chapter 1 with respect to energy metabolism in muscle. Creatine kinase can use ATP to phosphorylate creatine, forming creatine phosphate:

Table 3–2
Diagnostic Serum or Plasma Enzymes

Enzyme	Disease
Creatine kinase (CK)	
MB isoenzyme (CK-MB)	Myocardial infarction
MM isoenzyme (CK-MM)	Various pathologic states of skeletal muscle (e.g., Duchenne's muscular dystrophy)
Lactate dehydrogenase (LDH)*	Myocardial infarction
Aspartate aminotransferase (AST)	Myocardial infarction
Alanine aminotransferase (ALT)	Viral hepatitis
Amylase	Acute pancreatitis
Lipase	Acute pancreatitis
Acid phosphatase (AP)	Prostate cancer
Alkaline phosphatase (ALP)†	Bone disorders, liver diseases

* Specifically, a raised ratio of isoenzymes LD_1/LD_2
†Different isoenzymes of ALP can be used to distinguish bone and liver disease.

$$creatine + ATP \leftrightarrow creatine\ phosphate + ADP$$

Creatine phosphate serves as an energy reserve in muscle, and when concentrations of ATP are decreasing, creatine kinase can reform ATP from creatine phosphate and ADP. Creatine kinase can exist in three different molecular forms or isoenzymes. Isoenzymes are closely related enzymes that catalyze the same reaction but differ slightly from each other in amino acid sequence, and possibly in other properties, such as substrate affinity and Vmax. Isoenzymes of creatine kinase are made up of two subunits, each of which is a polypeptide. Thus, creatine kinase exists as dimers of subunits. The two subunits found in creatine kinase are called B and M. The BB dimer is found in the brain, and this dimer has a net negative charge. The MM dimer is the principal form of creatine kinase in skeletal muscle and also in cardiac muscle. However, cardiac muscle is distinctive because it also contains significant quantities of the mixed dimer or heterodimer, MB (20 to 40% of the total enzyme). In MI, with damage to cardiac muscle, there is a release of creatine kinase into the blood. About 6 hours after the MI, the activity of creatine kinase rises in the blood and peaks at about 36 hours. When cardiac muscle is damaged, there will be a specific rise in the levels of the MB heterodimer in blood. Because the M and B subunits differ in their net charges, the MM and MB dimers can be separated by electrophoresis. (Recall the principles of electrophoresis that we discussed in Chapter 2 with regard to the separation of plasma proteins.) The profile for the MM and MB dimers in the blood 24 hours after an MI is shown in Figure 3–18. Note that there is a small component of creatine kinase normally present in the blood as the MB heterodimer; thus, it is the increase in the MB peak that is used diagnostically for MI. Damage to skeletal muscle will result in increased levels of the MM dimer in blood, and this is also seen with certain muscle diseases, such as Duchenne's muscular dystrophy.

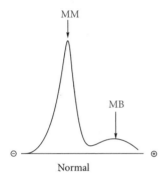
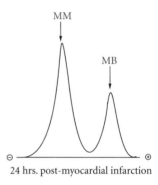

Figure 3–18 Serum creatine kinase isoenzymes and myocardial infarction (MI). The creatine kinase heterodimer MB is particularly enriched in cardiac muscle, while the homodimer MM is found in both skeletal and cardiac muscles. Following an MI, the serum values for creatine kinase increase as a result of leakage from damaged heart muscle cells. In particular, after the MI, the levels of the MB heterodimer increase substantially and serve as a diagnostic enzyme marker for MI. Elevations of the MB heterodimer can be detected a few hours after the MI and are shown at 24 hours in the diagram. The isoenzymes MB and MM are separated by electrophoresis (as shown) or by ion exchange chromatography (using a column filled with beads that have positively and negatively charged groups), as the M and B subunits differ in their net charges. Adapted from Marks DB, Marks AD, Smith CM. Basic medical biochemistry. Baltimore (MD): Williams and Wilkins; 1996.

Lactate Dehydrogenase

This is another cytoplasmic enzyme that can be released from cells into the blood in certain pathologic states. This enzyme catalyzes the reversible conversion of pyruvate into lactate, making use of the coenzyme NADH.

$$pyruvate + NADH \leftrightarrow lactate + NAD^+ + H^+$$

Lactate dehydrogenase (LDH) is present in red blood cells; thus, it is desirable to prepare plasma or serum from blood without excessive delay for a true serum/plasma value. The enzyme exists as tetramers of two types of polypeptide subunit. H is the subunit found primarily in heart muscle, while the M subunit is found in liver and skeletal muscle. The tetrameric make-up of the isoenzymes of LDH is H_4, H_3M, H_2M_2, HM_3, and M_4. These are also known as LD_1, LD_2, LD_3, LD_4, and LD_5, respectively. Like the isoenzymes of creatine kinase, these LDH tetramers can be separated by electrophoresis. Heart muscle is particularly rich in LD_1 with smaller quantities of LD_2. Again, LDH is found in normal serum or plasma, but the normal distribution shows a predominance of LD_2 over LD_1. In MI, this serum pattern is reversed as cardiac LDH is released into the extracellular fluid (Figure 3–19). Activities of LDH in serum will rise and peak about 3 days after the MI. In hepatobiliary disease, LD_5 is found to increase most prominently in serum samples, as the M_4 tetramer predominates in the liver.

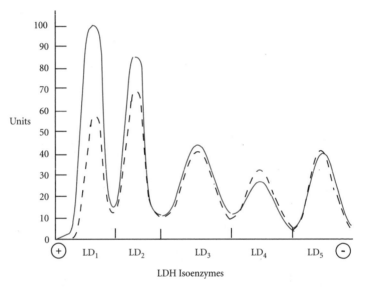

LDH Isoenzymes

Figure 3–19 Serum LDH isoenzymes and MI. Heart muscle is particularly enriched in the LD_1 isoenzyme, followed by the LD_2 isoenzyme. However, in normal blood, the LD_2 isoenzyme predominates. Following MI, there is a shift in the relative values of these two isoenzymes so that there is a predominance of LD_1 to LD_2 in serum. The five isoenzymes of LDH can be separated electrophoretically as shown, numbered LD_1 to LD_5, on the basis of their order of migration. (Dotted line = normal pattern; solid line = 12–24 hours after MI). The elevation of LDH in the blood develops more slowly following an MI than does the elevation of creatine kinase. As well, the elevated LDH levels persist longer in blood, making LDH a useful tool in the diagnosis of an MI that occurred a week previously. Adapted from Gornall AG. Applied biochemistry of clinical disorders. 2nd ed. Philadelphia (PA): Lippincott; 1986.

Aminotransferases: Aspartate Aminotransferase (AST) and Alanine Aminotransferase (ALT)

These enzymes catalyze the reversible transfer of the amino group from the amino acids aspartate or alanine. For AST or ALT, the amino group is transferred to α-ketoglutarate, with the formation of the amino acid glutamate. In older texts, you may see the acronyms SGOT (serum glutamate oxaloacetate transaminase) and SGPT (serum glutamate pyruvate transaminase), other terms for AST and ALT, respectively.

aspartate + α-ketoglutarate ↔ oxaloacetate + glutamate

alanine + α-ketoglutarate ↔ pyruvate + glutamate

Oxaloacetate and pyruvate are the C-skeletons that are produced after the removal of the amino groups from the two amino acids. We will discuss these aminotransferase reactions in more detail in Chapter 7, but for the time being, you should know that aminotransferases are important both in the removal of amino acid N for its ultimate disposal in urea and in the synthesis of amino acids using glutamate as the amino donor.

AST is particularly abundant in the liver, heart, and skeletal muscles, while ALT is found in highest concentration in the liver. Levels of AST in serum are elevated 6 to 12 hours after MI, rising to a peak at about 20 to 48 hours. ALT, in contrast, is not useful in diagnosing MI. In viral hepatitis, serum values of both AST and ALT are elevated, and this is also the case with many types of hepatobiliary diseases.

Lipase and Amylase

The pancreas generates a variety of digestive enzymes for secretion into the duodenum via the common bile duct. Damage to the pancreas, which can occur in alcoholics, can be accompanied by a release of pancreatic enzymes and their detection in serum or plasma. The father of one of the authors (RB) experienced a blocked bile duct (likely due to a stone) on a trip to Portugal and was promptly rushed to a hospital (founded by Wellington during the Napoleonic Wars when it largely specialized in amputations, a fairly common procedure following the effects of cannon balls on British [and Scottish!] regulars). On seeing the blood work and diagnostic enzymes from this Canadian patient, one of the first questions the Portuguese internist asked was "Are you an alcoholic?" Somewhat ironic, as RB's father was a teetotaller, who often played the piano at Temperance Union parties during his retirement.

Diagnosis and Disease Progression

While the diagnosis of a myocardial infarction can be confirmed by noting an elevation and peaking of creatine kinase (MB) and LDH (LD_1) in serum, it is also possible to monitor the course of diseases in which there are longer lasting periods of cellular damage. For example, viral hepatitis can result in elevated serum levels of ALT, indicating liver damage. If the elevated ALT activities remain high over time, it is possible that a chronic form of hepatitis may be present. Thus, serum enzyme levels can be used in the diagnosis of both acute and chronic diseases. By a similar token, serum enzymes can be used to monitor the effects of therapeutic treatments for disease. For example, a patient with breast cancer may develop metastases to bone, with subsequent bone destruction shown by elevated serum alkaline phosphatase. (Alkaline phosphatase is an enzyme that removes phosphate groups and shows an optimum pH in the alkaline range.) Chemotherapy for the patient with breast cancer may result in decreased serum alkaline phosphatase as bone destruction declines or is halted. Analysis of serum alkaline phosphatase following remission of the cancer would be advisable to rule out the possibility of recurrence of the disease.

Origin of Serum Enzymes

Enzymes present in serum can have a variety of origins. Some serum enzymes are released from cells by secretion. Platelets are small anucleate cells in the blood that can aggregate to form a thrombus or participate in arresting blood loss from a damaged vessel. Platelets, when stimulated, can release certain enzymes into the blood. For example, an enzyme called **phospholipase A$_2$** (sPLA$_2$) is secreted, and this enzyme can attack phospholipids in cellular membranes. Remember that we mentioned phospholipids in Chapter 2, when we discussed lipoproteins. Of course, there will be enzymes in blood that are released from normal aging cells that are at the end of their life span. However, pathologic states affecting the heart, liver, skeletal muscle, pancreas, bone, and other tissues can result in rising levels of diagnostic enzyme markers. In cell injury and cell death, the first enzymes to be lost from the cell are soluble enzymes of the cytoplasm. These are followed by mitochondrial and then nuclear enzymes as the cells lose their structure. There are several general pathologic situations in which cells will show an accelerated loss of enzyme markers. One of these is ischemia, in which blood flow to a tissue is compromised, and the cells are damaged by lack or diminished supply of oxygen and glucose (e.g., MI and stroke). Necrosis, or cell death, can follow ischemia, viral infection (e.g., viral hepatitis), or liver cirrhosis in alcoholism. Another situation is inflammation, which is mediated by the release of biologically active molecules coming from blood cells, such as platelets and white blood cells, following stimulation (e.g., the response of the lungs of asthmatics to irritation, such as air pollution). One final circumstance is the spread of cancerous cells within a tissue, releasing enzymes themselves or bringing about the demise of other cells.

Enzyme Clearance from Blood

Once in the blood, an enzyme can be removed in a number of ways. Serum proteases can break down these serum enzymes. Similarly, the enzymes may pass through the renal glomeruli, if they are relatively small in size. Other cells may take up the enzymes in the blood and degrade them (e.g., cells of the reticuloendothelial system, such as Kupffer's cells and macrophages).

Use of Serum Enzymes in Diagnosis

The simple presence of a diagnostic enzyme in serum does not constitute evidence for a specific disease. There will be low levels of these enzymes in serum samples that originate from the normal turnover of cells in the body. What is important is the level of these serum enzymes, the ratio of component isoenzymes (when applicable), and the timing of their appearance during or following a specific pathologic state. The normal levels of these enzymes will depend on age, gender, and race. Thus, it is very important to compare patient values with the appropriate reference ranges of these enzymes in serum before a diagnosis can be made. As can be seen, it is also useful, when possible, to monitor more than one enzyme that may be diagnostic for a disease (e.g., the use of creatine kinase and LDH isoenzymes following MI).

Inevitably, this raises the question: what degree of elevation for a serum diagnostic enzyme indicates a positive diagnosis? There are published ranges to assist you, but you should be aware that such ranges were established by careful examination of two criteria: **sensitivity** and **specificity**. In an ideal situation, you would have reference values that would prevent the occurrence of false positives, that is, the mistaken identification of a particular pathologic condition. For example, Mr. Jones has had chest pain and is exhibiting levels of creatine kinase, which are somewhat elevated above normal by reference values. Yet, by other criteria, say an electrocardiogram, Mr. Jones did not experience an MI. Your diagnosis of MI based simply on one enzyme level could precipitate a real heart attack for this unfortunate patient! The other aspect of enzyme diagnosis is the false negative, where the serum enzyme indicates values within a normal range, but unfortunately, the disease or pathology is present. Thus, while serum levels of alkaline phosphatase for Mrs. Cheng indicate that her bone cancer is still in remission, unfortunately, this may not be the case. As you can see, it all depends on where you set the reference limits for the enzyme levels. If the bar is set too high, you will avoid false positives but will inevitably miss a significant number of patients who, indeed, have the disease. If the bar is set too low, there will be no false negatives, but a corresponding number of erroneous diagnoses for disease will be made.

On the basis of these criteria, the *sensitivity* of a diagnostic enzyme is defined as

[True Positives/All those who have the disease] × 100.

If the sensitivity for a diagnostic enzyme is 90%, it means that 10% of those tested would be considered not to have the disease, while, in fact, these 10% are false negatives, missed by the standard levels set.

Similarly, *specificity* for a particular diagnostic enzyme is defined as

[True negatives/All those without the disease] × 100.

If the specificity for the enzyme is 90%, there would be 10% who would be considered to have the disease but who are, in fact, disease-free (i.e., these are false positives).

Other considerations for the usefulness of diagnostic enzymes are the time it takes for a serum enzyme to appear during or following a pathologic state. An enzyme that appears early in the course of a disease would obviously allow you to make a therapeutic intervention that much earlier in an effort to arrest or ameliorate the condition. Another factor is the use of isoenzymes (as we discussed earlier for creatine kinase and LDH) that would indicate the involvement of a specific tissue and make diagnosis that much more accurate. Thus, prior to introducing a new enzyme diagnostic test, it should meet the following criteria. The enzyme should be stable so that a refrigerated sample may still show the enzyme activity. (Usually, samples for assay are not frozen.) The enzyme should be easily and cheaply assayed. It should have reasonably high activity so that it can be detected at relatively low levels. It should have a degree of tissue specificity, directing you to a likely pathology in a particular tissue. The level of the enzyme in serum should also reflect the severity of the pathology.

One other consideration is the source of the enzyme. Usually, plasma or serum samples derived from blood are used in diagnosis. It may also be possible to assess blood cells for enzyme levels, for example, red and white blood cells or platelets. Urine may be used for enzyme determination (particularly, in renal and urinary tract diseases), as may other fluids, such as amniotic fluid or gastric juice, although these are not as easily accessible. It is also possible to take biopsy tissue, homogenize a portion to break open the cells, and assay the liberated enzymes.

Enzymes in Genetic Disease

We have so far discussed elevated levels of enzymes as diagnostic indicators for various pathologic states and diseases. Another possibility is the lack of an enzyme resulting from a genetic error that is found within a family. Disease genes are discussed in greater depth in Chapter 8, but you should know that a defective gene can result in the lack or deficiency of a specific enzyme activity. These problems are caused by genetic mutations so that the codes for specific proteins have errors that compromise protein folding and function. Most proteins are made at the endoplasmic reticulum and are then sorted and shipped to various organelles within the cell and the plasma membrane. An incorrectly folded protein may not even leave the endoplasmic reticulum and can thus be degraded without reaching the proper destination. This kind of genetic defect can be passed from parents to children, and if the child is unfortunate to inherit the same defective gene from each parent, she or he can show an absence of a particular enzyme activity. Commonly cited examples are degradative enzymes found in lysosomes, subcellular particles that are really the "garburettors" of cells. Lysosomes have a wide variety of different hydrolytic enzymes that allow the breakdown of lipids, proteins, nucleic acids, phosphate- and sugar-containing compounds, and a variety of others. The smaller breakdown products can be released from the cell or reused in the synthesis of new compounds. A deficiency of one of these lysosomal activities, because of a defective gene inherited from each parent, generally leads to the build-up of nondegradable material, lysosomal swelling and possible leakage, and cell death. One example is Tay-Sachs disease, in which there is a deficiency in the enzyme hexosaminidase A that removes the sugar N-acetylgalactosamine from sugar chains attached to complex lipids called gangliosides. Tay-Sachs disease is an autosomal recessive disorder; thus, if each parent is a carrier for the disease gene, there is a 25% chance that a child will have both copies of the defective gene and manifest the disease. In Tay-Sachs disease, the nondegraded lipid byproduct accumulates, with lysosomal and cellular swelling and cell death. The disease causes severe neurologic signs and symptoms, and blindness, retardation, and death can occur by a very early age. There are a number of these lysosomal storage diseases, each usually caused by the absence or deficiency of a specific hydrolytic enzyme through a specific genetic defect. For Tay-Sachs disease, the enzyme can be tested by an assay for hexosaminidase utilizing a substrate containing N-acetylgalactosamine and white cells isolated from blood samples. The white cells are lysed to free lysosomal enzymes, and the lysates used in the enzyme assays. This is another example of the use of enzymes in diagnosis, and individual assays can be carried out for a variety of enzyme deficiencies. If you suspect a genetic defect, family history will be a very important indicator of such a possibility, as another family member (in the immediate family or among cousins, aunts, and uncles) may likely have shown the disease.

USE OF ENZYMES AS THERAPEUTIC AGENTS

With the development of recombinant DNA technologies (discussed in Chapter 8), it is now possible to produce large quantities of human proteins and enzymes ex vivo. These recombinant enzymes can be used in various replacement therapies. It is often not possible to alleviate intracellular enzyme deficiencies by exposing cells to the purified enzyme (i.e., intravenous delivery of recombinant enzyme), but it is possible to increase levels of extracellular enzymes by this approach. For example, platelet-activating factor (PAF) is a lipid made by many different cell types and is also an extracellular mediator of inflammation in a variety of diseases. PAF can be inactivated by the removal of its acetyl group, catalyzed by a plasma enzyme known as **PAF acetylhydrolase**. In order to reduce the half-life of PAF within the blood or extracellular fluids in inflammatory states, recombinant human plasma PAF acetylhydrolase has been used and has been reported to ameliorate the damage associated with high levels of PAF.

Recombinant human enzymes can be used in other extracellular applications. For example, patients with cystic fibrosis often have respiratory difficulties because of the increased viscosity of secretions within the lung. DNA from dying neutrophils trapped in mucus plays a role in this increased viscosity, and recombinant human DNase (an enzyme that degrades DNA) can be used in inhalants to reduce this problem.

Other uses of enzymes include the proteolytic enzyme papain that can be used to clear away dead cells from an area of necrosis. A somewhat similar approach is the use of the enzyme streptokinase, urokinase, or tissue plasminogen activating factor as "clot busters" in stroke or MI. These proteins activate the plasma protease plasmin, which can dissolve thrombi blocking the cerebral or coronary vessels, thereby restoring blood flow and ending ischemia. We will talk of these more in the next chapter, when hemostasis is discussed.

4

Hemostasis

In this chapter, we want to understand, at a biochemical level, hemostasis, the mechanism that stops bleeding following vascular injury. One of the processes involved in hemostasis is coagulation, leading ultimately to the formation of a seal supported by the protein fibrin, which assists in closing a bleeding vessel. Coagulation involves an important sequence of enzyme activation steps, triggered by injury to blood vessels, in which enzymes are converted from inactive to active forms. Injury to blood vessels also prompts cellular events that involve platelets, which are small anucleate cells that become sticky when activated and participate along with fibrin in sealing broken vessels. We will discuss coagulation and the steps in platelet activation that allow both proteins and cells to come together to plug a leaking blood vessel in hemostasis.

Another significant and related process is thrombosis, in which a thrombus, or blood clot of fibrin and blood cells, is produced. Thrombosis can be initiated by damage to the endothelial lining of vessels (e.g., the damage associated with the rupture of an atherosclerotic plaque) and is important as thrombi can block off or reduce blood flow to specific tissues. Thrombi may also travel as emboli within the circulation, ultimately producing the same effect. This reduction or blockade in the blood flow can initiate ischemic events, such as myocardial infarction (MI) and transient ischemic attacks (TIAs) in the brain and the more severe loss of neurologic function associated with a stroke.

COAGULATION PATHWAYS

Among the plasma proteins (introduced in Chapter 2) are a number of inactive enzymes known as **zymogens**. With damage to blood vessels or in vascular disease, these proteins can be activated by limited hydrolysis within a sequence of enzymatic steps referred to as the coagulation cascade. The activated enzymes in the coagulation cascade are relatives of trypsin (discussed in Chapter 3) and have the amino acid residue serine at their active site. Collectively, this family of enzymes is known as serine proteases. Each activated serine protease in the cascade can, in turn, activate another zymogen by removing one or more specific peptides by hydrolysis. You will remember that enzymes can act on a relatively large number of substrate molecules within a short period of time (our turnstile analogy from Chapter 3). Consider then the remarkable degree of amplification when each product of an enzyme-catalyzed reaction is another active enzyme. Coagulation can be compared to an avalanche, in which a relatively small but significant event (say, a footstep on an overhanging snow ledge) leads to a massive crescendo of snowfall that submerges the town in the valley below. Understanding the coagulation sequence will allow you to appreciate how defects in individual members of the sequence can lead to bleeding disorders, how anticoagulants work, and how anticoagulants are used in clinical situations to prevent coagulation or the formation of thrombi. We will also discuss the steps involved in the dissolution of a thrombus and how thrombi or emboli can be removed therapeutically to re-establish blood flow to ischemic tissue following a heart attack or stroke.

Note that proteins participating in the coagulation sequence are called **coagulation factors** and are numbered using Roman numerals I to XIII. The clotting factors are mostly zymogens, but there are some factors that are not enzymes. You will likely find the sequence of clotting factors to be somewhat like a maze, and it is important to achieve an overview of the whole cascade. If you find your eyes glazing over, take a break, and refer to Figure 4–1 for a comprehensive picture. We will try to take you through this process as gently as possible. We take no responsibility for the numbering system or its inherent logic but assure our readers that whatever its defects, the use of numbers is considerably less confusing than the older system that used names for the factors. As our readers likely can appreciate, each division within medical and health science biochemistry has its own language, and each language can be further complicated by the existence of differing dialects coming from different laboratories, each of which supports its own lingo as the official medium of communication. With time, a certain consensus is reached that attempts to simplify the swamp that has been created.

Tissue Factor Pathway

Also known as the extrinsic pathway, this is the important initiating pathway within the coagulation sequence. This is shown in Figure 4–1. The first step in this pathway is the exposure of a specific tissue-bound glycoprotein to blood. Glycoproteins carry sugar chains, and tissue-bound glycoproteins are found in the plasma membranes of cells, oriented so that their sugar components are exposed on the exterior cellular surface. The specific glycoprotein of the extrinsic pathway is called **tissue factor** (TF), also referred to as factor III or thromboplastin, and is found in the plasma membranes of the cells of the subendothelium. These cells lie below the single layer of endothelial cells lining a blood vessel. TF is not normally accessible to proteins found in the circulation. In addition, TF is found in membranes of damaged endothelial cells and in membranes of stimulated macrophages. On exposure to blood, TF binds with coagulation factor VII. This leads to the formation of active factor VIIa from factor VII. Note that activated clotting factors usually have the "a" designation. The presence of calcium ions and a negatively charged phospholipid surface provided by the membrane greatly accelerates this activation step. We will discuss phospholipids in more detail in the context of platelet activation later in this chapter. The association of TF and VIIa is called tissue factor complex (TFC), and TFC converts several coagulation factors into their active forms in the presence of calcium ions, including the conversion of IX to IXa, X to Xa, and additional factor VII to VIIa.

Factor Xa participates in the activation of factor II to form thrombin (factor IIa). Factor II is also known as prothrombin. As noted in Figure 4–1, thrombin can amplify the coagulation sequence greatly by promoting the conversion of factor V to Va, VIII to VIIIa, and XI to XIa. This is a positive feedback reaction in which thrombin can accelerate its own production from prothrombin. Note that factors Va and VIIIa are not serine proteases, but these active factors will form complexes with other active clotting factors to accelerate specific enzymatic activation steps. Factor XIa enzymatically activates factor IX to IXa in the presence of calcium ions, and IXa associates with VIIIa at a membrane surface. Specifically, it is the negatively charged phospholipid at the membrane that interacts with calcium and the active factors VIIIa and IXa to form a complex called "Xase." As the name suggests, the complex activates factor X to Xa (in addition to the activation of factor X carried out by TFC). In a similar manner, active factors Va and Xa interact through calcium ions with negatively charged phospholipids of a membrane surface to form the complex "prothrombinase." This complex generates thrombin from prothrombin. From Figure 4–1, you can appreciate the cyclic nature of the coagulation cascade that is largely mediated by thrombin. Thrombin is a key component in the cascade. By converting the plasma protein fibrinogen to fibrin, thrombin generates fibrin monomers, which assemble into cross-linked fibrin polymers, the basis of the fibrin seal in hemostasis.

Intrinsic Pathway in the Coagulation Cascade

The initiating steps in this pathway are also shown in Figure 4–1. These steps can be referred to as the contact system, as exposure to a negatively charged surface will activate this pathway within the coagulation cascade. This is the readily observed blood clotting that takes place when blood is exposed to a glass surface (e.g., within a test tube). This pathway is of less importance in

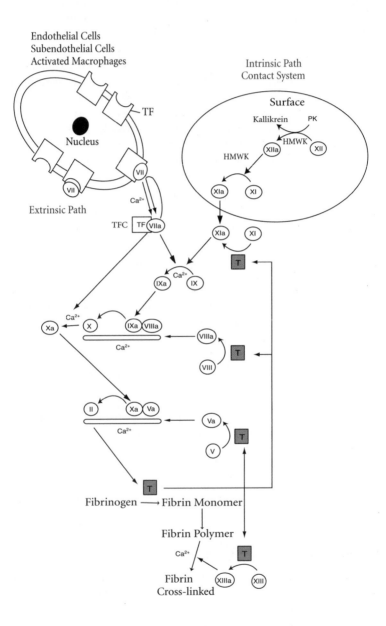

the initiation of the coagulation cascade in vivo. In the intrinsic pathway, factor XII is converted to XIIa at a phospholipid surface. This activation of factor XII is associated with the conversion of prekallikrein to kallikrein (an active proteolytic enzyme). Kallikrein and XIIa are also believed to activate each other. In turn, factor XIIa converts factor XI to XIa in the presence of the protein high-molecular-weight kininogen (HMWK), and XIa participates in the activation of factor IX. You can see that both the intrinsic pathway and the tissue factor pathway lead to the activation of factor X through the conversion of factor IX to IXa (see Figure 4–1). Thus, there is a convergence of the extrinsic and intrinsic pathways, and both paths share the activation step that converts prothrombin (factor II) to thrombin (IIa), the conversion of fibrinogen to fibrin, and the polymerization and cross-linking of fibrin monomers.

The intrinsic pathway may also amplify the strength of the tissue factor pathway by providing more factor IXa for the Xase complex. This amplification is of importance as it is possible that the tissue factor pathway to coagulation may not provoke a full hemostatic response because of the presence of an inhibitor (tissue factor pathway inhibitor) that can limit the actions of the tissue factor complex. We shall discuss the inhibitors of coagulation in greater detail later in this chapter.

It is also of interest that factors XIIa, XIa, and kallikrein can take part in fibrinolysis, the degradation of polymerized fibrin. Thus, the intrinsic pathway has an important role in vivo in the breakdown of the fibrin clot.

Testing for Abnormalities in the Cascade

You can see that there are a variety of factors involved in the coagulation cascade, and, thus, defects in individual factors (brought about by genetic

Figure 4–1 The coagulation cascade. The extrinsic or tissue factor pathway is initiated when the glycoprotein tissue factor (TF) in the plasma membrane of the damaged endothelium is exposed to the circulation (upper left in figure). The TF complex (TFC) arises from the association of TF with factor VII, resulting in the conversion of the zymogen VII to its active form VIIa. Many of the clotting factors (with the exception of V and VIII) are serine proteases that can activate the inactive or zymogen forms of other clotting factors by discrete hydrolytic reactions. TFC can catalyze the formation of factor Xa directly or via the activation of IXa, which, in turn, associates with VIIIa to form the active complex called the Xase complex. In turn, Xa associates with Va to form the prothrombinase complex that produces the dynamic clotting factor thrombin (T, factor IIa from prothrombin, factor II). Thrombin is not only involved in the production of fibrin but also participates in the activation of factors V, VIII, and XI, thus amplifying the coagulation response. The contact system (upper right) is so called because it is activated at surfaces where factor XII is converted to XIIa, and XIIa activates factor XI (as does thrombin). XIa can support and strengthen the sequence triggered by the extrinsic pathway by providing a second route for the activation factor IX. The bars below the Xase and prothrombinase complexes indicate the need for a negatively charged phospholipid surface for the reaction. PK = prekallikrein; HMWK = high-molecular-weight kininogen; T = thrombin (factor IIa). Adapted from Israels LG, Israels ED. Mechanisms in hematology. 2nd ed. Bayer Publishing; 1997.

flaws in the DNA codes for individual proteins) can compromise coagulation. It is possible to investigate the presence of defective elements in the cascade by testing clot formation using plasma samples in vitro. For example, thrombin time (TT) measures the formation of fibrin from plasma fibrinogen when thrombin is added to plasma. Prolonged values of TT can arise from abnormalities in fibrinogen, low levels of fibrinogen, or the presence of the anticoagulant heparin.

Prothrombin time (PT) is the time taken for clot formation after the addition of calcium and TF to plasma. PT will test for the presence and function of factors II, V, VII, and X. Thus, PT tests the efficiency of the coagulation cascade initiated by the extrinsic pathway. If you remember our introduction of the mad monk Rasputin in Chapter 1, you may recall that he rose to influence as a spiritualist/healer in the last czarist court, prior to World War I. Rasputin's rise to fame occurred largely because the heir to the Russian throne, Prince Alexis, suffered from hemophilia A. Hemophilia A and B are bleeding disorders that arise from defects in factors VIII and IX, respectively. The PT is not prolonged in these diseases because TFC can activate factor X without the intervention of factors VIIIa and IXa (see Figure 4–1). A normal PT is about 10 seconds, which is considerably shorter than the time (about 30 seconds) needed for clot formation initiated by the intrinsic pathway, following the exposure of plasma to a negatively charged contact surface. PT is prolonged by the presence of oral anticoagulants, and PT is generally reported as a ratio (the international normalized ratio [INR]), normalizing clotting times to a standard TF preparation. INR values are >1 in the presence of anticoagulants.

Activated partial thromboplastin time (APTT or PTT) is the clotting time following exposure to a negatively charged surface, as initiated by the intrinsic pathway. The APTT/PTT will measure defects in clotting factors leading up to fibrin polymerization, with the exception of factor VII. The APTT/PTT is about 30 seconds. Heparin and insufficient or abnormal fibrinogen can also increase APTT/PTT.

Need for Vitamin K in Coagulation

The K in vitamin K is taken from the Danish "koagulation." If there is insufficient vitamin K in the diet, bleeding disorders are observed. One form of vitamin K occurs in green leafy vegetables as phylloquinone, and a related form (menaquinone) is made by intestinal bacteria. Several of the clotting factors (II, VII, IX, and X) are synthesized in the liver and are vitamin K-dependent. Vitamin K is needed as a cofactor for the modification of these proteins following protein synthesis. This important modification involves the conversion of glutamate residues in the proteins to γ-carboxyglutamate via a carboxylation reaction (Figure 4–2). Note the side chains of γ-carboxyglutamate

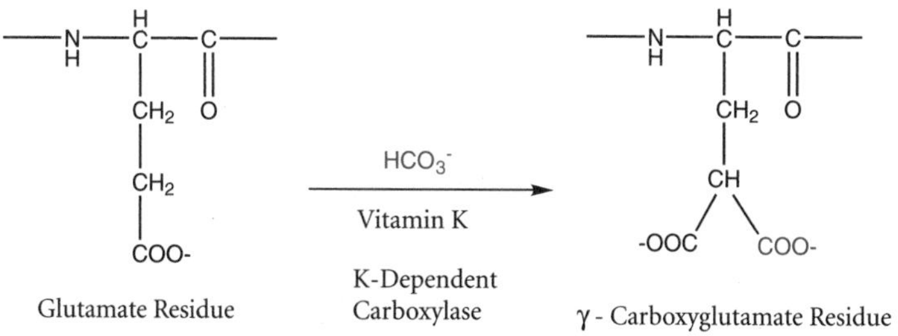

Figure 4–2 The production of γ-carboxyglutamate. This is a vitamin K–dependent reaction that carboxylates the side chain of glutamate residues found in several coagulation factors. The double carboxylate groups facilitate interactions with phospholipids in membranes via the divalent cation calcium.

have two carboxyl groups, and these are involved in binding calcium and in the calcium-mediated association of the clotting factors with phospholipid surfaces in membranes. In the absence of vitamin K, these clotting factors cannot undergo carboxylation. The compounds dicoumarol and warfarin can interfere with this carboxylation and result in abnormal prothrombin, abnormal factors VII, IX, and X, and defective formation of thrombin.

INHIBITION OF COAGULATION

Given the power of the coagulation cascade (remembering our image of the small mountain village engulfed in the avalanche), there must be natural controls to restrict coagulation to a site of injury. The alternative would be a fatal, spreading wave of coagulation that would solidify the circulatory system. As well, in diseases caused by thrombosis (blood clots that block vessels), there are drugs that can be used therapeutically to prevent coagulation.

Protein C and Thrombomodulin

As we have seen, thrombin is a powerful coagulation factor that is responsible for fibrin formation and has multiple activation effects within the coagulation cascade. We will also see that thrombin very effectively activates platelets. Thus, mechanisms that neutralize thrombin are of particular importance. A membrane protein called **thrombomodulin** is found in endothelial cells, and this membrane protein can bind and deactivate thrombin (Figure 4–3). In this complex, thrombin also binds protein C, a circulating plasma protein. This binding activates protein C and leads to the further binding of protein S, which serves as a cofactor in the protein C–mediated inactivation of factors Va and VIIIa. Both proteins C and S are vitamin K-dependent, contain γ-carboxyglutamate, and require calcium ions for their binding to this membrane complex.

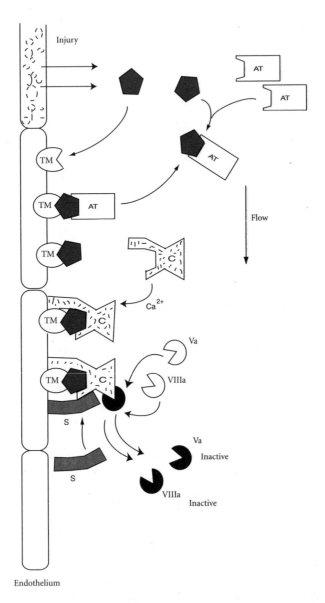

Figure 4–3 Inhibition of the coagulation cascade. The figure represents the contents of the lumen of a medium-sized artery. Thrombin (pentagon symbol) can be inhibited by binding with the plasma protein antithrombin (AT). The endothelial protein thrombomodulin (TM) can also bind thrombin and neutralize its activity. The thrombin–TM complex can be joined by AT, with subsequent liberation of a thrombin–AT complex. Thrombin complexed with TM can also bind protein C and protein S (both of which have γ-carboxyglutamate residues to facilitate membrane binding). The large thrombin–TM–protein C–protein S complex cleaves and inactivates clotting factors Va and VIIIa.

Antithrombin

Many of the coagulation factors are serine proteases, and there are natural inhibitors to control these enzymes. "Serpin" is an acronym for serine proteinase inhibitor, and antithrombin (AT) is a member of the serpin class of proteins. AT principally inhibits thrombin and Xa, but VIIa, IXa, XIa, and XIIa can also be inactivated. The inhibition begins slowly, but the effects increase as more of the activated forms of the clotting factors become available during cascade activation. The inhibitor–clotting factor complexes do not dissociate easily, and these complexes are readily removed from the circulation by the liver. AT can also bind to thrombin immobilized in the complex with thrombomodulin, with the subsequent release of the AT–thrombin complex and its uptake by the liver. This increases the effectiveness of AT in the plasma. As levels of thrombin fall, further activation of protein C also declines.

The effectiveness of AT can also be greatly enhanced by the binding of the anticoagulant heparin to AT. Heparin is a sulfated glycosaminoglycan (a polysaccharide or polymer of pairs of simple sugars) that is produced by mast cells. Heparin binds at a specific site on antithrombin, and this binding leads to a conformational change in the inhibitor that increases its affinity for thrombin and the other coagulation factors previously noted. Preparations of heparin can also be given therapeutically as anticoagulants. Because of the numerous roles of thrombin within the coagulation cascade, the inhibitory effectiveness of the AT–heparin complex is seen at several levels.

Tissue Factor Pathway Inhibitor (Lipoprotein-Associated Coagulation Inhibitor)

This is a protease inhibitor that can limit the effectiveness of the coagulation cascade initiated through the tissue factor pathway, if there is not an extra source of IXa, coming from the intrinsic pathway. This inhibitor binds to both VIIa and Xa, neutralizing both activities.

ANTIBODIES TO COAGULATION FACTORS

As certain bleeding disorders arise from deficiencies in specific clotting factors, the administration of the appropriate factor to alleviate the problem appears a logical solution to the disease. Unfortunately, in some cases, likely because an individual does not have the natural circulating clotting factor (and thus does not recognize it as an endogenous protein), antibodies can be made against the therapeutically administered factor. This is seen in patients with hemophilia A and B, who receive factor VIII or IX, respectively. Antibody formation is more commonly found following administration of factor VIII.

THROMBOPHILIA

This indicates a predisposition toward blood clotting and thrombosis and may be caused by deficiency in AT, resistance of factor Va to degradation by protein C, deficiencies of proteins C and S, and increased levels of circulating homocysteine (an amino acid relative of cysteine) within the blood. Homocysteine may promote coagulation by increasing activity of factor V or expression of TF and by decreasing the effectiveness of inhibitors of coagulation. Hyperhomocysteinemia (and homocystinuria) is also associated with atherosclerotic lesions and occurs likely because of deficiencies of vitamins B_6, B_{12}, and folic acid. We will discuss homocysteine in more detail in Chapter 6 (in association with cobalamin and folic acid).

THERAPEUTIC ANTICOAGULANTS

As we have noted, heparin complexed with AT is a very effective anticoagulant, inhibiting thrombin, factor Xa, and a variety of other coagulation factors. Unfractionated heparin is a mixture of molecules of different sizes that are sulfated glycosaminoglycans (polymers of pairs of simple sugars that have negatively charged sulfate groups). The sizes of the molecules in this preparation of heparin may vary from 3,000 to 30,000 in molecular weight. Heparin is usually given intravenously and boosts the power of AT, resulting in rapid anticoagulation. The effectiveness of heparin can be assessed by APTT/PTT. The use of unfractionated heparin can result in thrombocytopenia (low platelet levels), as heparin can trigger an immune response that promotes the formation of platelet aggregates and increases the potential for thrombosis. Unfractionated heparin can be replaced by other anticoagulants. These include heparinoid, a glycosaminoglycan cocktail of smaller mean molecular weight that provokes little immune response, or hirudin, a polypeptide from leeches that inhibits thrombin in a rather unique way, without the preliminary formation of a heparin–AT complex. Hirudin is a very potent, natural anticoagulant that binds very tightly to thrombin. Leeches produce this anticoagulant to assist them in sucking blood, and indeed blood letting by this mode was a rather routine medical practice in the treatment of a variety of diseases up to the 19th century. Without meaning to offend those of you en route to medical degrees, the term "leech" was also used to describe medical practitioners, for this very reason. Leeches also have a long and perhaps stereotyped association with novels and films with tropical settings. If you are an old-film buff, you may remember Humphrey Bogart in "The African Queen" covered in leeches following a sortie into a rather murky tropical stream. We believe that a burning cigarette was used to remove these rather resourceful creatures from our hero; however, the predisposition to the cure in this case may well be more dangerous than the ailment.

Low-Molecular-Weight Heparins

The fractionated, low-molecular-weight heparin (LMWH) binds to AT. Its advantages over the mixed unfractionated heparin include a lesser binding to plasma proteins, a considerably longer half-life, the maintenance of adequate coagulation by fewer doses (subcutaneous), and a much lower incidence of thrombocytopenia. The therapeutic use of LMWH is increasing.

Vitamin K Antagonists

These anticoagulants are dicoumarol and warfarin and are given orally to produce a vitamin K deficiency. They do so by blocking the carboxylation reaction that produces γ-carboxyglutamate residues in the vitamin K–dependent clotting factors II (prothrombin), VII, IX, and X, as well as protein C and protein S. Administration of vitamin K can reverse this form of anticoagulation. Warfarin is also known as a rat poison, although some species of rats can tolerate this compound remarkably well. There are certainly more effective poisons that might be used to control rodents, but the possibility of lethal poisoning of pets and children by mistake likely has diminished the enthusiasm for their application.

HEMOPHILIA A AND B

Coagulation factor VIII is a cofactor in the conversion of factor X to Xa by factor IXa. Factor VIII is made in the liver and released into blood, where it binds with another protein called von Willebrand's factor (vWF). In the complex, factor VIII is resistant to proteolytic degradation, except that catalyzed by thrombin. Thrombin acts both to free VIII from the complex and to activate VIII to VIIIa, which can participate in the coagulation cascade. Hemophilia A is a genetic disorder that is produced by deficiency of factor VIII. Hemophilia A is an X-linked recessive disorder and occurs with a frequency of about 1/10,000 male births. A variety of genetic defects in the gene for factor VIII can result in factor VIII deficiency. Indeed, the gene for factor VIII is quite large, and this likely accounts for the large number of mutations (alterations in the genetic sequence) that are seen. Male children of female carriers with a defective gene for factor VIII have a 50% chance of having the disease. There are no male carriers, as there is only one X-chromosome in the male genome. The female carriers do not usually show symptoms, as they have levels of factor VIII that are about 50% of normal. Carriers can be identified by DNA testing (see Chapter 8). The blood level of factor VIII in severe bleeders is <1% of normal.

Before the advent of recombinant DNA technologies (as described in Chapter 8), hemophiliacs were treated by the administration of preparations enriched in factor VIII, isolated from donated blood. However, there was the risk of hepatitis C, human immunodeficiency virus (HIV), and other blood-borne infections. Now, recombinant factor VIII can be given, although there is the possibility of development of antibodies to this factor.

A deficiency of functional coagulation factor IX (serine protease zymo-gen, which is also vitamin K-dependent) is the cause of hemophilia B. Like factor VIII, the gene for factor IX is carried on the X-chromosome. Hemo-philia B can be caused by a number of defects in the gene for factor IX, including single mutations and also relatively large deletions of the genetic sequence. Carriers of the mutated gene usually have about 50% of normal levels of the clotting factor.

Of the two hemophilias, hemophilia A is the more common, account-ing for some 80% of the cases. While PT is normal, APTT is prolonged. Patients with hemophilia B show a considerably lower occurrence of immune reaction to replacement therapy (factor IX) than do patients with hemophilia A given factor VIII. The hemophilias are characterized by pro-longed bleeding in response to significant injury or surgery, ready bruising, and spontaneous hemorrhage at joints and muscles.

FIBRIN POLYMERIZATION AND CLOT FORMATION

The initial formation of fibrin monomers, which spontaneously assemble into polymers, comes from the attack of thrombin on fibrinogen. While not in as high concentration as albumin or the γ-globulins, fibrinogen is one of the more abundant plasma proteins (2 to 5 g/L), and its structure is perhaps the most complex of these. Fibrinogen is a large protein (340 kD) and is com-posed of three different polypeptides, each occurring as a pair (Figure 4–4). The nomenclature is understandably confusing, as fibrinogen can be repre-sented as $(A\alpha)_2 (B\beta)_2 \gamma_2$. It's a little easier when you appreciate that $A\alpha$, $B\beta$, and γ are the names of each of the three polypeptide subunits. A and B rep-resent 16 and 14 amino acid sequences at the N-terminal ends of the α- and β-polypeptides, and thrombin releases these fibrinopeptides A and B in the conversion of fibrinogen to fibrin. This produces the fibrin monomer desig-nated $\alpha_2\beta_2\gamma_2$ (see Figure 4–4). Often, the term "monomer" refers to an indi-vidual polypeptide subunit, but for fibrin, the monomer or subunit structure is more complex, consisting of these six polypeptide chains. Each polypep-tide chain is covalently linked to its duplicate chain by disulfide bridges. The six chains are believed to be oriented so that each fibrin monomer has three node domains: two D-node domains at the ends of the six-chain monomer and one E-node domain at the center of the six-chain monomer. The term "node domain" simply specifies a region of the fibrin monomer that accom-modates the ends of the six chains. Within the E node domain, the matching chains are linked by disulfide bridges. The loss of the fibrinopeptides A and

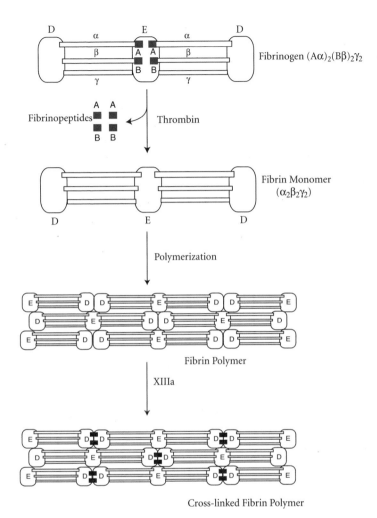

Figure 4–4 Formation of fibrin. The attack of thrombin on fibrinogen releases the fibrinopeptides A and B and produces the fibrin monomer composed of pairs of α-, β-, and γ-chains. This modification of the chain structure within the E-domain of the monomer allows the association of the fibrin monomers into polymers during the formation of the "soft clot." Factor XIIIa then cross-links pairs of γ-chains and pairs of α-chains to stabilize polymeric fibrin by covalent bonds,

B occurs at the E-node, and this peptide loss is believed to expose sites at the ends of these polypeptide chains that allow the polymerization of the fibrin subunits. The monomers spontaneously form a polymer of subunits by association of D-domains between subunits and also an association of central E domains with D-domain dimers. Each E-domain can associate with two D-domain dimers, further linking the fibrin monomers into a growing polymer. This ultimately leads to the formation of a fibrin fiber.

Most of this initial fibrin structure is based on noncovalent interactions (i.e., there are relatively few strong linkages holding this intricate polymerized network together). The clot formed by this association of fibrin monomers is rather delicate and is called a "soft" clot. To increase the durability of this polymer, covalent links are needed. These are supplied by the action of another coagulation factor, XIII. Factor XIII is another factor that is activated by thrombin, forming XIIIa. XIIIa is also called the fibrin-stabilizing factor. Factor XIIIa is a transglutaminase that introduces covalent cross-links between neighboring polypeptides within the soft clot. The reaction requires calcium ions and creates an amide bond between the R-groups of the amino acid residues lysine and glutamine (Figure 4–5). This creates an isopeptide bond that links nearby chains within the clot. Initially, this stabilization occurs between the γ-chains, although with time some α-chains may bind with each other in this manner. Almost all the γ-chains cross-link covalently in this way, and this greatly increases the strength of the fibrin clot (the "hard" clot). Such a cross-linked clot is less susceptible to fibrinolysis or clot breakdown. Two proteins, α_2-antiplasmin and fibronectin (a protein of the subendothelial matrix), can also associate with the clot and increase stability and resistance to breakdown of fibrin.

Genetic mutations can result in low levels of circulating fibrinogen, its absence, or the presence of dysfunctional fibrinogens. Structural changes in abnormal fibrinogens can result in changes in the polymerization and cross-linking processes. Interestingly, these changes often make polymerized fibrin less susceptible to breakdown. These dysfibrinogenemias are frequently seen in thrombotic disease. Deficiencies in factor XIII are also known, and if individuals are homozygous for the mutated gene, clotting is severely compromised. Factor XIII has a relatively long half-life in the circulation, and XIII can be given therapeutically in such deficiencies. Deficiencies in factor XIII can be assessed by the stability of blood clots in vitro in the presence of concentrated urea (a chemical that disrupts noncovalent linkages).

FIBRINOLYSIS

While clot formation is, to say the least, vital in controlling bleeding, it is also of importance to remove the clot during the healing process. In addition, the formation of clots or thrombi has a distinctly dark side (conjuring up Skywalker and Vader images). Diseased vessels, such as the coronary or carotid arteries, showing atherosclerotic lesions can also accelerate the formation of thrombi. We will discuss the nature of these lesions later in this chapter. Thrombi can travel from their site of formation as emboli and ultimately block blood flow through a small vessel. This is the basis of MI and TIAs. TIAs usually involve a specific, transient loss of central neurologic

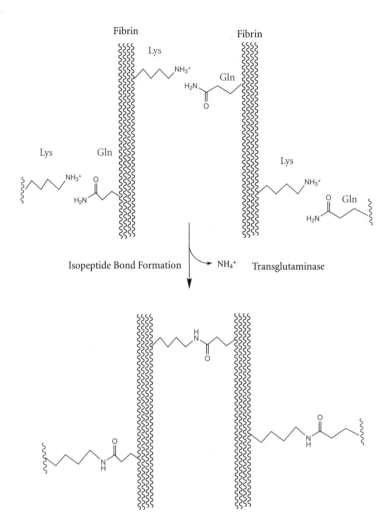

Figure 4–5 Action of factor XIIIa. This clotting factor forms covalent links between polypeptide chains in the fibrin polymer. This is catalyzed by a transglutaminase activity in XIIIa that forms an isopeptide bond utilizing the R-groups of lysine (Lys) on one chain of fibrin and glutamine (Gln) on another. This cross-linking greatly strengthens the fibrin polymer and is the basis of the "hard clot." Adapted from Devlin TM. Textbook of biochemistry with clinical correlations. 4th ed. New York: Wiley-Liss; 1997.

function as an embolus occludes a particular cerebral blood vessel. TIAs often precede ischemic (thrombotic) stroke. Thus, the mechanisms for clot dissolution are very important and are the basis for therapeutic intervention in heart attack and stroke.

Fibrinolysis is largely catalyzed by the enzyme plasmin, which is a remarkably good dismantler of fibrin polymers. Plasmin is formed from the zymogen plasminogen, and this conversion is mediated by several enzyme activities (Figure 4–6). These include urokinase- (urokinase-type plasminogen activator or u-PA) and tissue-type plasminogen activator (t-PA). Urokinase is made in the kidneys and, as suggested by its name, is also found in urine. Urokinase can also be made by macrophages and monocytes. Urokinase is initially made in an inactive form (acu-PA) that can be activated by plasmin or by kallikrein, a proteolytic enzyme that participates in the intrinsic pathway of the coagulation cascade. Thus, the intrinsic pathway makes a contribution not only to coagulation but also ultimately to fib-

Plasminogen - Plasmin System

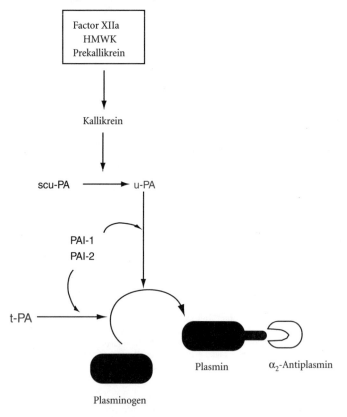

Figure 4–6 Activation of plasmin. Plasminogen can be activated by tissue-type plasminogen activator (t-PA) and by urokinase-type plasminogen activator (u-PA). Kallikrein, an active enzyme produced by the contact system of the coagulation cascade, converts single-chain urokinase (scu-PA) into the active u-PA. Both urokinase and t-PA can be inactivated by plasminogen activator inhibitors (PAI-1 and PAI-2). Antiplasmin is a plasma protein and the chief inactivator of plasmin.

rin dissolution. The extracellular matrix is the most important locus for the degradative action of urokinase. t-PA is a serine protease made by endothelial cells and is of principal importance in the activation of plasminogen in plasma. t-PA can be inhibited by binding to plasminogen activator inhibitors (PAIs). There are four of these, but PAI-1 and -2 are the most specific and accelerate the removal of t-PA from the circulation.

Plasminogen has an affinity for fibrin, and t-PA will bind to this complex of fibrin and plasminogen. This binding greatly increases the activity of t-PA and accelerates the conversion of plasminogen to plasmin. Plasmin can also promote the attack of t-PA on plasminogen, thus amplifying the generation of plasmin. When plasmin attacks mature cross-linked fibrin, two end-products of the hydrolysis include the E-domain and a dimer of D-domains (Figure 4–7). If fibrinogen, or fibrin that has not been covalently cross-linked, is attacked by plasmin, only E- and single D-domains are produced. Individuals suffering from thrombophilia may be identified by the persistence of D-dimers in the plasma. It may be appropriate to treat such coagulation problems with anticoagulants, such as dicoumarol.

Given the potential power of plasmin in fibrinolysis, there are inhibitors for its activity. α_2-Antiplasmin is a plasma protein that binds to plasmin and blocks the binding between fibrin and plasmin. α_2-Antiplasmin is a serine protease inhibitor that also has the ability to bind to cross-linked fibrin, strengthening the durability of the hard clot. Plasmin that has already bound to fibrin resists the inhibitor, while free plasmin can be easily inhib-

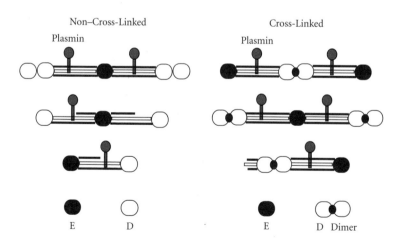

Figure 4–7 Fibrinolysis. Plasminogen binds to fibrin and is activated by tissue-type plasminogen activator (t-PA). Plasmin attacks the cross-linked fibrin and releases fragments, notably the E-domain and a dimer of the D-domain. Fibrin that has not been covalently cross-linked will release fragments containing single D- and E-domains. Adapted from Israels LG, Israels ED. Mechanisms in hematology. 2nd ed. Bayer Publishing; 1997.

ited by α_2-antiplasmin. α_2-Macroglobulin is a plasma protease that can disable urokinase, t-PA, and plasmin, although it has a relatively less specific and slower action than α_2-antiplasmin.

CLOT BUSTERS AND THERAPIES FOR CLOT LYSIS

Thrombi may provoke tissue ischemia by cutting off blood flow to areas of the brain or heart. The formation of thrombi can be triggered by damage to the endothelium lining blood vessels, by rupture of the endothelial lining caused by an atherosclerotic plaque, or by vessel malformation. It is possible to administer agents that promote clot dissolution (clot busters), in efforts to restore blood flow. You may remember the use of the "-buster" suffix that arose following the popular film "Ghost Busters" in the mid-1980s, and this suggests the time frame for the development of these therapeutic agents. Streptokinase (SK) is one of these. This is not an enzyme; rather, it is a protein obtained from certain bacteria (β-hemolytic *streptococci*) that can bind to plasminogen, and the SK-plasminogen complex can activate other plasminogen molecules (Figure 4–8). One drawback with SK is its ability to promote not only fibrin dissolution but also the breakdown of plasma fibrinogen, promoting the risk of bleeding. Thus, SK has no selectivity for plasminogen associated with fibrin but can activate free plasma plasminogen as well. Be careful in the use of SK, as its administration can promote the formation of antibodies and the potential for an allergic reaction should the drug be given on a second occasion. Thus, SK may be limited to a single regimen for each patient.

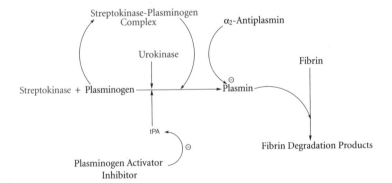

Figure 4–8 Clot busters. The actions of tissue-type plasminogen activator (t-PA), urokinase, streptokinase, and streptokinase-plasminogen complex are shown in the conversion of plasminogen to plasmin. If given soon enough following heart attack or stroke, these agents can restore circulation to ischemic tissues.

Recombinant DNA techniques have allowed the production of human proteins with greater specificity in clot dissolution. In particular, recombinant t-PA is now available. If given within a specific time frame following the onset of signs and symptoms of heart attack or stroke, t-PA can very effectively reduce mortality and damage associated with these diseases. As time is critical in the administration of clot busters during cardiovascular crisis, you may, as health-care professionals, encourage the use of emergency alert devices for your more senior patients who live on their own. These devices are often pendants worn around the neck that can be activated by pushing a button. This, in turn, alerts a surveillance service that will respond very quickly to the call for help. Certainly, this alert system can also be of assistance should an elderly patient fall or otherwise be made immobile. For similar purposes, you may, for a senior living alone, recommend that the doors be left open when the bathroom is in use. This may be considered a little radical, but there are precedents for single seniors in cardiovascular crisis, hastening to a washroom, only to collapse inside the door and, thus, block any attempts for initial rescue.

Naturally, when considering the use of clot busters in stroke, care must be taken to determine that the ischemia is produced by blood vessel occlusion and not by brain hemorrhage! Hemorrhagic stroke accounts for some 20% of strokes and can be associated with untreated hypertension (e.g., those individuals who proudly proclaim that they have not seen a physician in 20 years). Similarly, it is also harmful to administer clot busters outside the time frame indicated by the onset of heart attack or stroke. t-PA is superior to SK in its effectiveness in restoring blood flow, but at present, the great disadvantage in using t-PA is its price. t-PA has a certain prestige, as it was the first commercial drug made by recombinant DNA technology. We will discuss these techniques in detail in Chapter 8, but in brief, the procedure involves isolation of the DNA that codes for the production of human t-PA, its insertion into an expression vector (a double-stranded DNA that henceforth carries the t-PA genetic sequence), and the transfection of cultured mammalian cells with the vector. Cells that produce t-PA in considerable quantity can secrete this protein into the culture medium, which serves as a source for the purification of this recombinant protein.

Alteplase and Reteplase are two commercial types of t-PA. While Alteplase is a copy of natural t-PA, Reteplase is a modified version of the natural protein that retains certain of the functional domains of the natural protein. This alteration has extended the half-life of Reteplase in the circulation to 16 to 18 minutes, compared with 3 to 6 minutes for Alteplase. Reteplase is given as two bolus injections, while Alteplase is given as a continuous infusion over 90 minutes, with weight-adjusted dosages. Both drugs have similar efficacies in reducing patient mortality rates following heart attack.

PLATELETS IN HEMOSTASIS AND THROMBOSIS

While the coagulation cascade, which leads to the formation of polymerized, cross-linked fibrin, is an important event in controlling blood loss following vessel injury, platelets are also a very important component in hemostasis and thrombosis. Thrombosis occurs in vascular diseases, such as atherosclerosis, and is not necessarily initiated by a severed vessel. Both hemostasis and thrombosis involve platelet activation, the aggregation of platelets, and the formation of fibrin. Platelet activation leads to changes in the platelet plasma membrane that permit the association and adherence of platelets. For both hemostasis and thrombosis, platelets can aggregate at a site of injury, and fibrin can form a matrix to stabilize the platelet aggregate. This is the basis of a hemostatic plug that seals a broken vessel, or a thrombus that may form at a site of endothelial injury and then become the source of emboli that move downstream.

Platelets are small anucleate cells in the blood and are made by the break-up of large cells called **megakaryocytes** in bone marrow. While platelets lack nuclei and, thus, have little or no ability to synthesize new protein, they do have specialized secretory granules (Figure 4–9) that carry biologically active compounds and are themselves remarkably responsive to stimulation. ADP and ATP (ATP, the energy molecule, was discussed in Chapter 1), as well as serotonin and calcium, are found in platelet-dense granules. On platelet stimulation, these components are released, and some can provoke the activation of other platelets. Proteins, such as the adhesion molecules, vWF, and fibronectin, and the coagulation factors V, XI, and XIII, are found in platelet α-granules and are also released during platelet activation.

Platelets are sensitive to a variety of biologically active molecules. Thus, the platelet plasma membrane has a number of receptors, proteins that bind specifically to extracellular agents (ligands). The formation of a receptor–ligand complex leads to a chain of metabolic events within the platelets. These events lead to platelet aggregation. In certain cases, the binding of a specific ligand to its receptor will block platelet activation events.

The receptors in the platelet plasma membrane can bind to molecules found in the matrix below the endothelial cell layer (that will be exposed to the circulation following vessel injury) or to proteins in the plasma (Figure 4–10). One event in these interactions occurs between a vWF and the protein GPIb (GP stands for glycoprotein) found in the platelet plasma membrane. vWF is made in endothelial cells and megakaryocytes, found in platelet granules, and present in the subendothelium. vWF can bind to the platelet surface and can also bind to collagen found in the cellular matrix of the vessel wall. Thus, vWF can serve as a tether linking platelets to the exposed subendothelium. A genetic deficiency in vWF can lead to a bleeding disorder (von Willebrand disease), as vWF plays an important role in

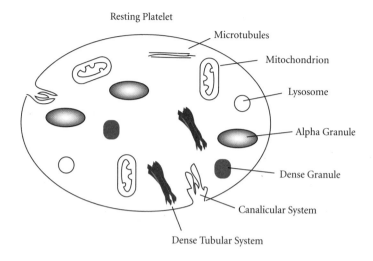

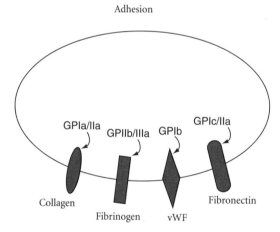

Figure 4–9 Platelet structure and surface binding molecules. Platelets are small anucleate cells of the blood that lack a nucleus but possess secretory granules (dense granules, alpha-granules) that contain a variety of compounds that can promote platelet activation and aggregation. Platelets are formed by the fragmentation of larger cells in bone marrow called megakaryocytes. The proteins collagen, fibrinogen, vWF (von Willebrand factor), and fibronectin can specifically interact with glycoproteins at the platelet plasma membrane.

platelet recruitment to areas of vessel damage. The interaction of collagen-linked vWF with GPIb leads to shape changes in platelets and to the activation of GPIIb/IIIa (this protein is also known as the integrin $\alpha_{IIb}\beta_3$, another component of the platelet plasma membrane). vWF also interacts with activated GPIIb/IIIa on different platelet surfaces, promoting the interaction and aggregation of platelets. Activated GPIIb/IIIa at two platelet surfaces can bind one molecule of fibrinogen, and this additionally facilitates the formation of platelet aggregates, which, along with fibrin polymerization, form a hemostatic plug sealing a severed blood vessel. Other molecules can bind to the platelet plasma membrane, including collagen (binding to GPIa/IIa) and fibronectin (to GPIc/IIa), and these interactions will also lead to platelet activation (see Figure 4–9). One additional, very important, biologically active molecule that initiates platelet activation is thrombin. Thrombin does have a receptor on the platelet plasma membrane and, on interaction, thrombin actually modifies its receptor by hydrolyzing a peptide bond and releasing a short N-terminal peptide (Figure 4–11).

Plasma Membrane of the Platelet

This membrane is very important in platelet activation and also in the coagulation cascade, as it provides a surface for the activation of coagulation factors X and prothrombin. As the platelet is activated, there are very significant changes in the distribution of phospholipids in the bilayer that is the core of membrane structure. We last described phospholipids in Chapter 2, with reference to lipoprotein structure. Recall that phospholipids in a monolayer surround these lipid-transporting particles. In cellular membranes, phospholipids make up a bilayer so that the hydrophilic head groups of phospholipids of the inner monolayer face the cytoplasm, while

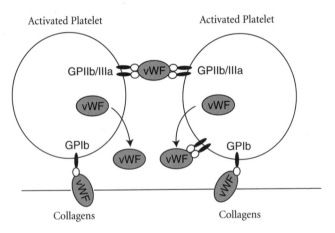

Figure 4–10 Platelet adhesion and vWF. Von Willebrand factor can bind to exposed collagen from the damaged subendothelium and, in so doing, can also bind to glycoprotein GPIb of the platelet plasma membrane. This helps to attach platelets to sites of injury. vWF can also interact with GPIIb/IIIa and facilitate surface interactions between activated platelets. Adapted from Israels LG, Israels ED. Mechanisms in hematology. 2nd ed. Bayer Publishing; 1997.

the head groups of phospholipids of the outer monolayer face the blood (Figure 4–12). The hydrophobic fatty acid chains make up the interior of the bilayer. When the platelets are activated, the hydrophilic groups of a negatively charged phospholipid, called **phosphatidylserine**, become exposed on the surface. In other words, platelet activation brings about a reorientation of phosphatidylserine from the inner monolayer (facing the cytoplasm) to the outer monolayer (facing the blood). This phospholipid, along with calcium ions, promotes activation events in the coagulation cascade.

Just as we considered the remarkable degree of amplification in the coagulation cascade, there is an equally remarkable amplification in the recruitment of platelets into an aggregate. This involves initial stimulation events, say, with exposure to collagen or thrombin, followed by release of platelet granule components, further platelet activation and recruitment to the aggregate, and coagulation factor activation at the platelet surface.

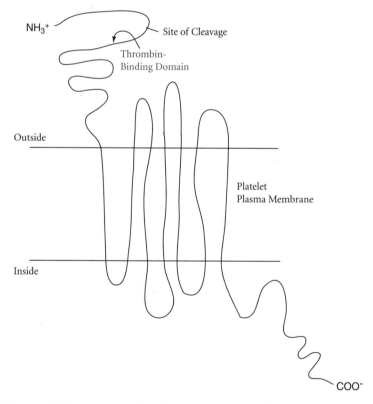

Figure 4–11 Thrombin receptor of the platelet plasma membrane. This membrane-bound protein has seven transmembrane spanning regions and a thrombin-binding domain facing the outside of the cell. Once thrombin binds, it cleaves its receptor at the site indicated, and remarkably, the new N-terminus binds to another portion of the protein, activating it.

Platelet Activation, Phospholipases, and Eicosanoids

When thrombin binds to its receptor, there follows a rather remarkable chain of events inside the platelet (Figure 4–13). The pathways involved are often referred to as intracellular signalling pathways. Initially, G-proteins are activated, which, in turn, switch on an enzyme called **phospholipase C** (PLC) at the inner face of the plasma membrane. This enzyme degrades a complex phospholipid (phosphatidylinositol 4,5-bisphosphate) located within the plasma membrane and often designated by the abbreviation PIP_2 (Figure 4–14). The result of this hydrolysis is the release of two products: a lipid called **diacylglycerol** and a hydrophilic compound called **IP_3** or **inositol trisphosphate**. This latter product provokes a rise in intracellular free calcium ions. Calcium, together with diacylglycerol, promotes the activity of protein kinase C (PKC). PKC can phosphorylate a protein called **pleckstrin**, and its phosphorylation promotes the release of the contents of secretory granules, thus promoting further platelet activation. In addition, the rising levels of calcium in platelets can activate calmodulin and thus myosin light chain kinase. The phosphorylation of myosin in platelets is associated with

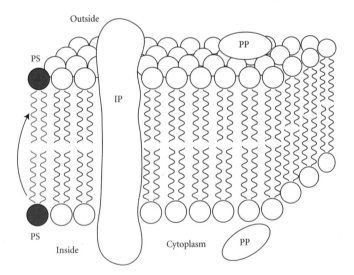

Figure 4–12 Phospholipid bilayer. In membranes, phospholipid molecules are oriented in a bilayer structure so that the polar head groups (represented by circles) face an aqueous environment outside or inside the cell, while the fatty acid chains form a hydrophobic layer at the core of the membrane structure. Also shown is a protein that traverses the bilayer (integral protein [IP]) and proteins associated with the two surfaces of the bilayer (peripheral proteins [PP]). For the platelet plasma membrane, activation can stimulate the movement of the negatively charged phospholipid, phosphatidylserine, from the inner monolayer, facing the cytoplasm, to the outer monolayer, where it can participate in events of the coagulation cascade.

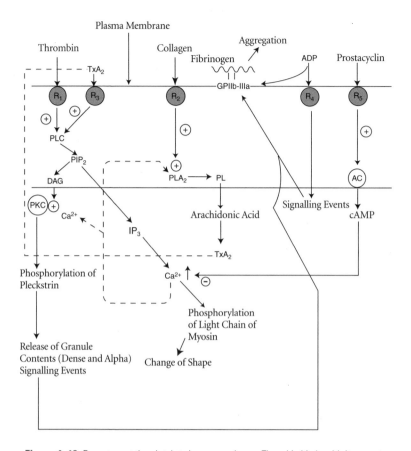

Figure 4–13 Receptors at the platelet plasma membrane. Thrombin binds with its receptor (R_1) and, in so doing, activates the platelet by a chain of events that activate phospholipase C (PLC), an enzyme that degrades the very polar phospholipid PIP_2 located in the platelet plasma membrane. This action liberates a smaller molecule, inositol trisphosphate (IP_3), which mediates a rise in the concentration of free calcium within the platelet. Calcium and the second product of PLC, diacylglycerol (DAG), activate a protein kinase, called PKC. PKC phosphorylates the protein pleckstrin and initiates granule-release mechanisms in activated platelets. Rising levels of free calcium will also activate the phosphorylation of the light chain of myosin, leading to shape changes in platelets. Collagen also interacts with its receptor (R_2) on the platelet plasma membrane and activates another phospholipase known as phospholipase A_2 (PLA_2). PLA_2 activity is increased by rising levels of calcium in platelets. This enzyme releases arachidonic acid from phospholipids of the platelet plasma membrane. By a chain of reactions, arachidonic acid is converted to the eicosanoid thromboxane A_2 (TxA_2), which is released from platelets. Via its receptor (R_3), TxA_2 stimulates PLC and the production of more IP_3 and DAG. The released granule component ADP can interact with its receptor (R_4) on the platelet plasma membrane, and this interaction initiates a sequence of events that leads to the exposure of more activated GPIIb/IIIa at the platelet surface. Prostacyclin (PGI_2) is an eicosanoid made by endothelial cells of the blood vessel wall. When prostacyclin binds to its receptor (R_5), adenylate cyclase (AC) is activated . The cyclic AMP (cAMP) product opposes platelet activation by blocking increases in levels of free calcium. Adapted from Murray RK, Granner DK, Mayes PA, Rodwell VW. Harper's biochemistry. 25th ed. Stamford (CT): Appleton and Lange; 2000.

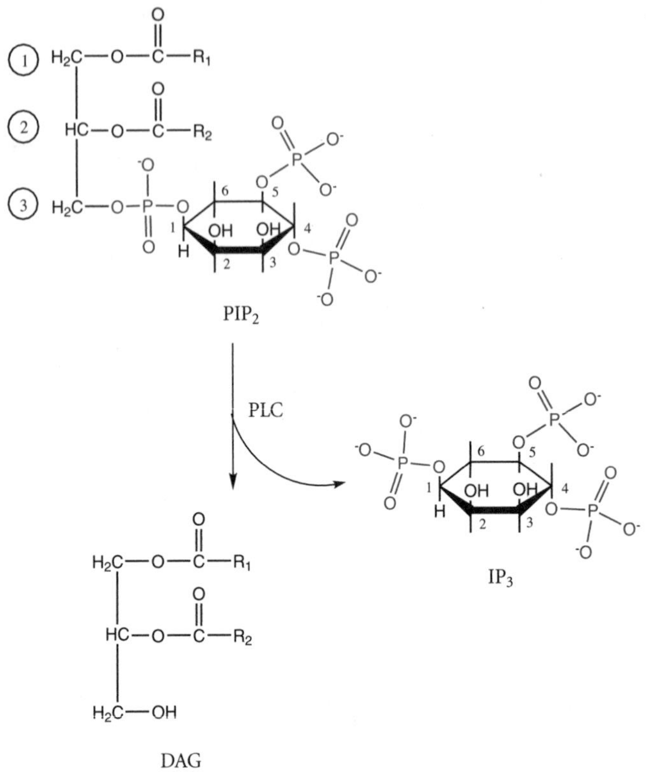

Figure 4–14 Phosphatidylinositol 4,5-bisphosphate. This phospholipid, given the abbreviation PIP$_2$, is involved in signalling events associated with the platelet plasma membrane, as noted in Figure 4–13. Like many other phospholipids, PIP$_2$ has a glycerol backbone and two long-chain fatty acids (-O-CO-R) in ester link at carbons 1 and 2 on the glycerol backbone. The head group in PIP$_2$ (located at carbon 3 on the glycerol backbone) is particularly highly charged because it has three phosphate groups. The enzymatic cleavage of PIP$_2$ by phospholipase C produces two products of very different polarity: the hydrophobic diacylglycerol (glycerol and the two attached fatty acids) and the highly water-soluble inositol trisphosphate (IP$_3$). Both these products play roles in signalling events, as shown in Figure 4–13.

cellular shape changes. Recall that we discussed in Chapter 1 the phosphorylation of myosin carried out by myosin light chain kinase in muscle.

The interaction of collagen with its receptor in the platelet plasma membrane is shown in Figure 4–13. In this path, a different type of phospholipid-degrading enzyme is activated. This enzyme is called **phospholipase A$_2$**, and with rising levels of calcium ions within the platelet, it releases the fatty acid arachidonate from phospholipids of the platelet plasma membrane. Arachidonate can serve as a precursor molecule for a variety of biologically active lipids called **eicosanoids** (Figure 4–15). In platelets, the principal eicosanoid formed is called **thromboxane A$_2$** (TxA$_2$), and from its name, you can likely guess that it plays a role in thrombosis. TxA_2 has its own receptor in the platelet plasma membrane, and on its release and interaction with platelets, a signalling path that involves degradation of PIP_2 by phospholipase C is activated (similar to that initiated by thrombin binding, noted in Figure 4–13). Thus, TxA_2 will trigger further platelet activation and aggregation. ADP, the component released from platelet-dense granules, also has a receptor on the plasma membrane, and its signalling pathway can contribute to the interaction of activated GPIIb-IIIa with fibrinogen at the platelet surface.

Given the remarkable diversity of agents and events that can trigger the activation of platelets, you may be excused for wondering why, say, following a particularly violent sneeze, every drop of your blood is not propelled into clot formation. Indeed, preparations of platelets isolated from blood are sensitive to physical stress so that excessive mixing of a suspension of platelets can lead to their aggregation. Naturally, given the potential strength of the responses in hemostasis and thrombosis, there have to be systems that control or counteract platelet activation and aggregation. One of these is initiated by the eicosanoid called **prostacyclin** (PGI_2). This is another compound formed from arachidonate, and prostacyclin has its own receptor at the platelet plasma membrane (see Figure 4–13). You may certainly think of the plasma membrane as some gigantic switchboard that will take an incoming compound into its appropriate niche and initiate a specific response pattern, rather like calling up customer service, technical service, the mailroom, the CEO, and so on. (That is, presuming you ever get to hear a human voice!)

Prostacyclin is made not by platelets but by the endothelial cells lining the blood vessel wall. Prostacyclin is a very potent inhibitor that will block platelet activation, and prostacyclin serves to counter the response to TxA_2. Following binding of prostacyclin, the signalling sequence involves the activation of an enzyme called **adenylate cyclase**, which leads to the formation of **cyclic adenosine monophosphate** (cAMP) from ATP. cAMP acts to oppose the rise of calcium within the platelet, and this effectively blocks platelet activation. Thus, prostacyclin will counter the formation of platelet aggregates on blood vessel walls. Endothelial cells can also break down ADP (released from platelets) and can synthesize the vasodilator nitric oxide (see Chapter 1) as well as plasminogen activators. Thus, you can appreciate that there is a balance between agents that promote and inhibit platelet activation and the coagulation cascade.

TxA_2 and prostacyclin are only two of the many eicosanoids that can be formed from free arachidonate. There are several major classes of these (see Figure 4–15), and unfortunately, many of these can be involved in pathologic responses. The first eicosanoids to be discovered were the prostaglandins, so called because they were first isolated from seminal fluid but later found in many cells and tissues. Prostaglandin E_2 (PGE_2) is an example, and this eicosanoid has its own receptor at the plasma membrane

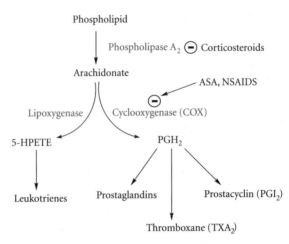

Figure 4–15 Conversion of arachidonate acid into eicosanoids. Arachidonate is liberated from membrane phospholipids by the action of PLA$_2$ (phospholipase A$_2$). This activity is stimulated during platelet activation. In nucleated cells, PLA$_2$ can be inhibited by the use of anti-inflammatory corticosteroids. Arachidonate can be used by two major metabolic routes. Cyclooxygenase can convert arachidonate to a cyclic precursor molecule PGH$_2$, which, in turn, can give rise to prostaglandins, thromboxane A$_2$ (TxA$_2$), or prostacyclin (PGI$_2$) by the action of specific enzymes. TxA$_2$ synthase is found in platelets, and PGI$_2$ synthase is found in endothelial cells. Alternatively, arachidonate can be converted by the enzyme lipoxygenase that produces 5-HPETE, a precursor for the compounds called leukotrienes. Some of these are important in the bronchoconstriction seen in asthma.

of responsive cells. The production of prostaglandin E$_2$ can be associated with pain and fever, among many other responses. Another class of eicosanoids includes the leukotrienes, some of which are involved in bronchoconstriction, as seen in asthma.

The eicosanoids are made through two principal metabolic pathways. The path first discovered utilizes an enzyme called **cyclooxygenase** (COX-1). This produces a compound that serves as a precursor for prostacyclin, thromboxane, and prostaglandin. One potent inhibitor of cyclooxygenase is aspirin (acetylsalicylic acid [ASA]). ASA will irreversibly modify cyclooxygenase (via acetylation) so that it can no longer function. Thus, platelets exposed to ASA cannot make TxA$_2$, and this drug very effectively reduces platelet activation and aggregation. Naturally, ASA also inhibits cyclooxygenase in endothelial cells and thus blocks the synthesis of prostacyclin. But the big difference for endothelial cells is their ability to make more cyclooxygenase and, thus, to recover from ASA, while platelets (as they have no nuclei) cannot regenerate their cyclooxygenase. Thus, ASA acts as an antiplatelet drug and is often given to individuals with cardiovascular disease to reduce the risk of heart attack or stroke.

One very important feature of cardiovascular disease is the atherosclerotic plaque, which can be found in arterial walls, such as those of the carotid or coronary arteries. These plaques develop following the infiltration of lipoprotein particles (low-density lipoprotein [LDL], Chapter 2) into the vessel wall (Figure 4–16). This can be facilitated by damage to the vessel endothelial cells caused, for example, by high blood pressure, diabetes, or smoking. The infiltrating LDL particles can elicit a response from circulating monocytes that enter the arterial wall in pursuit. LDL particles that have been altered by oxidation reactions (oxidized LDL) provoke a greater response and are thus more atherogenic. In Chapter 2, we noted the relatively high content of cholesterol in LDL and pointed out that defects in LDL uptake by the LDL receptor can elevate LDL levels within blood. This condition (hypercholesterolemia) can contribute to the formation of atherosclerotic plaques (atherogenesis). A prolonged half-life of LDL particles in the circulation may likely increase their chemical modification by oxidation. The potential involvement of oxidants derived from tobacco smoke cannot be emphasized enough.

Once inside the vessel wall, monocytes differentiate into macrophages that phagocytose the LDL particles. The macrophages often cannot escape and may die within the vessel wall, leaving behind accumulations of cholesterol and other lipids. LDL particles themselves may also aggregate within the wall. These processes lead to the formation of a lipid pool within the vessel wall that contributes to the distortion and reduction of the vessel lumen. Thus, blood flowing by may undergo turbulent flow patterns when passing through vessels with such distortions. This turbulence and the damaged endothelial surface can provoke the formation of thrombi on the vessel surface. If the thrombus is located in a carotid artery, the release of emboli from the thrombus may precipitate an ischemic event when an embolus occludes a small vessel in the brain. If this occlusion is temporary, a TIA will occur. A TIA can have very specific symptoms, such as blindness in one eye, that may last for 30 minutes to more than 6 hours. TIAs are particularly important as warnings of stroke (when the occlusion of a vessel in the brain can result in much more severe and lasting neurologic disability), and a neurologist should be consulted without delay. Often, ASA is prescribed as an antiplatelet drug to reduce the chance of thrombus formation. ASA is a member of a group of pharmaceuticals known as nonsteroidal antiinflammatory drugs (NSAIDs), which includes indomethacin. As suggested by the term NSAID, eicosanoids are often involved in inflammatory reactions accompanying various forms of injury, including stroke, heart attack, allergic response, arthritis, and responses to wounding. Arthritics and those with vascular disease can take ASA for prolonged periods, so you might well ask whether eicosanoids are necessary for cellular function.

There is one major problem associated with ASA, and that is gastric irritation and bleeding, seen in certain individuals. The stomach does require the synthesis of certain levels of eicosanoids to maintain integrity in the gastric lining, and this is blocked by the inhibition of cyclooxygenase by ASA.

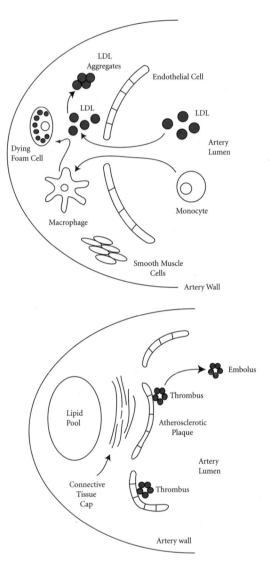

Figure 4–16 An atherosclerotic lesion. The generation of an atherosclerotic plaque is believed to be initiated by damage to the endothelial cells lining arteries, with subsequent infiltration of LDL particles. Within the wall, LDL can aggregate or be phagocytosed by invading monocytes that differentiate into macrophages. The macrophages may turn into foam cells, noted by their high content of lipid, highly enriched in cholesterol and cholesterol esters. Foam cells may die within the wall and contribute, along with LDL aggregates, to the formation of a lipid pool. There is also the generation of excessive connective tissue within the artery wall, often seen as a cap over the lipid pool. Together, the lipid pool and connective tissue cap bring about a distortion in the wall that can reduce the size of the lumen of the artery and promote the formation of thrombi. Emboli can be formed from thrombi and travel in the blood until they come to occlude a smaller blood vessel.

An important discovery was that cyclooxygenase activities increased during an inflammatory response, and this was due to the production of a new isoenzyme of cyclooxygenase called **cyclooxgenase 2** (COX-2). Thus, drugs (such as Celebra or Vioxx) have been developed as specific COX-2 inhibitors that block the inflammatory response, without compromising the synthesis of eicosanoids by the housekeeping cyclooxygenase COX-1.

Another class of antiplatelet drugs is the GPIIb/IIIa blockers. These have been developed as alternatives to ASA and cyclooxygenase inhibition. Activated GPIIb/IIIa is involved in the binding of fibrinogen and vWF, a critical step leading to platelet aggregation and thrombus formation. The GPIIb/IIIa blockers work by occupying the binding site for fibrinogen on this receptor protein. While ASA and heparin are the basic agents administered to block eicosanoid production by platelets and coagulation, the GPIIb/IIIa blockers can also be used in combination with other therapies, such as clot busters, which can then be used at lower doses.

The name NSAID implies that there are also steroidal anti-inflammatories. This is indeed the case, and corticosteroids, such as dexamethasone and budesonide, will stop eicosanoid production by blocking the synthesis of COX-2 at the level of nuclear transcription (transcription is discussed in Chapter 8). Corticosteroids have a wide range of action and inhibit the enzyme phospholipase A_2, thus blocking the release of arachidonate. It was found that these anti-inflammatories are also useful in the treatment of asthma. Asthmatics suffer from narrowed airways, produced by bronchoconstriction. This can be brought about by eicosanoids called **leukotrienes**. Interestingly, these eicosanoids are made from arachidonate in pathways that are controlled not by cyclooxygenase but by another enzyme called **lipoxygenase** (see Figure 4–15). Lipoxygenase is not sensitive to ASA. In fact, it can be dangerous for asthmatics to take ASA, simply because the inhibition of cyclooxygenase allows more free arachidonate to pass through lipoxygenase, supporting greater levels of production of leukotrienes. There are a variety of therapeutic interventions for asthma, including inhaled corticosteroids, smooth muscle relaxants, and antileukotrienes (which, yes, do block leukotriene receptors at the plasma membrane of sensitive cells). Nonetheless, the management of asthma and related respiratory disorders continues to be a challenge, largely because of side reactions found in the use of corticosteroids. It has been observed, at our local children's hospital, that the majority of emergency patients are there because of respiratory conditions. It would be very useful to have a drug like ASA with specificity for the lipoxygenase enzyme.

5

Hemoglobin, Porphyrias, and Jaundice

As our readers can appreciate by now, blood is a biological fluid of particular significance to doctors and other health-care professionals. It carries a variety of important compounds, often bound to transport proteins, including albumin, transferrin, and ceruloplasmin, as we described in Chapter 2. Blood can also be sampled to assess abnormal serum (or plasma) enzyme levels that are diagnostic for a variety of diseases (as noted in Chapter 3). In Chapter 4, we described the interplay of the coagulation cascade and platelet activation leading to the sealing off of severed blood vessels in the vital process of hemostasis and the formation of thrombi and emboli in the circulation, which are major players in heart attack, transient ischemic attacks (TIAs), and stroke. It should be apparent that blood is a highly accessible medium that can be used as a very rapid route for the administration of life-saving drugs (e.g., the clot busters and heparin, as described in Chapter 4). Perhaps more importantly, blood, by its relentless flow, supplying a wide variety of organs with nutrients, hormones, and oxygen and removing waste products, such as urea and carbon dioxide, is rather like a river or a highway connecting a series of interdependent major cities. Blood reflects the "state of the nation" or the condition of the body and has been the focus for a considerable number of biochemical studies of medical interest. In this chapter, we will broaden our knowledge of blood by focusing on the oxygen-transporting protein hemoglobin, the control of oxygen transport, and the genetic defects that compromise the function of hemoglobin. We will also discuss problems in the synthesis and disposal of heme, the prosthetic group in hemoglobin responsible for oxygen binding, that account for the porphyrias and various types of jaundice.

STRUCTURE OF HEMOGLOBIN AND OXYGEN BINDING

Hemoglobin is a protein that is made up of subunits. Hopefully, you remember our discussion of fibrin in the previous chapter and the way in which the rather complex fibrin monomers or subunits polymerize into the tough fibrin of hard clots. The assembly and cross-linking of subunits give fibrin its mechanical resilience and strength. Using a football analogy (the North American game that uses the ellipsoidal ball and usually accumulates large scores, for the benefit of readers from the United Kingdom), fibrin is a tough and massive frontline player. In contrast, the subunit structure of the soluble protein hemoglobin lends a remarkably dynamic quality to this protein that allows it to respond readily to its environment. In our football analogy, hemoglobin is the quarterback, superbly mobile and flexible, picking up oxygen, holding on to it in certain cases, while in other circumstances delivering it to other players by hand-offs or passing.

As subunit interaction is the key to understanding hemoglobin function, the first topic for discussion is subunit structure. It is quite common for textbooks to introduce the protein myoglobin before considering hemoglobin. This arises because myoglobin is very similar in structure to a hemoglobin subunit, yet myoglobin exists as a simple monomer, and thus shows many functional differences when compared with the more complex hemoglobin. Myoglobin is a protein of muscle cells and it can bind and store oxygen and also facilitate the distribution of oxygen within these cells. Remember oxygen is vital for cellular energy metabolism and oxygen is needed for the mitochondrial production of ATP, the nucleotide derivative that is a fundamental requirement for muscle contraction. We will discuss ATP in more detail when we outline metabolism in Chapter 7.

Myoglobin is a single polypeptide and is made up of 153 amino acids, with a molecular mass of 17 kDa. Myoglobin is a soluble, globular protein that consists of eight α-helical regions folded into a very compact, roughly spherical shape (Figure 5–1). Remember that globular proteins generally have amino acid residues with hydrophilic, charged, or polar side chains on the outside of the molecule, while those with hydrophobic or nonpolar side chains are found within the molecule. One remarkable feature of myoglobin is that it has a red color. You may recall that the plasma protein ceruloplasmin is blue in color because of its bound copper, and indeed, the red color of myoglobin is largely attributable to bound iron. Yet, in myoglobin, the iron is not bound simply by charge links; rather, iron is actually complexed into a heme group, which itself is covalently bound to the protein. The heme group is not composed of amino acids but is an organic ring system with an iron ion at its center. This is indicated in Figure 5–2, which shows a protoporphyrin ring composed essentially of four interlocking pyrroles and the iron, which is coordinated with four nitrogens of the ring. Ferrous iron normally has six binding or coordination sites, and thus two sites are available that extend at right angles from the plane of the porphyrin ring. In Figure 5–2, one of these sites would come out toward you from the Fe^{2+}, while the other would extend back into the page.

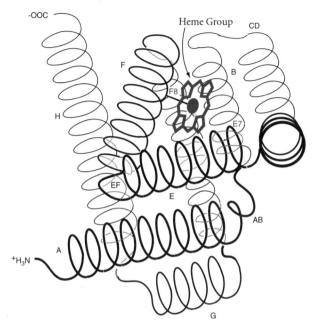

Figure 5–1 The three-dimensional structure of myoglobin. Myoglobin is a single polypeptide composed of eight α-helical segments, lettered A to H. Transition regions may show double letters, for example, AB, CD, EF. The heme group is coordinated with the side chain of histidine F-8 (i.e., the eighth amino acid in the F α-helix, also called the proximal histidine). Oxygen binds on the side of the heme group facing histidine E-7 (the distal histidine).

The iron ion can exist in two charged states. In high school, you likely encountered the litany of the periodic chart and the memorization of various valences of the different metal atoms. Doubtless, you found this as tedious as we did. For the medical sciences, however, metal ions play key roles and without them our lifestyles, and indeed our existence, would be in question. Chemistry teachers also tend to be quite forceful or memorable figures. One of the authors recalls that his chemistry master was a very dynamic individual, an environmentalist before his time, and an active opponent of second-hand smoke, who would hold his breath between bus stops until the bus door was opened by the driver. (This was in the 1960s when public transportation permitted smoking on board). If you had such a teacher, you can probably recall that iron exists in ferrous (Fe^{2+}) and ferric (Fe^{3+}) states. We will run into this again in our discussions of metabolism; so, please keep these forms of iron in mind. It is the Fe^{2+} in heme in myoglobin that binds oxygen. If this ferrous iron is oxidized to Fe^{3+}, this molecule is called metmyoglobin, which cannot bind oxygen. Thus, oxidation of the heme group is to be avoided at all costs. Yet, when heme itself is dissolved in water (without its attachment to myoglobin), the Fe^{2+} in heme

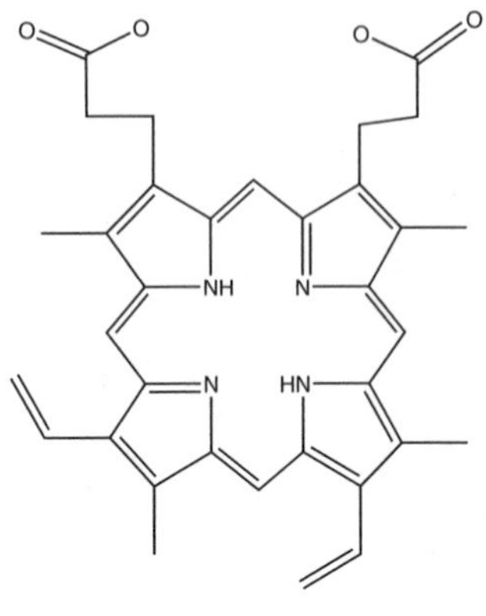

Protoporphyrin IX 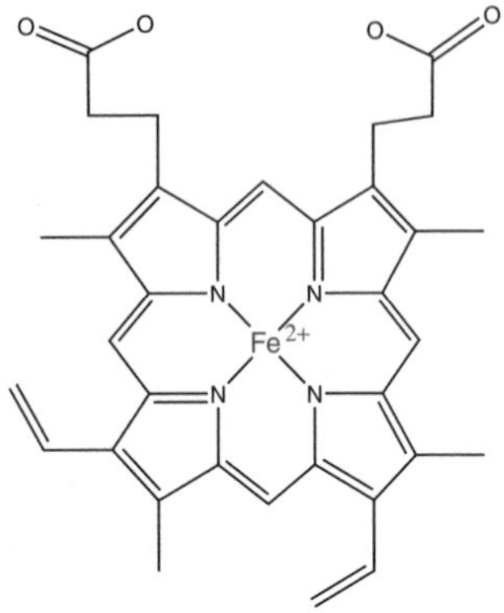   Heme (Fe²⁺-Protoporphyrin IX)

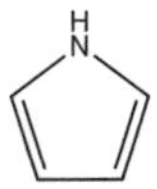

Pyrrole

Figure 5–2 Structure of the heme group. Heme is composed of the central iron ion (Fe²⁺), which is coordinately bound to four nitrogens of the tetrapyrrole ring system. The ring (without iron) is also known as protoporphyrin IX.

does oxidize very readily. How can this be prevented in myoglobin? Quite simply, by having heme in a hydrophobic crevice in the protein that is normally shielded from water but that allows oxygen to enter for an oxygenation reaction. Be careful to distinguish between oxidation (loss of electrons, remember the chemical rubric LEO GER?) as shown by the transition Fe^{2+} → Fe^{3+} and oxygenation, which is the uptake of O_2, with no change in valence of iron. The binding of oxygen at the ferrous ion in the heme of myoglobin also results in a dramatic color change (dark to bright red) as deoxymyoglobin becomes oxymyoglobin.

The heme group is rather like a shield, with iron at its center. One of the two coordinate binding sites extending at right angles from Fe^{2+} attaches to residue His F-8 in myoglobin (Figure 5–3). This nomenclature may be somewhat confusing, as we have noted in Chapter 1, that the amino acids in proteins are simply numbered in sequence starting from the N-terminus, which is amino acid residue number 1. Myoglobin (also known as a heme protein) was the first protein whose three-dimensional structure was studied, and its amino acid residues were numbered according to their positions within the eight different α-helices (lettered A to H) within the molecule.

Thus, His F-8 is the eighth residue within the F-helix (see Figure 5-1). Within the crevice in the protein, the heme group is oriented like a flat disc between the residues His F-8 and His E-7 (see Figure 5–3). An oxygen molecule enters the crevice and binds to the ferrous iron of the heme ring on the side facing the side chain of His E-7; the oxygen will also interact with the side chain of this histidine residue. As you can see, the heme group is the essential functional component within myoglobin. You can visualize heme as a red-colored dime within a much larger ball of dough or clay.

There is a story that might assist you in remembering the dime-like nature of heme structure and its buried orientation within the structure of myoglobin. This comes from the early 1950s, when a new practice was introduced in the preparation of birthday cakes. The cake was prepared with small "silver" money inside it. The money was first boiled to maintain hygiene (a large

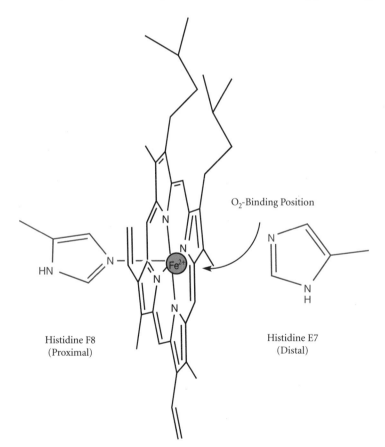

Figure 5–3 Structure of the oxygen-binding site in myoglobin. Heme is essentially a flat ring, with iron at its center. Oxygen binds at iron's sixth coordination position, close to histidine E-7.

domestic concept in the 1950s) and then inserted into the cake batter, prior to cooking and the application of icing. The member of the birthday party finding the most money in his or her piece of carefully dissected cake would be deemed a winner and would keep the found capital (a significant sum at that time period!). Unfortunately, in our story, after the customary blowing out of candles and distribution of cake, the mother was called out of the party room at a critical moment, before the rules of this rather new ritual were completely explained to the children. On seeing the empty plates on her return, she asked "Who is the lucky winner?" only to be met by puzzled expressions. In consuming the cake (likely at a great speed and without much decorum in the absence of an adult), not one of the children had encountered any of the hidden $2.50. The party was then quickly adjourned to the emergency room of the local hospital, but happily, as one might say, everything came out fine in the end. If you are a medical student, during your Pediatrics rotation you may be shown the astounding collection of materials (many, unhappily, not round and smooth) that children can ingest.

Turning from these medically oriented festivities back to myoglobin, recall that this protein is close in structure to a subunit of hemoglobin. While myoglobin is a single sphere-like structure, hemoglobin actually consists of four of these subunits, oriented within a cluster (Figure 5–4). There are two α-subunits and two β-subunits in adult hemoglobin, which is often designated $\alpha_2\beta_2$. The α- and β-subunits are somewhat smaller than myoglobin, composed of 141 and 146 residues, respectively. The polypeptide portions of these subunits are called **globins**. The α- and β-globins are the products of separate genes and do show some differences in amino acid composition. However, the three-dimensional shapes of myoglobin and the two subunits of hemoglobin are very similar. The subunits interact mainly by electrostatic bonds (the bonds between negatively and positively charged side chains of amino acids found at the surfaces of the subunits).

A hemoglobin tetramer has four heme groups, one residing in each subunit. Remember that hemoglobin, unlike myoglobin, is a travelling protein, as it is found within red cells circulating throughout the body. Hemoglobin certainly gives blood its red color, which can range from the darker red of venous blood, which carries deoxyhemoglobin, to the bright red of arterial blood, carrying oxyhemoglobin. From a physiologic point of view, you can understand the need for a circulatory system to supply efficiently the needs of organisms with different tissue and organ systems and the impossibility of delivering these by a simple process of diffusion (that serves the needs of much smaller and simpler life forms). Even with a circulating fluid, you would find a very limited capacity to carry oxygen in a warm medium, already carrying many solutes, in the absence of an oxygen-binding protein. Perhaps you have seen gas bubbles collecting on the sides of a glass of cold water allowed to warm to room temperature, indicating the decreased sol-

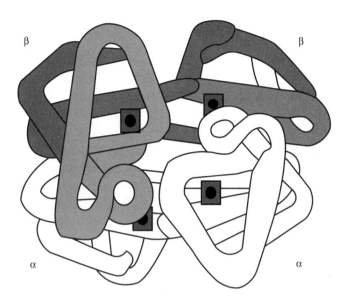

β   β

α   α

Hemoglobin

Figure 5–4 A three-dimensional model of hemoglobin structure. Adult hemoglobin (HbA) is a tetramer, made up of α- and β-subunits ($\alpha_2\beta_2$). Each subunit is similar in three-dimensional structure to myoglobin, and each subunit carries a heme group. There are four oxygen-binding sites on hemoglobin. Adapted from Mathews CK, van Holde KE, Ahern KG. Biochemistry. 3rd ed. San Francisco (CA): Addison Wesley Longman; 2000.

ubility of gases in a warm liquid. Carbonated soft drinks very readily release their carbon dioxide when you open a bottle or can or add more sugar to these beverages. These are examples of the limited capacity of fluids to carry dissolved gases.

Accepting the need for an oxygen-transporting protein, you might well question the need for hemoglobin and its subunit structure. Why not simply pack red cells with the monomeric, oxygen-carrying myoglobin? The answer lies in the truly dynamic nature of oxygen binding that is shown by hemoglobin. When you compare the abilities of myoglobin and hemoglobin to bind oxygen, you find that with rising oxygen concentration (or partial pressure of oxygen, pO_2, as they say in the gas business), myoglobin very rapidly and efficiently binds oxygen (Figure 5–5). For myoglobin, the curve of oxygen saturation of protein versus oxygen pressure is hyperbolic (rather similar to a substrate concentration versus velocity curve, as we noted for enzymes in Chapter 3). At low pO_2 (10 torr), myoglobin is almost fully saturated with oxygen. In contrast, the larger, tetrameric hemoglobin initially responds more slowly to pO_2, showing a curve that is sigmoid in shape (a slow start, followed by a rapid binding of oxygen

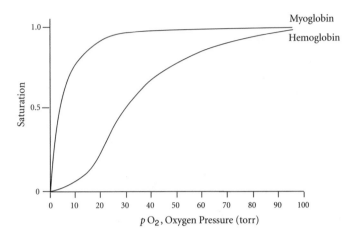

Figure 5–5 Curves of oxygen dissociation for myoglobin and hemoglobin. Note the hyperbolic curve for myoglobin and the sigmoid curve for hemoglobin. The sigmoid curve is indicative of cooperativity effects in oxygen binding to hemoglobin and is physiologically important, as oxygen is readily bound at high oxygen pressure (at the lungs) but is released at oxygen pressures (20 to 40 torr) seen at the tissues.

between 20 and 40 torr). Parenthetically, one torr corresponds to 1 mm Hg (torr is a new, not very helpful, metric unit, which is simply homage to an earlier scientist, Evangelista Torricelli, a big name in mercury barometers in the 17th century).

So, if myoglobin is a very efficient binder of oxygen, why not use it as an oxygen transporter in red cells? To see the problem with myoglobin in this hypothetical situation, consider this scenario. A bus (not carrying a chemistry teacher this time) with a high affinity for students in transit readily takes up its passengers at the subway (metro, train) station. Each passenger is delighted with the efficiency of the service. Yet, as each student approaches her or his stop, close to home, she or he cannot get out of the seat. The door opens, more passengers get on, the door closes and everyone travels back to the subway station. A rather nightmarish situation, but as myoglobin releases its oxygen at pO_2 values lower than those found near tissues, it is possible to envision a rapid saturation of myoglobin with oxygen at the lungs, and little or no chance for oxygen release at capillaries close to the tissues that need oxygen. Mind you, myoglobin is, in reality, found within muscle cells and is ideally suited to capturing oxygen released from the circulation and then releasing it within those cells in which relatively low oxygen pressures occur.

An oxygen carrier in the blood must effectively take up oxygen but, at the same time, be able to release oxygen to the tissues. Thus, there is the need for a graded response in oxygen binding over a physiologically significant range of oxygen pressures. Hemoglobin takes up oxygen effectively at the lungs (high pO_2, 90 to 100 torr) and efficiently unloads oxygen at the tissues (low pO_2, 20 to 40 torr) (see Figure 5–5).

How does hemoglobin do this? And more specifically, how can it exhibit this sigmoid binding curve? The answer lies within the subunit structure of hemoglobin and a phenomenon known as **positive cooperativity**. It appears that the affinity for oxygen actually increases rapidly in hemoglobin as each of the four heme sites is filled. This explains the rapid rise in oxygen affinity seen as pO_2 rises. In other words, hemoglobin with oxygen bound at one heme site (at one subunit) shows considerably higher affinity for the binding of the second oxygen. And this affinity increases again after a second and then again after a third oxygen molecule is bound. The affinity for the binding of the fourth and final oxygen molecule into the hemoglobin tetramer is some 300 times the affinity of unoxygenated hemoglobin (deoxyhemoglobin) for that first oxygen molecule. The implication is that oxygen binding at one subunit influences, in a positive way, the binding at a second subunit. This is known as an **allosteric mechanism** because a site filled with oxygen in one subunit is influencing the binding efficiency of oxygen at another binding site in a second subunit. "Allosteric" means other site. This comes from classical Greek, and it's not a bad idea to take a course in scientific and medical nomenclature if it is offered at your college or university.

To understand positive cooperativity in a hemoglobin tetramer, consider this image. Four children, say 7 years of age, two male and two female ($\alpha_2\beta_2$), are placed in a hollow square so that a shoulder of each child touches the shoulder of another child. They are all facing directly outward from the square and cannot see each other. Consider that they all enjoy chocolate bars (a reasonable, Willy-Wonka-style assumption). What happens if you place a piece of chocolate in the mouth (binding site) of one child (subunit)? Naturally, you get a reaction (jaws working convulsively, the sound of chops being licked, and a definite amount of body movement) from this one child. You will certainly expect a reaction from the other children who cannot see yet are likely very much influenced by what is going on. They too want chocolate (increased affinity). If a second child receives this treatment, the remaining two are that much more expectant for something at their binding site (mouths opened wide, higher affinity), as is the fourth if he or she is the only one without chocolate. This emphasizes the power of cooperativity in oxygen binding within hemoglobin.

The actual basis for this effect is explained by a change in the conformation of the hemoglobin tetramer with oxygen binding. When an oxygen molecule comes to interact with the Fe^{2+} of the heme ring, on the histidine E-7 side of heme, the iron ion actually moves from slightly above into the

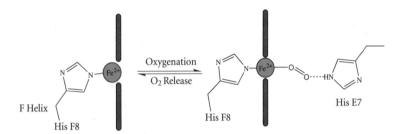

Figure 5–6 The change in iron orientation with oxygenation. With oxygen binding to a hemoglobin subunit, the iron of heme moves into the plane of the heme ring. Because of the attachment of iron to histidine F-8, there is a change in structure of the polypeptide. This, in turn, will promote shifts in structure in other hemoglobin subunits so that the tetramer changes from a tight (T) to a more relaxed (R) conformation.

plane of the ring (Figure 5–6). As the iron is linked to the side chain of histidine F-8, this movement promotes a change in the conformation of the tetramer. With oxygen binding, there is a transition from a tight (T) state to a relaxed (R) state for the hemoglobin tetramer. This is accompanied by a breakage of salt bridges between subunits (Figure 5–7), with a rotation or shifting in the position of the subunits and a progressive and substantial change in conformation of component subunits that facilitates further oxygen binding at other subunit sites. Thus, oxygen binding promotes structural change that, in turn, promotes further oxygen binding. This is the basis for the sigmoid response.

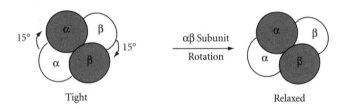

Figure 5–7 Shifts in subunit orientation with oxygen binding. The change in orientation from a tight (T) form of hemoglobin to a relaxed (R) form is associated with a rotation and shift of subunits. Here, one αβ pair rotates through 15°, relative to the second subunit pair, in the progression from a T to an R form of hemoglobin.

REGULATION OF OXYGEN BINDING TO HEMOGLOBIN

Not only is tetrameric hemoglobin well suited to oxygen pick-up and delivery, it can also respond to physiologic changes that control oxygen binding

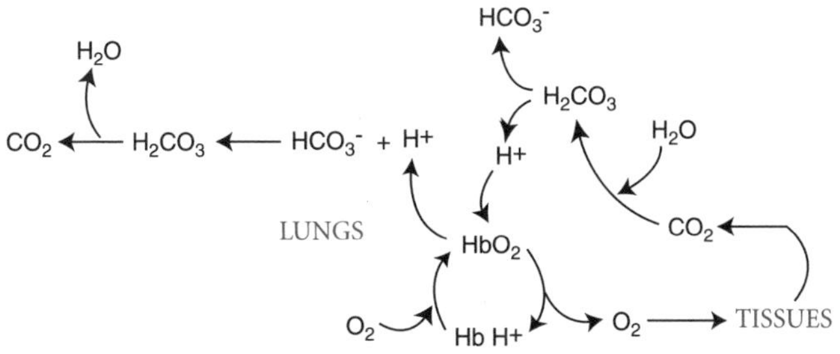

Figure 5–8 Carbon dioxide production and release. Carbon dioxide released by tissues is converted by the enzyme carbonic anhydrase of the red cells to carbonic acid. The acid dissociates, releasing a proton and the bicarbonate ion. Protons are taken up by deoxyhemoglobin (HbH+), stabilizing its structure. At the lungs, with the binding of oxygen to hemoglobin, comes a release of protons, a reformation of carbonic acid, and a release of carbon dioxide.

at the lungs or tissues. For example, carbon dioxide is produced by cellular respiration at the tissues and is in relatively high concentration near tissues (Figure 5–8). Carbon dioxide dissolves in extracellular fluid and plasma to form carbonic acid, which dissociates to release protons.

$$CO_2 + H_2O \leftrightarrow H_2CO_3 \leftrightarrow H^+ + HCO_3^-$$

The conversion of carbon dioxide to carbonic acid can also be mediated by the action of the enzyme carbonic anhydrase located inside the red cells. We noted the action of carbonic anhydrase in Chapter 3. Thus, inside the red cells, near the tissues, the liberation of protons leads to proton binding to hemoglobin. In turn, this protonation encourages interaction between the subunits in the hemoglobin tetramer, which helps the unloading of oxygen and the stabilization of the deoxy form of hemoglobin. This response to changing pH is noted by a shift to the right in the oxygenation curve for hemoglobin, indicating the reduced affinity for oxygen under these conditions (Figure 5–9). This response to pH is known as the **Bohr effect**. (Yes, this scientist was the father of the atomic physicist, Niels Bohr.)

A similar control is exerted by the actual interaction of carbon dioxide with the N-terminal amino acid residues of the four hemoglobin subunits.

$$CO_2 + NH_2\text{-}R \leftrightarrow {}^-OOC\text{-}NH\text{-}R + H^+$$

This forms structures called **carbamates**, which also stabilize hemoglobin in its deoxy form by electrostatic bond formation between subunits. Thus, at the tissues, once oxygen is lost from oxyhemoglobin, the deoxy form is relatively stable and returns within the red cells of the venous blood to the lungs. This stabilization of deoxyhemoglobin prevents the undesir-

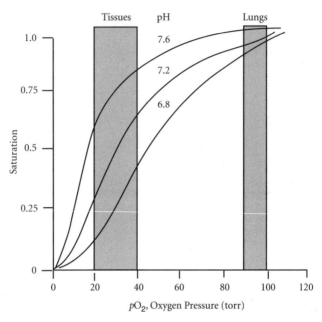

Figure 5–9 The Bohr effect. With the binding of protons to hemoglobin at low pH (at the tissues), there is a decreased affinity of hemoglobin for oxygen. Thus, oxyhemoglobin can more readily unload its oxygen at the tissues, and deoxyhemoglobin returns to the lungs for reoxygenation.

able reoxygenation of deoxyhemoglobin at the tissues, utilizing oxygen just released from oxyhemoglobin. In our bus analogy, this unfortunate situation would be equivalent to getting off the bus (hemoglobin) near your home (the tissues), only to be recaptured by the driver, placed back in your seat, and returned to the subway station (the lungs).

Again, setting aside this unfortunate "hostage" image for oxygen, the normal function at the lungs, with high oxygen pressure and relatively low carbon dioxide pressure, is the breakdown of carbamates in hemoglobin, the release of carbon dioxide, and the oxygenation of deoxyhemoglobin. This oxygenation promotes the release of carbon dioxide from the carbamate structure.

One further means of stabilizing deoxyhemoglobin at the tissues (and lowering the affinity of hemoglobin for oxygen) comes via the action of a small molecule called **2,3-bisphosphoglycerate** (Figure 5–10). This compound is produced from 1,3-bisphosphoglycerate, a molecule that is made in the red cells during glycolysis, a pathway involved in the breakdown of glucose to produce energy. We shall discuss glycolysis in more detail in Chapter 7. 2,3-Bisphosphoglycerate increases in concentration within the

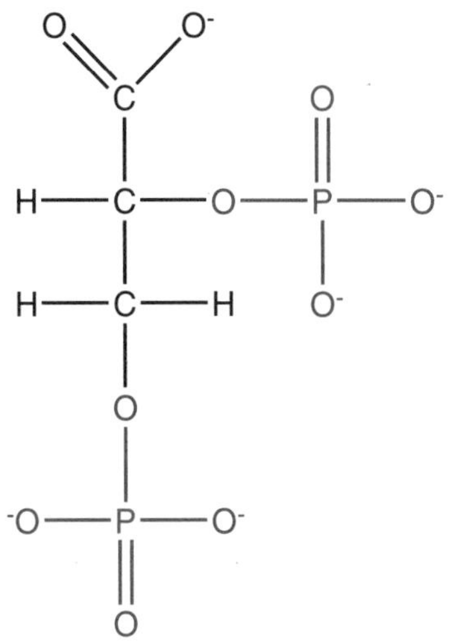

Figure 5–10 2,3-Bisphosphoglycerate, a highly negatively charged, allosteric effector for oxygen binding by hemoglobin.

cytosol of red cells when these are near the tissues. 2,3-Bisphosphoglycerate is highly negatively charged and can interact with deoxyhemoglobin within the central cavity of the tetramer in the space between the two hemoglobin β-subunits (Figure 5–11). Here, 2,3-bisphosphoglycerate forms electrostatic bonds (salt bridges) with positively charged side chains of β-subunit amino acid residues. This stabilizes the deoxyhemoglobin structure and again reduces oxygen affinity of hemoglobin. 2,3-Bisphosphoglycerate cannot enter the corresponding area of the oxyhemoglobin tetramer. This mechanism at the tissues again lowers the affinity of hemoglobin for oxygen and promotes the return of deoxyhemoglobin to the lungs. 2,3-Bisphosphoglycerate is known as an allosteric effector because it exerts its effects on oxygen binding at a site removed from the heme groups in the protein.

In low-oxygen environments, such as in chronic anoxia, levels of 2,3-bisphosphoglycerate are increased, favoring the unloading of oxygen from oxyhemoglobin. Effectively, 2,3-bisphosphoglycerate shifts the oxygen versus the saturation curve for hemoglobin to the right, expediting a more efficient unloading of hemoglobin at the tissues. Limitations in oxygen supply occur at high altitudes, and individuals arriving at such elevated locations adapt by the synthesis of more hemoglobin and an increased availability of 2,3-bisphosphoglycerate. 2,3-Bisphosphoglycerate is elevated in smokers, who also suffer from limited oxygen supply because of carbon monoxide intake. CO has a much higher affinity for hemoglobin than does

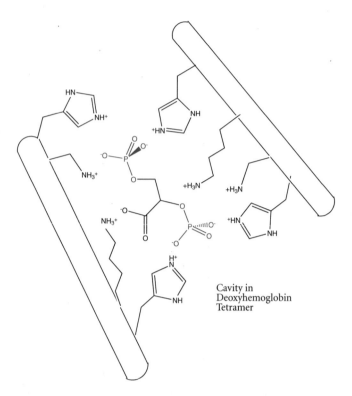

Figure 5–11 2,3 Bisphosphoglycerate (BPG) interactions with hemoglobin. BPG enters the central cavity of the deoxyhemoglobin tetramer, binding with eight positively charged side chains of amino acids of the two β subunits. This tightens the structure of deoxyhemoglobin and lowers its oxygen affinity.

oxygen, and CO (found in automotive exhaust fumes and produced in homes by inadequately vented natural gas furnaces) is a remarkably toxic gas. The toxicity is associated with quite low levels of CO—hence the importance of domestic CO detectors.

Interestingly, the storage of blood using the anticoagulant acid-citrate-dextrose (the citrate chelates calcium and thus blocks the coagulation cascade) will result in lower levels of red cell 2,3-bisphosphoglycerate and, consequently, poor oxygen unloading from hemoglobin. The shortcoming with this anticoagulated blood can be called an "oxygen trap."

One further role for 2,3-bisphosphoglycerate is found in the transfer of oxygen from maternal blood, across the placenta, to fetal blood. If the fetus is to receive adequate amounts of oxygen from the mother, there must be an efficient capture of oxygen by fetal hemoglobin. Fetal hemoglobin has a different subunit structure, compared with adult hemoglobin ($\alpha_2\beta_2$). Fetal hemoglobin has two α-subunits but possesses two γ-subunits per tetramer (hence $\alpha_2\gamma_2$). Fetal hemoglobin can be given the abbreviation HbF, while adult hemoglobin is HbA. As you can likely predict, following birth, there is a developmental change as HbF is replaced by HbA. The one important difference between HbF and HbA is that HbF has a considerably lower affinity for the binding of 2,3-bisphosphoglycerate to its deoxy form. This occurs because the γ-subunit has a serine residue instead of histidine found at the corresponding surface location in the β-subunit. This eliminates one of the positively charged residues that would bind to 2,3-bisphosphogly-cerate, and this greatly reduces the affinity of deoxy HbF for this molecule. The end result is that HbF shows a higher affinity for oxygen than does HbA, facilitating the flow of oxygen from mother to fetus (Figure 5–12).

This difference between HbA and HbF suggests that there may be other tetrameric forms of hemoglobin that differ on the basis of their subunits. This is, in fact, the case, and there exist for certain periods in the develop-

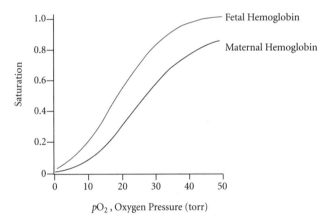

Figure 5–12 Oxygen dissociation curves for fetal ($\alpha_2\gamma_2$) and maternal hemoglobin ($\alpha_2\beta_2$). While maternal hemoglobin responds to 2,3-bisphosphoglycerate (BPG) with a decreased affinity for oxygen, this effect is not as prominent in fetal hemoglobin because it binds much less BPG. Thus, at the placenta, maternal oxyhemoglobin will surrender oxygen, and the fetal deoxyhemoglo-bin can more readily take it up.

ment of the embryo hemoglobins $\alpha_2\epsilon_2$, $\zeta_2\epsilon_2$, and $\zeta_2\gamma_2$. These also facilitate oxygen transfer to the embryo. In the adult, HbA ($\alpha_2\beta_2$) predominates, but there is a $\alpha_2\delta_2$ species found in a small quantity (about 2% of the total

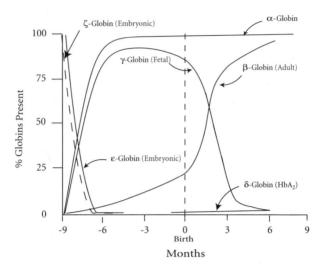

Figure 5–13 Human development and the production of globin polypeptides. While α-globin is predominant in adult life and most of fetal life, β-globin rises to prominence within a few months after birth. Thus, most adult hemoglobin (HbA) is $\alpha_2\beta_2$. In contrast, $\alpha_2\gamma_2$ is the predominant fetal hemoglobin, and the prominence of γ-globin declines after birth, matching the rise in β-globin. Embryonic hemoglobins are characterized by the presence of $\zeta_2\varepsilon_2$, $\zeta_2\gamma_2$, and $\alpha_2\varepsilon_2$ hemoglobin tetramers. Adapted from Beck S. Hematology. 5th ed. Cambridge (MA): MIT Press 1991.

hemoglobin tetramers). The change in predominance of subunits within hemoglobins as found with development is shown in Figure 5–13.

DISORDERS OF HEMOGLOBIN (HEMOGLOBINOPATHIES)

Just as there are mutations that give rise to dysfunctional coagulation factors VIII and IX in the hemophilias, there are also mutations that can lead to defective hemoglobins. Often, these mutations result in the replacement of one amino acid within the subunit structure by another. It should be noted that there are many hemoglobins that have substitutions that do not result in disease, the so-called **neutral mutations**. But if there is a change in an amino acid located near the heme pocket, a change in one of the two histidines involved in oxygen or heme binding (histidines E-7, F-8), or changes in residues important for subunit interactions, these can lead to decreased hemoglobin function and pathology. Interestingly, the genes for the β-, γ-, δ-, and ε-subunits lie within the so-called β-globin cluster on chromosome 11, while the genes for the α- and ζ-subunits lie within the α-globin cluster on chromosome 16. The temporal order of appearance of the globins in development matches the linear order of the genes on these chromosomes.

The most prominent of the hemoglobin disorders is sickle cell anemia. It was noted very early in the 20th century that erythrocytes from an African-American patient suffering from anemia (anemias are caused by low levels of red cells or hemoglobin in the blood) exhibited a curious, elongated, sickle-shaped cellular morphology. These cells break up readily (hemolysis) and have considerably less flexibility than normal red cells (the traditional biconcave disc structures). Anemia and painful vessel occlusion are attributed to these fragile, irregularly shaped cells. Sickle cell patients can experience episodes of chest, back, abdominal, or extremity pain. Cardiovascular, renal, and pulmonary ischemias (lack of blood supply) are noted. In children, growth can be delayed and decreased immune responsiveness is also found, with increased incidence of infection. As hemoglobin is the most prominent constituent of red cells, a problem with hemoglobin appeared to be a logical hypothesis for this disease. Linus Pauling may be known to some of you as the Californian scientist who supported megadoses of vitamin C as a cure for the common cold; he was also the investigator who originally supported a triple helix structure for DNA. Hopefully, you won't dismiss the work of this gentleman because he was a pioneer in chemistry and protein structure, a Nobel laureate, and an early investigator of the molecular basis for sickle cell disease.

Pauling and Itano reported in 1949 that hemoglobin from sickle cell patients was more positively charged than HbA (normal adult hemoglobin). This was shown during electrophoresis (remember how plasma proteins were separated, as discussed in Chapter 2), when hemoglobin from the patients was found to migrate more slowly toward the positive pole of the electrophoresis chamber (Figure 5–14). Hence, the new hemoglobin was called **HbS**, to distinguish it from the more quickly migrating HbA, and Pauling noted that sickle cell anemia was a truly "molecular disease." In 1957, Ingram discovered that the charge difference between HbS and HbA was the result of a change in amino acid sequence, in which a glutamate residue in HbA was replaced by a valine residue in HbS.

The genetics of sickle cell anemia indicated a recessive disease. A carrier (heterozygote) had one sickle cell allele and one normal allele and showed both HbA and HbS on analysis by electrophoresis (see Figure 5–14). This was called the **sickle cell trait**, and carriers did not usually show symptoms of sickle cell disease. The sickle cell mutation was subsequently shown to be the result of a single base change in the genetic sequence for the β-subunit of hemoglobin. We will discuss the genetic code more thoroughly in Chapter 8, but you should know that triplets composed of the bases A (adenine), G (guanine), C (cytosine), and T (thymine) within the genetic sequences in DNA determine the amino acid sequence in the coded protein. Thus, the triplet GAG encodes for the amino acid glutamate. A change in one base in one triplet within the genetic sequence can lead to the

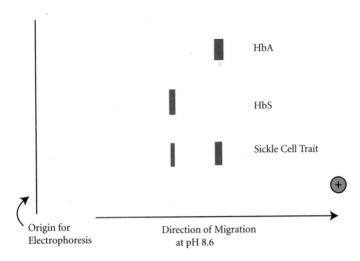

Figure 5–14 Migrations of normal and sickle cell hemoglobins. In electrophoresis at pH 8.6, normal hemoglobin (HbA) migrates more quickly to the positive pole than does the HbS found in sickle cell anemia. HbS has two fewer glutamate residues than does HbA (the two β^s-subunits each have a valine instead of a glutamate at position 6). Thus, HbS has a smaller negative overall charge, compared with HbA. Heterozygotes with the sickle cell trait can produce both HbA and HbS, and two bands are visible for these individuals.

substitution of one amino acid by another. For the sickle cell genetic sequence, the mutation results in the substitution of glutamate (with a negatively charged side chain) at amino acid position 6 in the β-subunit by a valine residue. The sickle subunit is often denoted as β^s. In the sickle cell mutation, GAG (in the normal code for the β-subunit) changed to GTG, the code for valine. Valine has a nonpolar, hydrophobic side chain. The sixth amino acid in the β-subunit is located on the surface of this polypeptide, where, normally, glutamate happily interacts with water molecules. Valine, however, is quite a different amino acid, and its exposure to water is unusual, promoting, under certain circumstances, a remarkable association of HbS tetramers into larger polymeric structures. Perhaps valine is a little like a friend who definitely does not want to be a public speaker. When she or he is forced to a podium in front of an audience, the results can be quite unconventional.

So what happens when the hydrophobic valine makes an appearance at the surface of the β^s-subunit? The conformational problem appears to arise after the HbS has unloaded oxygen. The deoxy HbS has a relatively low solubility within the red cells, and the valine residue at position 6 on the surface can function as a "sticky tab" that inserts into an accessible hydrophobic crevice on an adjacent tetramer. The result (because of the tetrameric structure of hemoglobin and the relatively high concentration of hemo-

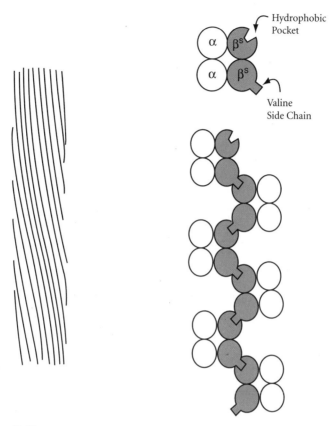

Figure 5–15 The polymerization of deoxy HbS. The deoxy form of HbS is rather insoluble within erythrocytes, and this promotes an interaction of HbS tetramers ($\alpha_2\beta^s{}_2$). Specifically, the valine residue at postion 6 in the β^s-subunits can interact with a hydrophobic pocket found in the structure of a second tetramer. Thus, HbS tetramers can link into polymers, which, in turn, can twist about each other to form sickle cell fibers composed of 14 such polymeric strands. It is these elongated fibers that are responsible for the cell distention noted in sickle cells.

globin within the red cells) is the assembly of deoxy HbS into long polymers (Figure 5–15). These polymers can also twist around each other, resulting in a 14-strand polymer (a sickle cell fiber). These polymers will distend the shape of the red cell, giving the sickle cell appearance, a little like a young person who successfully puts an entire chocolate bar into his or her mouth, causing considerable cheek distention. This abnormal shape accounts for the cellular fragility, the adhesion of these types of red cell, and the resulting painful occlusion noted in the blood vessels. There have been various therapies attempted to correct the problem. Desmopressin acetate administration leads to red cell swelling, increasing cellular water content and thus reducing HbS concentration (and hence limiting its ability to polymerize). Cyanate can reduce deoxy HbS concentrations and has decreased hemolysis but has not significantly limited the pain associated with crises in sickle cell disease. 5-Azacytidine or hydroxyurea, by interfering with DNA methylation and synthesis, respectively, activates HbF ($\alpha_2\gamma_2$) synthesis in the red cells of sickle cell patients, reducing the concentration of HbS and decreasing hemolysis of the red cells in sickle cell patients. Bone marrow transplantation (the insertion of normal progenitor cells from suitable donors within the marrow of sickle cell patients) or gene therapy (the addition of a normal β-subunit gene to the cells of patients, Chapter 8) is more likely to provide a cure for this genetic illness.

It is of interest to note that sickle cell anemia and HbS are prevalent in tropical countries. To those in these parts of the world, sickle cells actually offer an advantage because they are not favorable sites for the growth of the malarial parasite, which invades the red cells. Thus, the life cycle of this organism is interrupted, giving those with this genetic disease a degree of protection from infection.

There are many other hemoglobinopathies involving other individual amino acid mutations within the globin of hemoglobin (Table 5–1). The substitution of F-8 histidine by tyrosine in the α-subunit leads to decreased oxygen affinity and the tendency to form methemoglobin (water bound at Fe^{3+} in heme). The result of another mutation is the substitution of the F-8 histidine by glutamine in the β-subunit. In this case, heme cannot bind properly to the globin part of the molecule and the heme is lost from the β-subunit.

Table 5–1
Mutations Affecting Hemoglobins

Amino Acid Alteration	Functional Change	Explanation
Glutamate to valine at position 6 of the β-subunit	Red cell sickling	Polymerization of hemoglobin tetramers
Histidine to tyrosine at position F-8 of the β-subunit	Decreased O₂ binding Methemoglobin formation	Tyrosine now links iron and heme to globin
Histidine to glutamine at position F-8 of the β-subunit	Heme is lost in the β-subunit	Poor bonding between heme and globin
Phenylalanine to serine at position 42 of the β-subunit	Heme is lost in the β-subunit	Water enters heme pocket because of polar serine

In another mutation, the substitution of the hydrophobic phenylalanine at the β-subunit position 42 with serine (a hydrophilic, polar amino acid) alters the oxygen-binding pocket. Serine attracts water molecules into this pocket, which usually accommodates heme. This change destabilizes this region and leads to an absence of heme within the β-subunit of this hemoglobin.

These mutations and the sickle cell trait are the result of missense mutations that result in the change of a single amino acid residue. There can be other mutations that result in considerably more change in the amino acid composition of the globin molecule. For example, a base in the genetic sequence code for one of the globin subunits could be deleted, shifting the entire triplet coding sequence as a result. This is called a **frameshift mutation** (Table 5–2). Here, each amino acid in the code, downfield of the mutation, can be changed, producing a nonfunctional polypeptide chain that does not fold properly and may be destroyed by quality control mechanisms within the cell. A nonsense mutation, by a single base change, introduces

Table 5–2
Types of Genetic Mutation

Name of Mutation	Nature	Consequence
Normal genetic code	-GAG-AAG-TCT-	Functional protein is produced
Missense	-GTG-AAG-TCT- Substitution of a single base in the genetic sequence changes the code	Single amino acid substitution at a specific locus within the protein. Can lead to loss of function if the locus is in a critical region (e.g., sickle cell hemoglobin)
Nonsense	-GAG-TAG-TCT- Substitution of a single base gives a stop signal (TAG)	Protein synthesis is halted at the codon TAG, and a truncated protein is produced. Likely, the protein will not fold correctly and will be destroyed (e.g., some β-thalassemias)
Frameshift	-G ↓ GA-AGT-CT... Deletion of a base (A) shifts the coding sequence	Base deletion produces a completely new sequence of bases downfield and produces a new sequence of amino acids that will not be a functional protein

an aberrant stop signal within the genetic sequence so that the protein is not completed. Such mutations lead to very low or absent globin levels. Hemoglobinopathies of this type are known as **thalassemias**. β-Thalassemias involve the β-subunit. If only one gene is affected (heterozygotes), there can still be production of functional β-globin. However, individuals homozygous for the mutated gene cannot produce β-globin. These individuals can rely on the fetal hemoglobin ($\alpha_2\gamma_2$) after birth, but they rarely survive to maturity. Thalassemias involving the α-subunit (α-thalassemias) usually are not as serious as the defects found in the β-globin gene, simply because there are two copies of the α-globin gene on chromosome 16. This means that the pathologic effects are noted only when three or four α-globin genes are nonfunctional because of mutation.

BIOSYNTHESIS OF HEME AND THE PORPHYRIAS

While we have noted features of deficiencies in the production of the protein or globin component of hemoglobin, the assembly and breakdown of the heme group is equally important. Hemoglobin is certainly one of the most prominent of the proteins found in blood, and it is the most abundant of the iron-containing proteins in the body. And, of course, the red color makes hemoglobin particularly conspicuous. If human blood were colorless, arterial hemorrhaging would not be quite the spectacular emergency event that it is.

Metabolism will be covered in much more detail in Chapter 7, but it is useful now to use heme synthesis as an introductory example. It should be evident, particularly looking at a molecule like heme (see Figure 5–2), that one enzyme could not make this compound in one or even several steps, using the relatively simple molecules available in the body. The protoporphyrin ring has to be assembled, step by step, and ultimately iron has to be sequestered in the center of the molecule. We introduced the concept of enzyme pathways in Chapter 3, and indeed a number of enzymes participate sequentially in heme synthesis, each enzyme fulfilling a specific task in building the molecule. Remember our earlier image of an assembly line in the production of cars as end products.

There are diseases called **porphyrias** (see Table 5–3), which are associated with specific enzyme dysfunctions along the heme synthetic pathway; these diseases will bring us within the realm of the kings of England, and possibly we might uncover a vampire or werewolf along the way. Remember that a pathway, like a bucket brigade, is only as strong as its weakest link, and one enzyme deficiency along the path can have grave results.

The synthesis of heme takes place principally within the bone marrow and, to a lesser extent, within circulating erythrocyte precursors and other tissues, such as the liver. The first step in heme synthesis involves glycine,

Table 5–3
The Porphyrias

Type	Enzyme Affected	Symptoms	Increased Concentrations
Acute intermittent	UPG I synthase	Abdominal pain Neurologic	Urinary PBG, ALA
Congenital erythropoietic	UPG III cosynthase	Disfigurement	Urinary uroporphyrin
Cutanea tarda	UPG decarboxylase	Photosensitive	Urinary uroporphyrin
Hereditary coproporphyria	CPG oxidase	Photosensitive Neurologic Abdominal pain	Urinary PBG, uroporphyrin, coproporphyrin
Variegate	PPG oxidase	Photosensitive Neurologic Abdominal pain	Urinary PBG, uroporphyrin, fecal protoporphyrin
Protoporphyria	Ferrochetalase	Photosensitive	Fecal protoporphyrin

UPG = uroporphyrinogen; CPG = coproporphyrinogen; PPG = protoporphyrinogen.

the simplest of the amino acids. As shown in Figure 5–16, glycine reacts with the molecule succinyl-CoA (a compound formed during the breakdown of glucose) and requires the assistance of pyridoxal phosphate (a coenzyme derived from vitamin B_6). This reaction is catalyzed by the first enzyme, aminolevulinic acid synthase, sometimes referred to as ALA synthase. Lev-

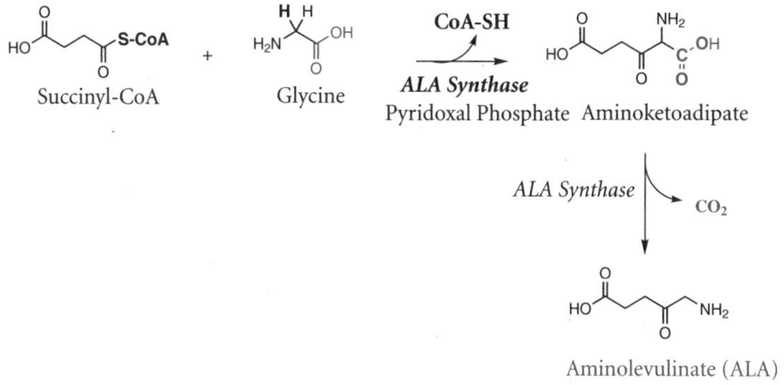

Figure 5–16 The ALA synthase reaction. Aminolevulinic acid synthase catalyzes the union of succinyl-CoA and the amino acid glycine. Coenzyme A is released during the reaction, and carbon dioxide is also liberated, as the —COOH group associated with the glycine end of the new molecule is lost in a decarboxylation reaction.

els of ALA synthase can be elevated by a variety of drugs, which induce increased synthesis of this enzyme. This enzyme brings together glycine and succinyl-CoA, releasing CoA and also liberating carbon dioxide from the glycine end of the new molecule. The product of ALA synthase is, perhaps not surprisingly, ALA. This new 5C molecule has two important functional groups, the amine ($-NH_3$) and the carbonyl ($-C=O$), which will be critical for the next reaction. ALA synthase is located within the mitochondria, which is logical because the succinyl-CoA substrate for the enzyme is also made within the mitochondria. ALA is used as substrate in the next enzyme-catalyzed step in the production of the pyrrole ring structures that are found within heme (Figure 5–17). Remember, there are four of these rings within the heme structure. In this step, two molecules of ALA interact to produce the five-member ring structure. This is a cyclization reaction, and two water molecules are liberated, as cross-bridges are formed between the two ALA molecules (see Figure 5–17). This enzyme is called ALA dehydratase, signifying the loss of water, and the product is porphobilinogen (PBG). ALA dehydratase is found in the cytoplasm of cells, indicating a diffusion of ALA to the outside of the mitochrondria. The dehydratase is an enzyme that contains zinc, and the enzyme activity can be inhibited by the presence of lead. We will discuss enzyme inhibition in greater detail in Chapter 7, but you

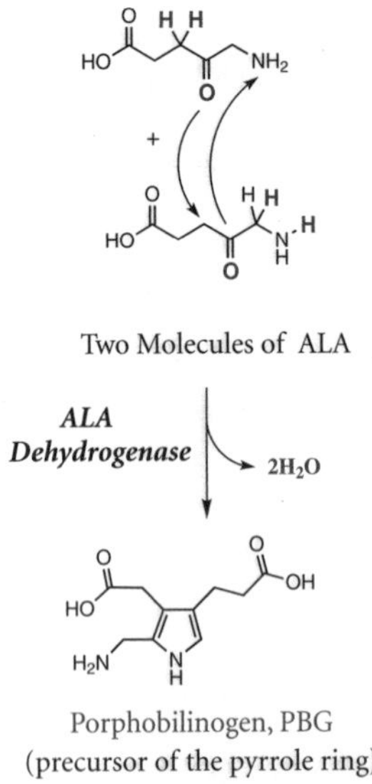

Two Molecules of ALA

ALA Dehydrogenase $2H_2O$

Porphobilinogen, PBG
(precursor of the pyrrole ring)

Figure 5–17 The ALA dehydratase reaction. As suggested by its name, this enzyme removes water from the structure of two molecules of ALA. This is fundamental to the formation of covalent links between two ALA molecules, producing the cyclic porphobilinogen (PBG), a pyrrole precursor.

should understand at this point that inhibitors can either interact at the active site of enzymes or cause conformational changes in enzymes, resulting in a temporary slowing down or permanent blockade of enzyme activity. Thus, lead poisoning can lead to a build-up of ALA. This can have a deleterious effect on the nervous system. Lead is found in paints used in houses dating back to the first half of the 20th century, and young children have been known to ingest flakes from these older painted surfaces. Lead poisoning was also believed to have been quite prevalent in the Roman Empire, because of its use in plumbing at that time.

Having formed the basic ring element in the heme structure, the rings must now be put together to allow the assembly of the larger and more complex protoporphyrin ring that is a tetrapyrrole. In this reaction, four PBG molecules are linked together by the enzyme uroporphyrinogen I synthase. This enzyme is a deaminase that catalyzes a loss of the amino groups, as links are made between the PBG molecules (Figure 5–18). The linear tetrapyrrole product (hydroxymethylbilane) then cyclizes either spontaneously or under the control of uroporphyrinogen I synthase and uroporphyrinogen III cosynthase to form uroporphyrinogen III. Uroporphyrinogen III has the complex ring structure that can be "fine-tuned" by subsequent reactions to form protoporphyrin. As you can see, the names of the products increase in complexity with the structures of these compounds. Uroporphyrinogen III is converted to coproporphyrinogen III by uroporphyrinogen decarboxylase. This reaction involves a release of carbon dioxide from the four acetyl arms ($-OOC-CH_2-$) of the uroporphyrinogen III structure to form simple methyl groups ($-CH_3$) (see Figure 5–18). Two further reactions catalyzed by coproporphyrinogen oxidase take place in the mitochondria (the coproporphyrinogen III substrate enters the mitochondrial matrix from the cytoplasm). This reaction modifies two of the four propionyl arms ($-OOC-CH_2-CH_2-$), converting them by decarboxylation and oxidation to vinyl groups, $CH_2=CH-$ (see Figure 5–18). This forms protoporphyrinogen IX, which is converted to protoporphyrin IX by protoporphyrinogen oxidase. (Note that protoporphyrin IX has a distinctly different double bond distribution than does protoporphyrinogen IX.) Finally, heme synthase or ferrochetalase facilitates the incorporation of Fe^{2+} into the protoporphyrin ring, coordinating the iron ion with each of the four nitrogens of the ring.

As you can see, heme synthesis is definitely not a one-step process (Figure 5–19)! It quite likely reminds you of the time you had to assemble a cabinet to hold your DVD and CD collections, using 35 arborite pieces (many of which were very similar), nuts, and bolts provided by a discount furniture warehouse. It also doesn't help that many of the names for substrates (and thus the enzymes that handle them) have upward of seven syllables each. Not to mention the Roman numerals. The numerals simply designate

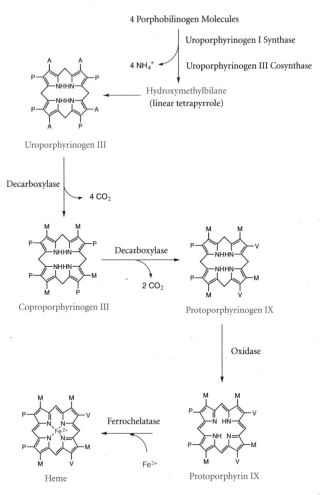

Figure 5–18 From porphobilinogen to heme. Four molecules of porphobilinogen (PBG) are used by the uroporphyrinogen I synthase to form a linear pyrrole called hydroxymethylbilane. In turn, the uroporphyrinogen I synthase and III cosynthase catalyze the cyclization of hydroxymethylbilane to form type III uroporphyrinogen. Also shown are the structures of coproporphyrinogen III (formed from uroporphyrinogen III by uroporphyrinogen decarboxylase), protoporphyrinogen IX (formed by coproporphyrinogen oxidase), and protoporphyrin IX (formed by protoporphyrinogen oxidase). A = acetyl ($-CH_2-COO^-$); P = propionyl ($-CH_2-CH_2-COO^-$); M = methyl ($-CH_3$); V = vinyl ($-CH=CH_2$). Adapted from Mathews CK, van Holde KE, Ahern KG. Biochemistry. 3rd ed. San Francisco (CA): Addison Wesley Longman; 2000.

a specific chemical isomer for individual tetrapyrrole ring structures found in the biochemical pathway. These isomeric forms are based on the number of different groups attached to the tetrapyrrole ring and their orientation. The type I and III isomers designate two specific arrangements of acetyl (or methyl) and propionyl groups. Type IX is used to designate one

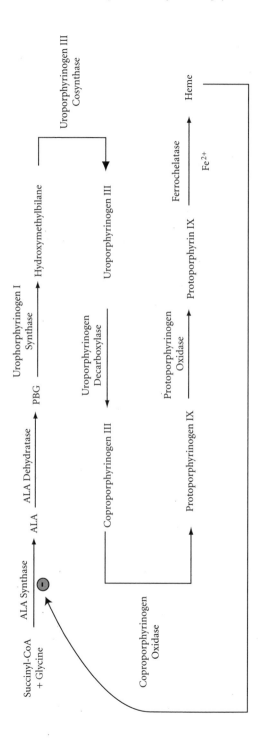

Figure 5–19 The metabolic pathway for heme synthesis. A summary of the sequential enzyme reactions, starting with ALA synthase and finishing with the insertion of Fe^{2+} into the protoporphyrin ring by ferrochetalase. The end product heme can regulate ALA synthase, repressing the synthesis of ALA. This is a feedback mechanism that attempts to maintain a steady level of heme production within cells.

isomer for the protoporphyrinogen and protoporphyrin rings, indicating a specific arrangement for the three groups: methyl, vinyl, and propionyl. The prefix "proto-" indicates one class of structure within a larger porphyrin family. The suffix "-inogen" usually denotes a precursor molecule. The prefixes "uro-" and "copro-" simply indicate the older and incorrect belief that these compounds were found only in the urine or stools, respectively.

Of course, as a come-on, to get you to read through all these enzyme sequences involved in heme synthesis, we did mention English royalty, vampires, and werewolves. One thing about royal houses, whether you love them or hate them, there is certainly well-documented evidence of genetic disease. Doubtless, introducing a few more commoners into the bloodline would have spared them considerable medical distress! In Chapters 1 and 4, we noted hemophilia among the Russian Romanovs and also traced the defective gene back to Queen Victoria, who really was the grandmother of much of European royalty at that time. Genetic mutations can also affect individual enzymes in the pathway for heme synthesis, resulting in the porphyrias. George III (grandfather of Queen Victoria and Elector of Hanover) suffered from bouts of insanity throughout his reign. There is evidence that George had porphyria, possibly the acute intermittent form (AIP) of the disease. Symptoms of AIP include acute abdominal pain and neurologic-psychiatric problems. This form of the disease stems from a deficiency in the enzyme uroporphyrinogen I synthase. Patients with the disease have elevated levels of PBG and ALA. This disease is not completely understood, but the pain and neurologic symptoms (derangement) are related to the increase in these intermediates of heme synthesis. Certainly, PBG can be detected in urine in these cases, and PBG at high concentration is converted to the derivative uroporphyrin nonenzymatically. It was recorded that the urine of George III at times changed to a blue or bloody color, which is seen in AIP, possibly because of the presence of increased quantities of oxidized pyrrole derivatives. In AIP, symptoms can be precipitated by a variety of drugs, including barbiturates, sulfonamides, clonazepam, nifedipine, and the use of alcohol. Many of these drugs exert their effects by inducing ALA synthase, thus increasing the rates of production of ALA. At this point in the discussion, most clinical biochemistry texts enter into speculation on medical-historical what ifs. For example, whether the United States would be part of the British Commonwealth had George III not had this disease, which may very well have influenced his unfortunate policies concerning the 13 American colonies. While this is interesting, it was also apparent that King George's autocratic decisions reflected the opinion of the majority of the English population at that time (who presumably were not collectively suffering the effects of porphyria). It was only the failure of the armies in the American colonies to enforce these royal decisions that was unpopular.

Another way to diagnose the condition of George III is to determine whether living descendants have porphyria and its nature. There is some evidence that two such royal patients of the House of Hanover showed symptoms of variegate porphyria (noted in Table 5–3). However, recent requests made to these patients for excretory samples, not surprisingly, were met by refusal. Thus, the precise identity of the malady of George III remains speculative.

Various kinds of porphyria are listed in Table 5-3. They result from specific enzyme deficiencies along the heme synthetic path. While porphyrinogens are not colored, porphyrins do have color and can fluoresce. Porphyrins (uroporphyrin and coproporphyrin) can be formed from the corresponding porphyrinogens by oxidation reactions catalyzed by light. Further, in the presence of light, these porphyrins can form derivatives that cause skin damage. The skin can very rapidly become inflamed and possibly even blister and scar. Thus, individuals with enzyme deficiencies at the level of uroporphorinogen decarboxylase and higher in the heme synthetic pathway will show photosensitivity. For example, the accumulation of uroporphyrinogen I can result in a red-colored urine, fluorescent teeth, and abnormal light sensitivity, as well as anemia because of poor heme production. Depending on the type of late night movies you prefer, you can envision individuals suffering from the photosensitive porphyrias as "night-people" and being classified by the more fanciful of earlier centuries as vampires or werewolves. One of the porphyrias does involve disfigurement. Blood drinking could even be proposed (again by the more fanciful) as an attempt to counter heme deficiency. Remember that, from a nutritional point of view, this is rather unlikely to occur given the size of heme or protoporphyrin and the biochemistry of digestion and absorption.

This being said, AIP can be treated by intravenous heme. This will, in turn, suppress ALA synthase and decrease levels of ALA and PBG. In many pathways, an end product can serve as an inhibitor for the first enzymatic step in the pathway. In the heme pathway, heme can actually take part in the repression of the nuclear expression of ALA synthase. We will discuss the details of protein synthesis directed by nuclear genetic blueprints in Chapter 8.

HEME BREAKDOWN, BILIRUBIN, AND JAUNDICE

As we noted in Chapter 2, the red cells have a limited life, and on aging, they are eliminated from the circulation and the component hemoglobin is degraded. Usually, the iron is carefully saved during this breakdown or catabolic procedure. Just as in heme synthesis, the catabolic pathway for heme proceeds via a sequence of enzyme steps. As considerable heme is degraded on a daily basis, and as derivatives flow through several body tissues and compartments, measurement of these various breakdown compounds is useful in the diagnosis of liver disease, obstructions in the flow of bile into the intestine, and abnormally accelerated heme degradation. These types of problems result in jaundice, which is manifested by a yellow color often seen in the skin or the sclerae of the eyes.

The traditional average adult male, 70 kg in weight, who is popular in medical texts (if not rather unrepresentative of the North American population) will degrade about 6 g of hemoglobin per day. That's a lot of colored protein and, as you might predict, there will be a generation of colored breakdown products as a result. Hemoglobin can be considered to be composed of two distinct parts. The globin protein is degraded to component amino acids by the actions of proteolytic enzymes. That leaves the brightly colored red heme group, which has its separate path for breakdown. When the heme is released from hemoglobin, its component iron is rapidly oxidized to Fe^{3+}, and the compound is called **hemin**. The first enzyme to deal with hemin is heme oxygenase. This enzyme is rather complex and is better called the **heme oxygenase system**, considering the variety of reactions it catalyzes. The overall reaction is the opening of the rather complex heme ring (Figure 5–20). The first step involves the reduction of the component iron back to its reduced form making use of the coenzyme NADPH. In a second step, oxygen and NADPH are used to generate an $-OH$ group attached to one of the bridges connecting two of the component pyrrole rings of heme. The iron is reoxidized and is lost from the ring, and the ring itself is opened utilizing another molecule of oxygen, with the loss of carbon monoxide from the ring in the process. The product of this reaction is biliverdin, which, indeed, is green (sometimes a knowledge of the Romance languages is a definite advantage in biochemistry).

A further enzymatic reduction of a double bond in biliverdin, by the enzyme biliverdin reductase, again making use of NADPH, generates the yellow compound bilirubin. You might now refer to any blond student in your class as el rubio or la rubia, as a small mnemonic. The degradation of various heme proteins will yield bilirubin, which is produced within the body at about 300 mg/d. This process of heme breakdown, with its rather prominent color changes, can be followed if you have a bruise. As we recall, hitting a volleyball repeatedly with your wrist, as opposed to your fist, does this quite nicely and allows you to study the process fairly readily without the need for disrobing. Bruising follows from blood vessel rupture, and the hemoglobin within the extracellular space will at first appear blue, changing to green and then yellow as the molecule is dismantled and degraded.

Albumin, that rather generic carrier of hydrophobic compounds (and others), can indeed carry bilirubin, which shows only a small solubility in plasma. In a decilitre (dL) of plasma, about 25 mg of bilirubin can be maximally transported by albumin in a tightly bound state. Certain drugs

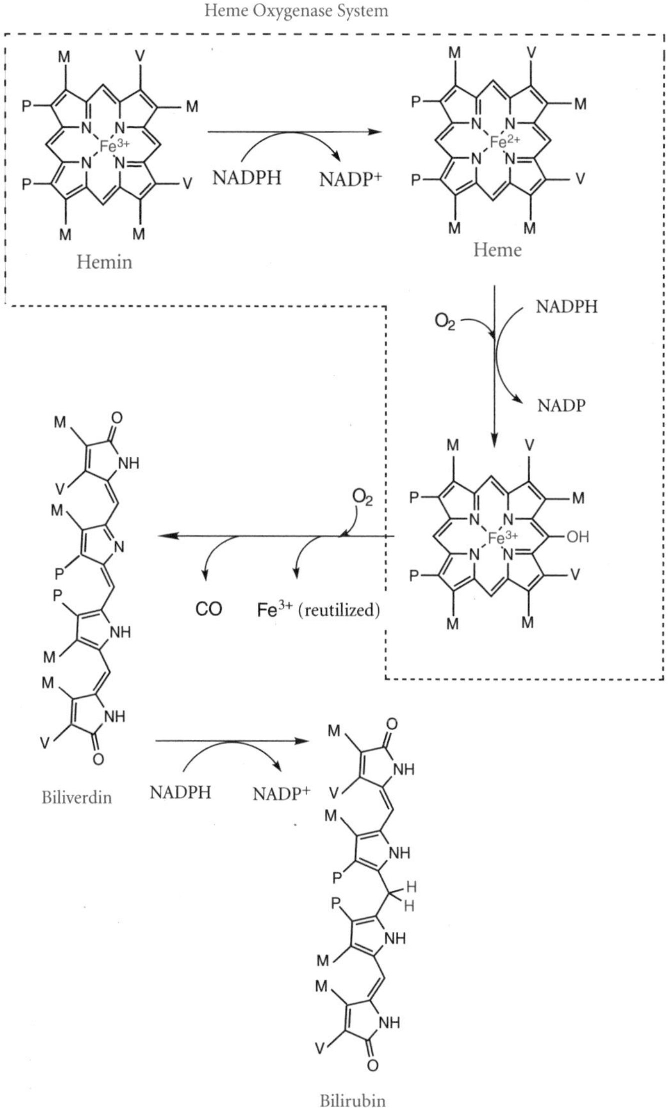

Heme Oxygenase System

Figure 5–20 The heme oxygenase system. This complex reaction reduces hemin using the cofactor NADPH for the reduction of Fe^{3+} and the subsequent use of oxygen and NADPH in the oxidation of Fe^{2+} with the insertion of an -OH group into the ring system. Next, a second molecule of oxygen is used as iron is removed from the ring (and the iron is carefully conserved), CO is lost, and the ring is opened into the linear biliverdin molecule. Biliverdin is then converted to bilirubin in a reduction reaction utilizing NADPH. Adapted from Beck S. Hematology. 5th ed. Cambridge (MA): MIT Press; 1991.

(including some antibiotics) that bind to albumin can displace bilirubin, which will enter the surrounding tissues. The liver, however, is the normal site for the uptake of bilirubin. This occurs at the plasma or boundary membrane of the hepatocytes. Newborns (particularly if they haven't gone completely to term) may have livers that are not able to handle bilirubin efficiently. Newborns can also show an accelerated rate of hemolysis and hemoglobin breakdown. These babies thus become jaundiced, as bilirubin builds up in the blood beyond the binding capacity of albumin and diffuses into surrounding tissues, giving them a yellow color. The danger here is that bilirubin can cross into the brain of these infants and cause damage, resulting in a form of encephalopathy called **kernicterus**. This can lead to mental retardation. The term **icterus** refers to jaundice or hyperbilirubinemia. Jaundiced newborns can be exposed to ultraviolet light (taking care to cover their eyes), and this phototherapy can chemically modify bilirubin to other molecules that can be excreted in the bile. Just a small word of caution with respect to diagnosis here. Medical students and students of other health disciplines are usually very observant and perceptive individuals, but with one exception. If you are a very close friend, close relative, or cohabitee of such a student, it would be wise for you to seek independent medical advice, as medical students and medical professionals have been known to miss symptoms of jaundice (or other maladies) in those very close to them.

Returning to the liver, you will find a carrier system in the plasma membrane that facilitates the entry of bilirubin (Figure 5–21). This transport system performs what is called facilitated diffusion. In this process (which can describe the passage of many different compounds across membranes), a specific protein binds bilirubin and brings it across the membrane. It is still considered diffusion because a gradient of bilirubin from outside the liver cell to the inside is required to drive the process. This bilirubin carrier normally has a considerable capacity for bilirubin transport. Thus, it is rare for individuals to be jaundiced because of inadequate bilirubin uptake by the liver. Following uptake, one problem faced by the liver cells is the difficulty in handling this rather hydrophobic compound, as bilirubin can associate with membrane lipids. To facilitate further metabolism of bilirubin, this molecule is made more water soluble by the addition of the highly polar and charged molecule glucuronate. This compound is a carboxylic acid derivative of glucose. Glucuronate is first converted into UDP-glucuronate (a nucleotide-sugar acid), which effectively energizes this glucose derivative. Liver enzymes, named glucuronosyl transferases, then transfer glucuronate to two positions on bilirubin (Figures 5–22 and 5–23). This is done in a stepwise manner, first producing bilirubin monoglucuronate and then bilirubin diglucuronate (see Figure 5–22). You may also see these compounds noted as mono- or diglucuronides. This conversion of bilirubin to

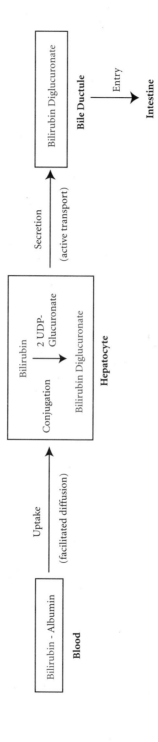

Figure 5–21 The processing of bilirubin. Bilirubin is carried in the blood by albumin and is taken into the liver by a process called facilitated diffusion that utilizes a specific carrier within the hepatocyte plasma membrane. Once inside the liver cell, bilirubin is converted into its conjugated (and more water-soluble) form by the addition of glucuronic acid residues. The bilirubin diglucuronate is secreted from the liver cells by an active transport mechanism that employs a specific carrier within the plasma membrane and utilizes ATP to drive the conjugated bilirubin against a concentration gradient into a bile ductule. Conjugated bilirubin subsequently enters the intestine in the bile.

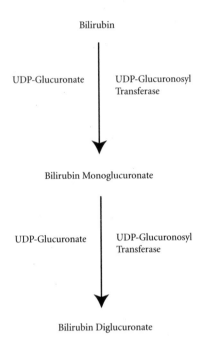

Bilirubin

UDP-Glucuronate | UDP-Glucuronosyl Transferase

Bilirubin Monoglucuronate

UDP-Glucuronate | UDP-Glucuronosyl Transferase

Bilirubin Diglucuronate

Figure 5–22 The production of conjugated bilirubin. UDP-glucuronosyl transferase activity transfers two glucuronate molecules to bilirubin, first forming bilirubin monoglucuronate and then bilirubin diglucuronate.

a more water-soluble compound is known as **conjugation**, and neonatal jaundice can arise from low glucuronosyltransferase activity. Phenobarbital is a drug that can induce the synthesis of this enzyme and is sometimes given to newborns for this purpose.

Bilirubin diglucuronate can be secreted from hepatocytes into the bile by another transport mechanism (see Figure 5–21). This process is known as active transport and involves a specific membrane protein carrier but works to pump out the conjugated bilirubin into an environment that has a higher bilirubin diglucuronate concentration. For this type of transport, energy is required. Recall the Na^+, K^+-ATPase of the plasma membrane of muscle cells that requires ATP to pump these ions against concentration gradients across this membrane (see Chapter 1). Once in the bile (a secretion made by the liver that contains pigments, inorganic salts, cholesterol and bile salts, derivatives of cholesterol used in the digestion of dietary fats), conjugated bilirubin passes to the duodenum via the gallbladder and common bile duct. When it reaches the intestine, the conjugated bilirubin is attacked by bacterial glucuronidases that convert the bilirubin diglucuronate back to bilirubin. You should be aware that there is a considerable

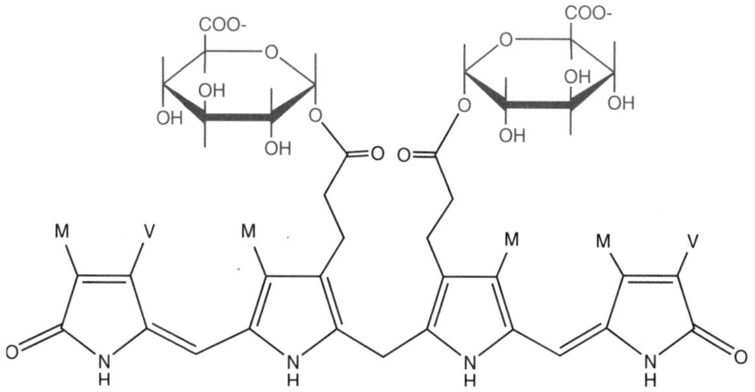

Figure 5–23 The structure of conjugated or direct bilirubin (bilirubin diglucuronate). M indicates a methyl group (-CH$_3$), and V indicates a vinyl group (-CH=CH$_2$). Adapted from Mathews CK, van Holde KE, Ahern KG. Biochemistry. 3rd ed. San Francisco (CA): Addison Wesley Longman; 2000.

amount of intestinal flora, which make many contributions to nutrient processing within the intestine. The bilirubin is now further converted to the colorless **stercobilinogen** (Figure 5–24). When found in urine, this compound is known as **urobilinogen**. An enterohepatic cycle exists for these compounds, as they can again be taken up by the intestine, enter the blood, and be taken up and resecreted by the liver. In certain pathologic states, the level of these compounds can rise in blood, with significant quantities of urobilinogen entering urine. If the stercobilinogens remain within the intestine, they can be further oxidized by bacteria to give stercobilins (see Figure 5–24), which give stools their characteristic color.

Given the hepatic site of conversion of bilirubin to conjugated bilirubin, it is useful to distinguish between these two compounds, as an indicator of potential problems along the path of bilirubin metabolism. The **Ehrlich reaction** is used to measure total bilirubin (conjugated and unconjugated) by the production of a reddish-purple derivative formed from bilirubin. The solvent methanol is used in this test to facilitate the solution of the hydrophobic bilirubin. However, if methanol is omitted from the test procedure, the more water-soluble conjugated bilirubin alone reacts to produce the color. This second method is known as the **van den Bergh reaction** and measures conjugated or **direct-reacting bilirubin**. By taking the difference in color between the Ehrlich and van den Bergh reactions, the quantity of **indirect bilirubin** (unconjugated) can be calculated:

Total bilirubin (with methanol) – Direct-acting bilirubin (no methanol)
= Indirect bilirubin (unconjugated)

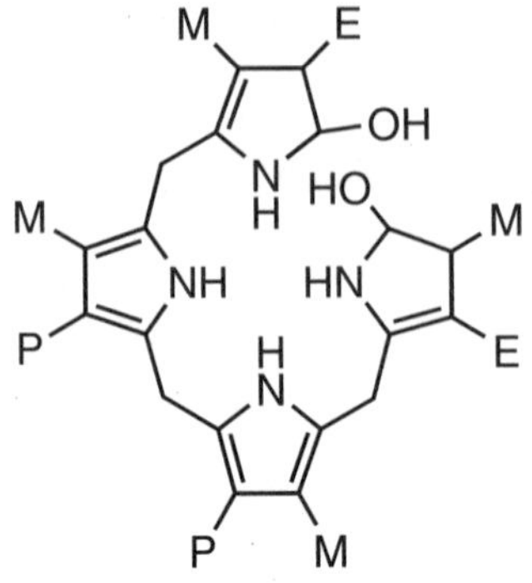

Stercobilinogen
(Urobilinogen)

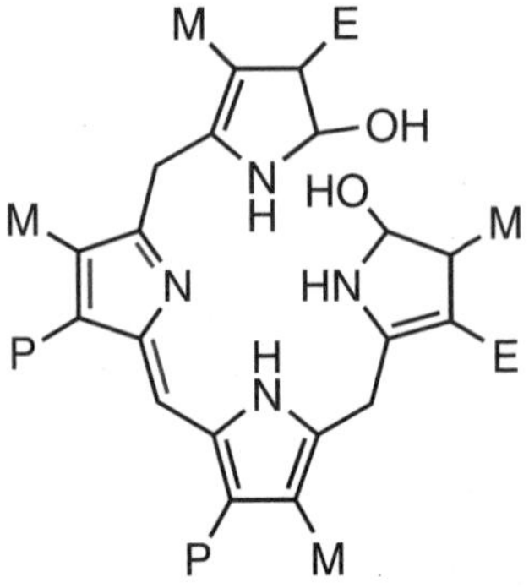

Stercobilin
(Urobilin)

Figure 5–24 The structures of urobilinogen (also known as stercobilinogen) and stercobilin (urobilin). When bilirubin diglucuronate enters the intestine, bacterial enzymes convert this conjugated or direct bilirubin back to bilirubin by the removal of the glucuronate residues. A subsequent reduction can form the colorless stercobilinogen (urobilinogen) from bilirubin. The intestine can take up the stercobilinogen (urobilinogen), in an enterohepatic cycle, for further processing by the liver. In this cycle, urobilinogen can make its way into urine. Further bacterial oxidation of stercobilinogen (urobilinogen) in the intestine results in the formation of the colored stercobilin (urobilin).

This is a very useful test, as a problem in the processing of bilirubin by the liver (and build-up of bilirubin in blood) would be shown by high levels of indirect or nonconjugated bilirubin. In contrast, a blocked bile duct (say, by a gallstone) would lead to the back-up of conjugated bilirubin into blood, leading to elevated levels of blood (direct) bilirubin.

There are various causes of **jaundice**, with hyperbilirubinemia existing at levels of bilirubin in blood in excess of 1 mg/dL. When this level increases above about 2 mg/dL, bilirubin is in the tissues in sufficient quantity to produce a yellow, jaundiced color. Jaundice is also referred to as icterus.

Let's consider the diagnosis of various types of jaundice, resulting from different problems along the bilirubin metabolic route that stretches from blood to the liver to bile to the intestine and back into blood. As shown in Figure 5–25, normally, bilirubin is processed by the liver, enters the intestine via bile, and passes out in feces as stercobilin, with some stercobilinogen (urobilinogen) being retaken up by the enterohepatic cycle. Bilirubin is absent from urine, although a small amount of urobilinogen may be present. Levels of normal serum bilirubin are 0.2 to 0.7 mg/dL indirect and 0.1 to 0.4 mg/dL direct.

If there is a liver problem, say, an immature liver in some neonates (neonatal jaundice), there may be an abnormally low hepatic processing of bilirubin. Thus, there is a rise in indirect bilirubin (unconjugated) in plasma, as the level of delivery of direct bilirubin to the intestine is inadequate. Stools may be pale in color. Levels of urobilinogen in urine will be decreased, as there is less direct bilirubin in the intestine and less stercobilinogen available for uptake.

In infectious hepatitis, viral infection may produce swollen, damaged cells that obstruct the bile ductules, and a less efficient handling of blood bilirubin (indirect) and a poorer secretion of bilirubin (direct) result. Thus, an increased level of both direct and indirect bilirubin may be seen in plasma. Levels of urobilinogen will be decreased in urine (because of an inefficient release of conjugated bilirubin into bile), while levels of direct bilirubin will increase in urine. These findings may vary with the stage of the viral infection and the extent of hepatocyte damage and ductule obstruction. Stool color may be pale (decreased stercobilin), and the level of the serum enzyme ALT may be elevated (see Chapter 3). This jaundice may be called choluric jaundice, as conjugated bilirubin "regurgitates" into the circulation.

Liver dysfunction can also be seen following hepatocyte damage caused by poisoning with choloroform, carbon tetrachloride, acetaminophen, and other drugs, or natural toxins. This damage can also be associated with poor functioning of the bile ductule. There are also genetic disorders, in which mutations lead to dysfunctional proteins that impair bilirubin processing in the liver. These are linked to inefficient conjugation of bilirubin, poor uptake of bilirubin, or poor secretion of conjugated bilirubin.

Complete obstruction of the common bile duct may be caused by a stone or cancer at the head of the pancreas. As the liver machinery for bilirubin metabolism is not impaired, this situation leads to specific increases in direct bilirubin in plasma, an absence of urinary urobilinogen but the presence of direct bilirubin in urine, and lowering or absence of stool stercobilin.

Hemolytic anemias are caused by the destruction of fragile, abnormal red cells, which will increase the levels of heme available for breakdown. Thus, jaundice associated with hemolytic anemias may show elevated indirect bilirubin in plasma, but remember that the liver, if functioning normally, has a high capacity to handle elevated indirect bilirubin. Stool stercobilin will be elevated, as indicated by darker stool color. This is the result of abnormally high quantities of direct bilirubin entering the intestine. In turn, this leads to elevated urine urobilinogen but not to elevated urine bilirubin (as indirect bilirubin is water insoluble). The hallmarks of hemolytic jaundice are elevated levels of plasma bilirubin (indirect) and increased levels of certain bilirubin products.

To summarize, the laboratory findings in various conditions that cause jaundice are listed in Table 5–4. Jaundice may be classified as prehepatic

Normal

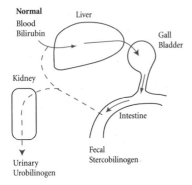

Neonatal Jaundice
Inadequate Liver Processing, Increased Hemolysis

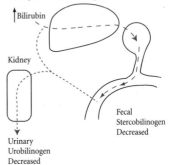

Hemolytic Anemia
Increased Bilirubin Production

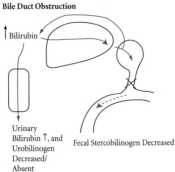

Viral Hepatitis
Damaged Hepatocytes, Decreased Ductule Function

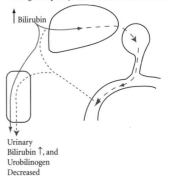

Bile Duct Obstruction

(e.g., hemolytic anemias, including sickle cell anemia caused by HbS, a hemoglobinopathy), hepatic (infectious hepatitis, liver poisoning), or posthepatic (blockage of the common bile duct, pancreatic cancer).

Table 5–4
Findings with Jaundice Caused by Different Conditions

Pathology	Bilirubin (serum)	Bilirubin (urine)	Urobilinogen (urine)	Sterco-bilinogen
Neonatal jaundice	↑Indirect	—	↓	↓
Hepatitis	↑Indirect, direct	↑	↓	↓
Hemolytic anemia	↑Indirect	Absent	↑	↑
Obstructive jaundice*	↑Direct	↑	Absent	↓

*Complete blockage of bile duct (e.g., tumor). A stone may allow intermittent flow of bile, giving changing levels of urinary urobilinogen and stool stercobilinogen

Figure 5–25 Mechanisms involved in jaundice in a variety of conditions. Several pathologic states are presented in comparison with normal bilirubin metabolism. Neonatal jaundice arises because an immature liver cannot adequately handle bilirubin and its accelerated formation resulting from increased levels of hemolysis. There is, thus, an increase in serum indirect (nonconjugated) bilirubin and possible declines in direct bilirubin secretion and in fecal stercobilinogen and urinary urobilinogen levels, compared with normal infants. In hemolytic anemia, liver function is normal, but there is increased metabolic traffic of bilirubin coming from premature red cell breakdown. Serum indirect bilirubin increases and, with a larger secretion of direct bilirubin into the bile, come elevated levels of urine urobilinogen and fecal stercobilinogen. Urinary bilirubin is absent, as indirect bilirubin is not particularly water soluble. For hepatitis, viral damage to the liver cells and adjacent bile ductules results in decreased excretion of direct bilirubin, decreased fecal stercobilinogen, and decreased urinary urobilinogen. Urobilinogen levels may depend on the stage of hepatitis, on the basis of the extent of damage to hepatocytes and micro-obstruction of biliary ductules. Serum levels of direct and indirect bilirubin rise, and bilirubin is detectable in the urine. Obstruction of the common bile duct by a tumor can result in complete blockage of bile flow into the intestine and a regurgitation of bile into the circulation. In this case, levels of serum direct bilirubin are increased, urinary urobilinogen is absent while bilirubin is found in urine, and levels of fecal stercobilinogen are depressed. A stone in the bile duct may lead to fluctuating delivery of bile and can be reflected in changing levels of fecal stercobilinogen and urinary urobilinogen.

In general, while bilirubin measurements and stool color provide important information in the diagnosis of jaundice and its cause, changes in urinary urobilinogen levels are, in practice, not very definitive. Thus, urinary urobilinogen is not commonly used in the diagnosis of specific forms of jaundice. Adapted from Krupp MA, editor. Physician's handbook. 21st ed. Los Altos (CA): Lang Medical Publications; 1985.

6

Vitamin B₁₂, Folic Acid, and Megaloblastic Anemia

In our earlier discussion on enzymes (in Chapter 3), we noted the importance of vitamins in the diet. Vitamins, or compounds derived in the body from these important biochemicals, play very important roles as coenzymes in enzymatic reactions. We mentioned in Chapter 3 the importance of vitamin C in the synthesis of connective tissue proteins and also the central role played by coenzymes derived from the B vitamins niacin, riboflavin, and thiamin. These coenzymes (NAD⁺, FAD, thiamin pyrophosphate) participate in a variety of reactions that are at the heart of intermediary metabolism (those enzyme pathways that are involved in the production of energy). In this chapter, we wish to explore in detail the actions of two other B vitamins: vitamin B₁₂ and folic acid, whose deficiencies result in megaloblastic anemia. Thus, this chapter has a definite nutritional focus and will hopefully encourage you as health professionals to carefully evaluate possible links between the medical problems your patients experience and the adequacy of their diets. We shall also see, in the case of vitamin B₁₂, that deficiencies can also arise from poor absorption of this vitamin.

Megaloblastic anemias are associated with enlarged bone marrow cells (megaloblasts) and enlarged red cells (macrocytes), the former serving as precursors to the latter. The enlarged red cells can be oval in shape and are in reduced numbers. There are various types of anemia (as outlined in Table 6–1). Anemias result in reduced red cell numbers in blood (producing a lowered hematocrit) and reduced levels of hemoglobin within the red cells. In Chapter 5, we described the genetic disease sickle cell anemia, in which sickle cell hemoglobin (HbS) contributes to the distorted shape of the red cells and their fragility in the circulation. In comparison, the megaloblastic anemias, arising from deficiencies of vitamin B₁₂ and folic acid, also cause symptoms and signs associated with anemia: weakness, fatigue, shortness of breath, and even heart failure. In addition, these vitamin deficiencies can

Table 6–1
Types of Anemia

Problems in red cell production (erythropoiesis)
- Megaloblastic anemias
  - Vitamin B_{12} deficiency
  - Folic acid deficiency
  - Vitamin C deficiency (some cases)
- Microcytic-hypochromic anemias
  - Deficiencies in dietary iron
  - Deficiencies in iron transport or utilization
  - Thalassemias
- Normocytic-normochromic anemias
  - Aplastic anemias

Red cell hemolysis
- Autoimmune hemolysis
- Mechanical injury (infection, trauma)
- Genetic red cell defects
  - Membrane structural problems
  - Metabolic deficiencies (glucose-6-phosphate dehydrogenase, pyruvate kinase)
  - Hemoglobinopathies
    - Sickle cell disease
    - Thalassemias

give rise to neurologic problems, such as neural tube defects in fetal development (folate deficiency) and degenerative changes within the adult nervous system (B_{12} deficiency).

VITAMIN B_{12}

This vitamin is also called **cyanocobalamin**, and its structure was determined in 1964 by Dorothy Hodgkin, in her Nobel Prize–winning research. As shown in Figure 6–1, cyanocobalamin has a large, planar ring system, referred to as the corrin ring system. This structure is certainly reminiscent of the porphyrin ring structure for myoglobin and hemoglobin (noted in Chapter 5), as the corrin ring is also made up of four pyrrole rings. However, instead of the iron found in heme proteins, cobalt is linked by coordinate bonds at the center of the corrin ring. The two remaining coordinate positions about cobalt are taken up by a cyano group (shown above the corrin ring) and a dimethylbenzamidazole group (the nine-member ring structure made up of joined six-member and five-member rings, shown below the corrin ring). The cyano group (-CN) found in cyanocobalamin

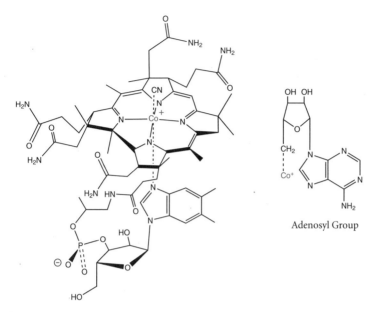

Adenosyl Group

Figure 6–1 The structure of cyanocobalamin. Note the corrin ring system with its four pyrrole rings. Cobalt is centrally coordinated in the ring system and has a -CN group and dimethylbenzamidazole in the other two coordinate positions above and below the ring system, respectively. Other forms of cobalamin (OH-Cbl, AdoCbl, and MeCbl) replace the -CN group with -OH, adenosine, and a -CH$_3$ group, respectively.

is a result of the purification procedure used for this vitamin. There are certainly examples of organically bound cyanide in nature (e.g., in almonds), and cyanocobalamin found in the relatively small quantities in the diet or in supplements does not pose a risk.

There can be other groups besides the -CN group found in cobalamins, and indeed, there are four kinds of cobalamins. Cyanocobalamin has the -CN group, as indicated, while hydroxocobalamin has an -OH group; methylcobalamin (MeCbl), appropriately enough, has a -CH$_3$ group, and adenosylcobalamin (AdoCbl) has adenosine. Adenosine is part of the structure of adenosine triphosphate (ATP), consisting of the nine-member, N-containing adenine ring, which is chemically linked to the sugar ribose (Figure 6–1). Essentially, adenosine is ATP without the three attached phosphate groups. AdoCbl and MeCbl act as coenzymes in certain reactions that we will discuss, and AdoCbl is the principal storage form of cobalamin in the liver.

Inevitably, when we discuss vitamin deficiencies, you will likely run through the composition of your own diet (possibly a very sobering exercise) and come to the conclusion that you are in the early stages of certain of these conditions. This is probably not the case, but nonetheless, your diet likely could benefit from fewer fast foods and the insertion of foods that you may only remember from distant parental guidelines of your youth. Vitamin B_{12} is produced by some microorganisms, and animals consuming these or having them within their intestines or rumen (in the case of the common farm animals) can serve as good sources of vitamin B_{12}. Vitamin B_{12} is found in meat, fish, eggs, milk, and liver. This vitamin is not found in plants; thus, strict vegetarians are wise to consider the use of supplements of this vitamin. Within North America, daily consumption of vitamin B_{12} is within a range of 5 to 30 µg (micrograms), of which some 20% is absorbed (1 to 5 µg). Presuming an adequate diet, the human liver holds about 1 mg of the vitamin, with kidney as another good source. The total body content of the vitamin is in the range of 1 to 5 mg. About 0.1% of this stored pool is lost on a daily basis, and the store of vitamin B_{12} in the liver is enough to supply the body's needs for 1 to 2 years, if B_{12} is no longer available in the diet. Thus, if an individual has the signs and symptoms of megaloblastic anemia caused by a deficiency of vitamin B_{12}, the lack of this vitamin in the diet is inevitably a problem that has existed for some time.

Roles of Vitamin B_{12} in Metabolism

AdoCbl-Dependent Reaction

So what does this vitamin do? There are two cobalamin-dependent enzyme reactions within the body. The first depends on AdoCbl and involves an isomerization reaction. This type of enzymatic reaction does not change the nature of the chemical groups within a molecule but can alter their locations or dispositions within the molecule. Remember, in Chapter 3, we gave the example of maleate isomerase, which changes the orientation of groups about a double bond (a cis→trans isomerization). The AdoCbl-dependent reaction is methylmalonyl-CoA mutase. We will discuss the malonyl groups and coenzyme A (CoA) (also a coenzyme derived from an essential dietary component, pantothenic acid) in more detail in Chapter 7. The methylmalonyl group is formed during the metabolism of propionic acid (Figure 6–2). Propionic acid is a simple carboxylic acid with three carbons and is, thus, a relative of acetic acid (two carbons). Propionic acid can be formed during the digestion of cellulose within the large stomachs of ruminants, such as cattle. Never underestimate the size of the four chambers of the bovine stomach or the involvement of bacteria within this great space (which can be as large as 70 liters). Methane is certainly one product of the bacterial breakdown of foods within the rumen, and it is advisable never to light a match within an enclosed space (e.g., a barn in winter) that might hold both yourself and a significant number of livestock. In ruminants, fer-

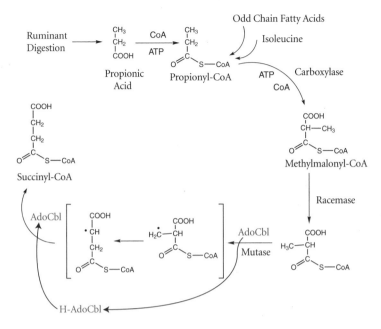

Figure 6–2 The metabolism of propionic acid. Propionic acid is metabolized to propionyl-CoA, which, in turn, is carboxylated to form methylmalonyl-CoA. An isomeric form of methylmalonyl-CoA is converted to succinyl-CoA by AdoCbl-dependent methylmalonyl-CoA mutase. The AdoCbl serves to transfer hydrogen (H) during the mechanism of this reaction. Structures in brackets are proposed intermediates. The •CH$_2$- group is a free radical (a single electron • is involved) that facilitates the insertion of this group into the malonyl three-carbon chain. Adapted from Beck S. Hematology. 5th ed. Cambridge (MA): MIT Press; 1991.

mentation reactions can take place using glucose derived from cellulose, and these reactions can produce the three-carbon propionic acid (see Figure 6–2). Propionate is enzymatically converted to its CoA derivative (propionyl-CoA), which is also made during the breakdown of the amino acid isoleucine or the degradation of fatty acids with an odd number of carbons. Propionyl-CoA links the -COOH group of propionate to the -SH group of CoA to form a thioester bond. In a reaction similar to that catalyzed by acetyl-CoA carboxylase (described in the next chapter), the enzyme propionyl-CoA carboxylase adds a carboxyl group to the propionyl-CoA substrate and forms methylmalonyl-CoA.

The next enzymatic step involves the use of AdoCbl. Normally, in organic chemistry, it is a difficult proposal to break a C-C bond. However, by utilizing AdoCbl as a coenzyme, the enzyme methylmalonyl-CoA mutase (an isomerase) can do this by the removal of a hydrogen from the -CH$_3$ group of the substrate, and this permits the incorporation of the -CH$_2$ group into the three-carbon malonyl group of the substrate. As shown in

Figure 6–2, after the hydrogen is removed, the -CH$_2$ has a single electron and is thus a very reactive chemical species that is known as a **free radical**. The AdoCbl picks up this hydrogen from the -CH$_3$ and transfers it back, once the -CH$_2$ group has been inserted to form the linear four-carbon succinyl-CoA molecule (see Figure 6–2).

You may or may not find this a fascinating mechanism, but your more pertinent question may very well be how does vitamin B$_{12}$ deficiency and, more specifically, an impaired methylmalonyl-CoA mutase reaction result in disease? Usually, methylmalonyl-CoA is an intermediate that does not accumulate but is converted to succinyl-CoA, which can be readily metabolized within the body. If methylmalonyl-CoA builds up, it may enter into other reactions. For example, the synthesis of fatty acids employs the compound malonyl-CoA (as noted in Chapter 7). It is possible that methylmalonyl-CoA could take the place of malonyl-CoA and disrupt the process of fatty acid synthesis or produce fatty acids with a rather unusual structure. In turn, these fatty acids, when incorporated into more complex membrane lipids, could hinder membrane function. And nowhere is membrane function more important than in the brain and nervous tissue, particularly in the multilamellar myelin membranes surrounding the axons of the nerve cells. This is one possible explanation for the neurologic problems seen with vitamin B$_{12}$ deficiency. Remember this mechanism because a block in a normal enzymatic pathway leads to a build-up of unused intermediates, which may participate in undesirable ways in different reactions. In vitamin B$_{12}$ deficiency, there can be an accumulation of methylmalonate and propionic acid in the urine.

MeCbl-Dependent Reaction

In this reaction, the methyl form of cobalamin plays an important role, as shown in Figure 6–3. This pathway utilizes not only MeCbl but also derivatives of the vitamin folic acid. Here MeCbl and N^5-methyl FH$_4$ (the folic acid derivative) are used as methyl donors. MeCbl-dependent methyltransferase (also known as **methionine synthase**) will convert the compound homocysteine into the amino acid methionine. The enzyme transfers the methyl group from MeCbl to the terminal -SH of homocysteine to form methionine. Methionine is an essential amino acid (i.e., an amino acid needed in the diet), but it can be formed if homocysteine is available. Homocysteine itself is an interesting amino acid, and elevations in the levels of homocysteine have been linked to cardiovascular disease. Thus, it is advantageous to remove homocysteine and form methionine (a needed constituent of body proteins). Once the methyl group is removed from MeCbl in the formation of methionine, a reaction is needed to restore a methyl group to this cobalamin. MeCbl can be formed from cobalamin by

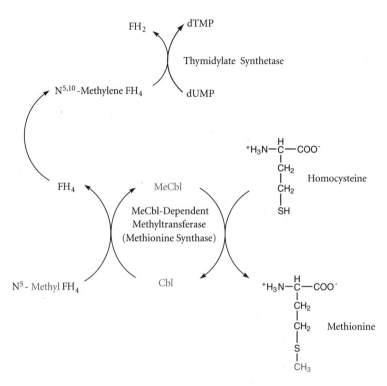

Figure 6–3 The involvement of cobalamin and folate in the MeCbl-dependent methyltransferase reaction. This enzyme catalyzes the methylation of homocysteine to form methionine. MeCbl serves as the methyl donor and is simultaneously converted to Cbl. To regenerate MeCbl, N^5-methyl FH$_4$ serves as methyl donor. FH$_4$ is thus produced and can be metabolized to the folate derivative N^{5,10}-methylene FH$_4$, which participates in the synthesis of dTMP from dUMP by the enzyme thymidylate synthase. Adapted from Beck S. Hematology. 5th ed. Cambridge (MA): MIT Press; 1991.

the use of another methyl donor, the coenzyme N^5-methyl FH$_4$. Thus, the fates of the coenzymes derived from vitamin B$_{12}$ and folic acid overlap. The regeneration of MeCbl is accompanied by the equally important formation of FH$_4$ (tetrahydrofolate) (see Figure 6–3). FH$_4$ can be converted to another folate derivative known as **N^{5,10}-methylene FH$_4$**, and this coenzyme participates in the formation of the nucleotide dTMP (deoxythymidine monophosphate or deoxythymidylate) by the enzyme thymidylate synthetase. We will discuss folate metabolism in more detail later in this chapter and nucleotides and nucleic acids in Chapter 8. However, you should realize that dTMP is a nucleotide that carries deoxyribose and also the base thymine. This nucleotide is vital for the synthesis of DNA (as is the availability of the other three deoxynucleotide derivatives needed for DNA synthesis: dATP, dGTP, and dCTP).

The importance of this enzymatic pathway is certainly evident. A deficiency in MeCbl will translate into an impairment of DNA synthesis. There are at least two explanations for this effect: (1) the folate trap hypothesis and (2) the misincorporation of uracil. A deficiency of MeCbl traps folic acid in its N^5-methyl FH_4 form, and this form of folic acid cannot participate in the thymidylate synthetase reaction. Thus, there is a reduction in the formation of dTMP and an impaired synthesis of DNA. The misincorporation of uracil into DNA is another effect linked to a deficiency in the thymidylate synthetase. The substrate used by this enzyme is deoxyuridine monophosphate (dUMP), a nucleotide that has structural similarities to the product dTMP. Uracil is a base that is usually found in RNA and not in DNA. If levels of dUMP rise, it may be used in place of dTMP during DNA synthesis. Impairment of DNA synthesis, produced by one or both of these mechanisms, is likely the basis for the megaloblastic anemia associated with vitamin B_{12} deficiency. Because of the impairment of DNA synthesis, the maturation of precursor cells into blood cells is hindered, with the production of fewer red cells, with unusual shapes and large sizes. In severe megaloblastic anemia, even nucleated red cells may be present in the circulation, underlining the associated problem with blood cell maturation within bone marrow.

The folate trap linked with vitamin B_{12} deficiency limits the production of FH_4 (tetrahydrofolate). This limitation not only compromises $N^{5,10}$-methylene FH_4 production and thymidylate synthetase but also the conversion of FH_4 into a variety of other folate derivatives (Figure 6–5), which we will describe when we outline the importance of folate later in this chapter. As well, deficiency in vitamin B_{12} slows the production of methionine, hinders protein synthesis (which relies on the availability of all 20 of the common amino acids), and, thus, may contribute to the neurologic symptoms noted. A final problem due to a poor supply of vitamin B_{12} is likely an elevated level of homocysteine in the circulation (hyperhomocysteinemia), which is believed to contribute to cardiovascular pathology. Of course, the uses of vitamin B_{12} and folate within this pathway are interdependent. Thus, a lack of folic acid can also impair the regeneration of MeCbl and the production of dTMP and cell division.

Pernicious Anemia

You should be aware that there are a variety of anemias, as outlined in Table 6–1. However the term "pernicious anemia" is used to describe a specific condition associated with vitamin B_{12} deficiency. A deficiency can be produced simply by a dietary insufficiency of this vitamin (although, given the consumption of meat products by the general North American population, you may find such a deficiency rather rare, except among vegetarians who do not consume eggs or dairy products). It has also been found that the use of nitrous oxide ("laughing gas") as an anesthetic can produce a B$_{12}$ deficiency by oxidizing the cobalt ion in cobalamin. Yet, B$_{12}$ deficiencies are not uncommon, and it is apparent in many cases that even though sufficient B$_{12}$ is present in the diet, some individuals do manifest the disease. Pernicious anemia is found in 40- to 70-year-old Caucasian as well as African North Americans, whose ages can be under 40 years.

An early clue to the nature of pernicious anemia came in 1926 from the demonstration that patients with this disease could be kept alive by the consumption of relatively large quantities of raw liver. This was prior to the discovery and isolation of B$_{12}$. Those of you who are not crazy about cooked liver can perhaps appreciate the lack of enthusiasm for this dietary intervention. Indeed, sad to say, there were those who literally would rather die than eat raw liver. Liver was later replaced by liver extracts. Yet, the high quantities of vitamin B$_{12}$ in liver provided a clue to the nature of the disease. As the consumption of very high quantities of B$_{12}$ could prevent megaloblastic anemia, this suggested that there may be a defect in the absorption of this relatively high-molecular-weight vitamin.

Indeed, this proved to be the case. Before vitamin B$_{12}$ was chemically defined as cobalamin, it was called extrinsic factor (EF), and it was determined, in 1929, that there was an intrinsic factor (IF) needed for the absorption of EF from the diet. In humans, IF is a glycoprotein (44 kDa molecular mass) that can bind EF. IF is secreted by the stomach and binds cobalamin released from the diet. Thus, IF is a component of the normal gastric juice. The IF–EF complex enters the intestine, and in the ileum, there are receptors that recognize the complex. The complex is internalized by endocytosis, the process (as described in Chapter 2) for transferrin and LDLs (low-density lipoproteins). Pernicious anemia is caused by gastric atrophy that leads to a deficiency in IF and a consequent decrease in vitamin B$_{12}$ absorption. This gastric atrophy can be a consequence of the production of autoantibodies to IF. There are other causes of cobalamin deficiencies, as noted in Table 6–2 (gastric dysfunction, gastrectomy, intestinal disease), and the associated anemias are generally referred to as B$_{12}$-deficieny anemias.

Once absorbed, cobalamin is released within the intestinal cells and makes its way to the portal circulation. Much of the cobalamin is stored as AdoCbl within the liver. A plasma protein called **transcobalamin II** (TC II) transports most of the cobalamin newly arriving in the circulation and is believed responsible for most of the cobalamin uptake by the cells of the body. There is a type of megaloblastic anemia caused by a deficiency in this protein. Transcobalamin I (TC I, haptocorrin) is another plasma protein that binds cobalamin, but this bound cobalamin has a longer half-life within the circulation. Most of the circulating cobalamin is complexed with TC I.

Table 6–2
Causes of Megaloblastic Anemias

Cobalamin deficiencies
- Inadequate diet
- Inadequate absorption
  — Pernicious anemia (IF deficiency)
  — Gastrectomy, gastric malfunction or injury
  — Intestinal disease
  — Competitive parasites (bacterial overgrowth or fish tapeworms can take up dietary cobalamin)
- Poor utilization
  — Deficiencies in cobalamin transporting proteins
  — Enzyme deficiencies
  — Nitrous oxide (oxidation of the cobalt ion in cobalamin)
- Increased need
  — Pregnancy, hyperthyroidism, neoplasia

Folic acid deficiencies
- Inadequate diet
- Hemodialysis
- Alcoholism
- Inadequate absorption
  — Intestinal disease
  — Oral contraceptives, anticonvulsants
- Poor utilization
  — Folic acid antimetabolites (methotrexate)
  — Enzyme deficiencies
- Increased need
  — Pregnancy, hyperthyroidism, neoplasia

Test for Anemias Caused by Poor Vitamin B_{12} Absorption

This is known as the Schilling test. Here, radioactive cyanocobalamin is given by mouth, followed by a "flushing dose" of unlabeled cyanocobalamin administered intramuscularly 2 hours later. If there is radioactive vitamin B_{12} uptake at the intestine and entry into the circulation, this unlabeled vitamin B_{12} serves to decrease the amount of radioactive vitamin B_{12} further taken up from the circulation by the tissues of the body. Urine samples are collected, and poor recovery of radioactivity in urine indicates poor intestinal absorption of the vitamin and possible deficiency of IF. The test is repeated with radioactive cyanocobalamin given orally with hog IF. Normal radioactive excretion of cyanocobalamin indicates that vitamin B_{12} has entered the circulation.

A positive Schilling test indicates a logical therapy for B_{12}-deficient anemias: the administration of vitamin B_{12} by injection. Frequent intramuscular injections of vitamin B_{12} are given, and once the symptoms of anemia subside, these individuals receive monthly injections of vitamin B$_{12}$ for the rest of their lives.

An important test more specifically associated with pernicious anemia is the lack of gastric production of HCl (achlorhydria) caused by gastric mucosal atrophy. Patients with pernicious anemia should be followed up regularly, as they have an increased incidence of gastric carcinoma.

In Table 6–3 are presented the clinical and hematologic features of this vitamin deficiency. Hematologic changes include red cell size, shape, and number as well as the occurrence of megaloblasts in bone marrow. Note that neutrophils can also show morphologic changes when vitamin B$_{12}$ is deficient. Laboratory signs include increased plasma bilirubin and lactate dehydrogenase (LDH), a serum enzyme marker discussed in Chapter 3, which result from hemolysis and poor red cell formation. There are also the more common signs and symptoms of anemia, such as weight loss and fatigue. These signs and symptoms of anemia are also found in other forms of anemia, including folic acid deficiency. More specific for vitamin B$_{12}$-related anemia are the neurologic symptoms, associated with the decreased activities of methylmalonyl-CoA mutase and MeCbl-dependent methyltransferase, discussed earlier. Here, the lab signs can include methylmalonic aciduria and increases in serum methylmalonate and homocysteine, coupled with low levels of serum cobalamin. The neurologic effects may involve cerebral malfunction (sometimes referred to as "megaloblastic madness"), spas-

Table 6–3
Clinical and Hematologic Features of Folate and Vitamin B$_{12}$ Deficiencies

Megaloblastic anemias	General: Weakness, shortness of breath, easily fatigued, light headed, heart failure, pallor, and slight jaundice Hematology: Macrocytic red cells, oval-shaped red cells, low hematocrit, nucleated red cells, hypersegmentation of neutrophils (i.e., multilobed nucleus), increased hemolysis, elevated serum LDH, and indirect (nonconjugated) bilirubin
Vitamin B$_{12}$ deficiency	Decreased cobalamin absorption, as monitored by Schilling test, responsiveness to vitamin B$_{12}$ therapy, neurologic changes may be seen as may elevated levels of urinary methylmalonate
Folate deficiency	Low levels of serum and red cell folate, rapid uptake of administered folate, excretion of FIGLU with histidine loading, rapid responsiveness to dietary or therapeutic folate, lack of neurologic changes, normal urinary methylmalonate

tic ataxia, paresthesias in feet and fingers, and degeneration of specific areas of the spinal cord. Of course, one ultimate test for vitamin B_{12}-associated megaloblastic anemia is a successful response to injections of vitamin B_{12}.

It must be emphasized that it is very important to diagnose unequivocally the cause of megaloblastic anemia, as folate and vitamin B_{12} deficiencies share many signs and symptoms. If vitamin B_{12} deficiency is involved, misdiagnosis and the administration of folate can temporarily improve the blood signs in the anemia without improving the neuropathology.

FOLIC ACID

This vitamin is much more important in one-carbon metabolism than is vitamin B_{12}. Folate deficiencies that may arise from dietary shortcomings also lead to megaloblastic anemia. One very significant result of folate deficiency is seen in neural tube defects and spina bifida. Thus, folate supplements are very important, particularly early in pregnancy, and folate must be available in fetal development to avoid these pathologic lesions.

Folic acid is found in a variety of dietary plant and animal sources (green leafy vegetables, lettuce, broccoli, spinach, asparagus, mushrooms, kidney, liver, and yeast). Folate is also made by many different bacteria. Folate can be removed or degraded by excessive cooking in water. A minimum daily requirement of 50 µg of folate in adults is cited in older texts, but higher daily requirements (400 µg) have been suggested more recently. The adult carries enough folate for a period of about 4 months (when folate is not provided by the diet). This is a much smaller bodily reserve than that of vitamin B_{12}, which is sufficient for several years if cobalamin is deficient.

The structure of folic acid is shown in Figure 6–4. It is easier to remember the structure by considering the parts that make up the whole. The 10-member double ring is known as **pteridine** (and this is where the molecule can be reduced or oxidized). The middle portion is para-aminobenzoic acid (PABA), a chemical also found in certain sunscreen preparations that reduce sunburn. The last part of the molecule (far right) is glutamic acid, an acidic amino acid found in proteins. Together, pteridine and PABA can be called pteroic acid, and folate is referred to as pteroylglutamate. Folates must have at least one glutamate (the monoglutamate form), but they can have up to seven glutamate residues linked to one another by peptide bonds (the polyglutamates). The monoglutamate form can be represented by the abbreviations F or PteGlu. Inside the cells, folates are usually found as polyglutamates, while folate circulating in blood is monoglutamate. The polyglutamate forms facilitate the retention of folates inside the cells. In nature, folate is found principally as polyglutamates, while the folate in supplements is PteGlu.

To participate in metabolism, folates must be reduced. This occurs within the pteridine part of the molecule, specifically at N5, N8, C6, and C7 (see Fig-

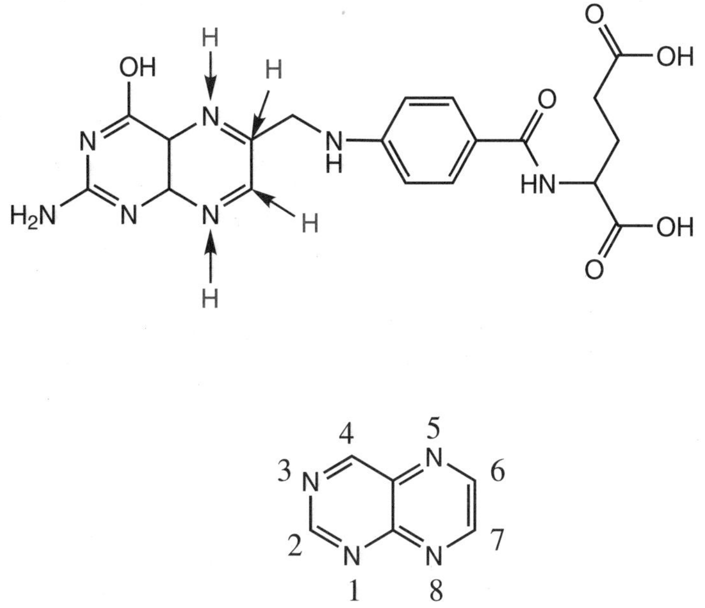

Figure 6–4 The structure of folic acid. Note the three parts making up the molecule: the pteridine ring (left side) that has the sites for reduction, p-aminobenzoic acid (middle), and glutamic acid (right side). Folic acid is also known as pteroylglutamic acid. This form of folic acid (or folate) can be reduced and methylated to form N^5-methyl FH$_4$, which is the principal form found in the circulation. Sites of reduction (producing FH$_4$) are shown by H→. Adapted from Beck S. Hematology. 5th ed. Cambridge (MA): MIT Press; 1991.

ure 6–4). The enzyme that catalyzes these reductions is dihydrofolate reductase (DHFR), and NADPH is used as the reducing cofactor in these reactions. F is first converted to FH$_2$ (dihydrofolate) and then to FH$_4$ (tetrahydrofolate). The metabolism of folate involves the addition of single-carbon components to the folate structure. Remember that folate functions as a one-carbon donor in enzymatic reactions, and these single-carbon additions to folates will, in turn, serve as the source of these transferred carbons.

The gallery of folate derivatives produced by one-carbon additions is shown in Figure 6–5. Again, don't be overwhelmed by these, but use your "metabolic" bird's eye perspective to focus on differences between individual molecules. These compounds are essentially identical, with the exception of those single-carbon additions. You can see that these single carbons exist as -CHO (formyl), -CH$_2$OH (hydroxymethyl), -CH$_3$ (methyl), -CH$_2$- (methylene), -CH= (methenyl), and -CHNH (forminino) groups within the FH$_4$ structure. Some of these derivatives can be interconverted by specific enzyme reactions. For example, the N^5-methyl FH$_4$ (used to methylate cobalamin, and thus to drive methionine synthesis from homocysteine) can

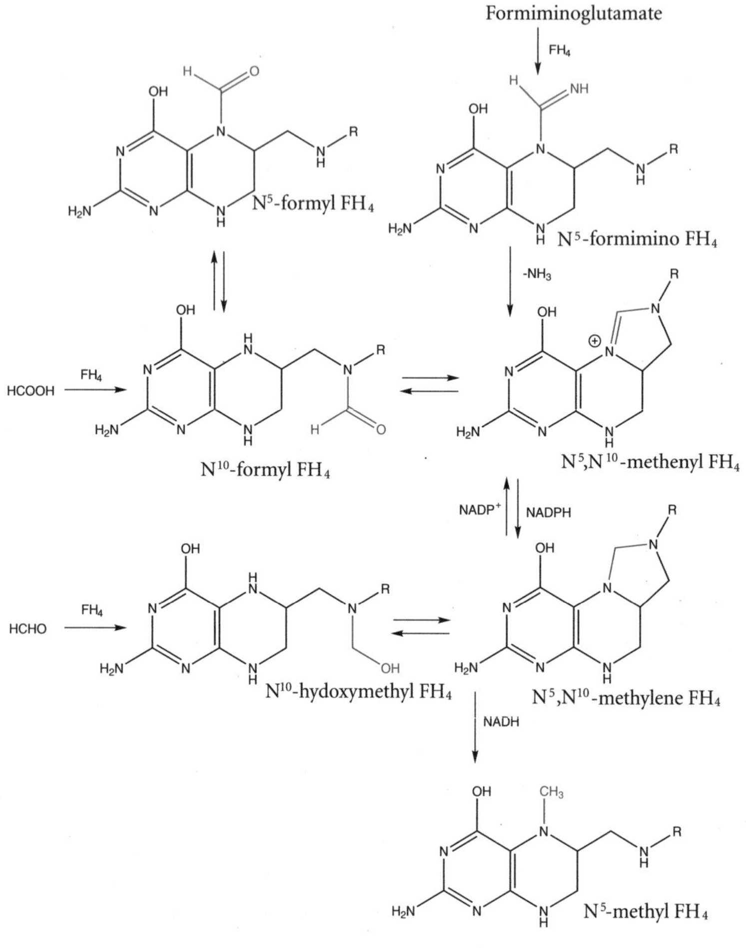

Figure 6–5 The derivatives of folic acid. FH$_4$ (liberated from circulating N^5-methyl FH$_4$) can be metabolized to form a variety of intracellular derivatives that can serve as carriers for single-carbon groups. These are shown as -CHO, -CH$_2$OH, -CHNH, -CH=, -CH$_2$-, and -CH$_3$. These will participate in a number of reactions, where individual compounds gain one carbon. Thus, folic acid is a donor of one-carbon groups. Adapted from Beck S. Hematology. 5th ed. Cambridge (MA): MIT Press; 1991.

be formed by the generation of a -CH$_2$OH group at the N of the PABA constituent (to form N^{10}-hydroxymethyl FH$_4$). The -CH$_2$OH group is provided by the amino acid serine, which loses its R-group during its enzymatic conversion to the simpler amino acid glycine. In turn, N^{10}-hydroxymethyl FH$_4$ is converted into N^5, N^{10}-methylene FH$_4$, as the single carbon added now bridges both N^{10} (the N in the PABA group) and the N^5 of the pteridine ring. This folate derivative can be enzymatically reduced using NADPH to form a methyl group (-CH$_3$) at N^5 as the one-carbon substituent. This generates

N^5-methyl FH$_4$, which can be used by the MeCbl-dependent methyltrans-ferase (see Figure 6–3).

You should view FH$_4$ as a cycling intermediate that transfers single car-bons via the variety of folate derivatives and then requires reactivation by the acquisition of new single-carbon units. Overall, this cycling of the cofactor can be generalized as

$$FH_4 + Y\text{-}C \rightarrow FH_4\text{-}C + Y$$
$$FH_4\text{-}C + Z \rightarrow FH_4 + Z\text{-}C$$
$$\overline{Y\text{-}C + Z \rightarrow Y + Z\text{-}C \text{ (Summation equation)}}$$

In the equations above, the single transferred C is shown as -C. Thus, the net effect of the intervention of folate derivatives is the transfer of C from a donor, noted as Y-C to an acceptor, noted as Z. FH$_4$-C is the folate derivative that serves as the single-carbon intermediary. Again, note that the folate derivatives that are active within cellular metabolism are the poly-glutamyl forms of FH$_4$.

To study one such reaction in more detail, consider the synthesis of dTMP that we noted during the discussion of MeCbl-dependent methyl-transferase. The folate derivative required for dTMP synthesis by the enzyme thymidylate synthase is N^5, N^{10}-methylene FH$_4$ (remember, this was the folate derivative with the bridging -CH$_2$- group we noted previously). You can see in Figure 6–6 that the one-carbon constituent of N^5, N^{10}-meth-

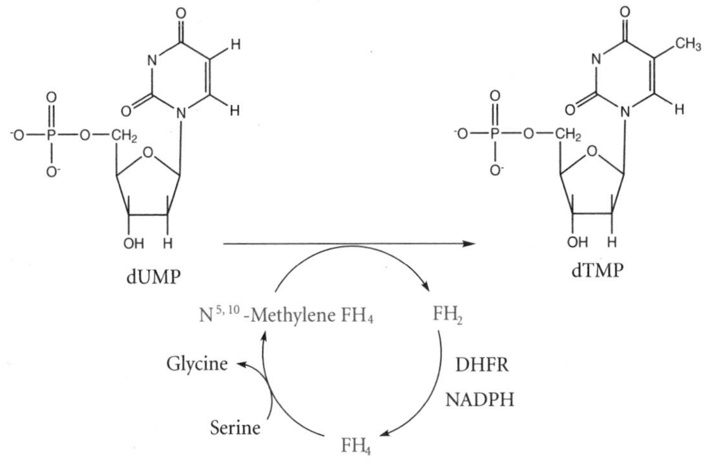

Figure 6–6 The thymidylate synthase reaction. dUMP is converted to dTMP using a single car-bon donated by N^{5,10}-methylene FH$_4$. Note the -CH$_3$ group difference between the uracil and thymine rings in the two compounds. At the same time, the folate derivative is converted to FH$_2$. Thus, DHFR (dihydrofolate reductase) using NADPH as coenzyme is required to regener-ate FH$_4$. In turn, the enzymatic conversion of serine to glycine provides the necessary carbon for the conversion of FH$_4$ to N^{5,10}-methylene FH$_4$.

ylene FH_4 is transferred to dUMP (deoxyuridylate) to make dTMP, as the only difference between dUMP and dTMP is the extra $-CH_3$ group on the thymine ring of dTMP. However, this reaction also generates FH_2 instead of FH_4; thus, DHFR and NADPH are required to restore FH_4.

Thymidylate synthase: N^5, N^{10}-methylene FH_4 + dUMP $\rightarrow$ dTMP + FH_2
DHFR: FH_2 + NADPH $\rightarrow$ FH_4 + $NADP^+$

Just as cobalamin deficiency could limit dTMP synthesis and, thus, lead to impaired or faulty DNA synthesis, so too can folate deficiency impede correct DNA synthesis in cells. Thus, deficiency of either vitamin is associated with an accumulation of DNA within the precursor cells, the generation of megaloblasts, and the resulting megaloblastic anemia. While folate can be absorbed without the need of a factor (such as IF required by vitamin B_{12}), nonetheless, folate deficiency is found not only with poor diet but also as a result of poor absorption associated with alcoholism, intestinal disease, and the use of oral contraceptives or anticonvulsants.

Therapies can be used to limit the amount of FH_4 available within the body. Folate analogues called **aminopterin** (4-aminofolate) and **amethopterin** (4-amino-10-methylfolate) (Figure 6–7) were found to be antimetabolites for folate. Antimetabolites block reactions involving the natural compounds. In this case, the two antimetabolites for folate (noted above) could bind much more tightly than folate to the enzyme DHFR. The result was a slow-down in DNA synthesis. The application was the control of cancer cell proliferation. Thus, amethopterin (also known as methotrexate) and aminopterin could produce remissions in leukemias and in other cancers. The chemotherapeutic natures of these compounds was discovered in 1948, well before the biochemical mechanism was elucidated. This antimetabolite concept had been applied to folate metabolism even before World War II, when A.D. Woods, a biochemist, used sulfanilamide as an antimetabolite for PABA. Bacteria make their own folate but need PABA for this biosynthesis. Thus, the sulfa drugs (containing this antimetabolite or its derivatives) could retard bacterial growth and were among the first effective antibiotics. Human tissues and cells were not affected by this antimetabolite, as they relied on the dietary supply of folate, rather than making them from PABA. This exploitation of differences in bacterial and human metabolism became a very useful approach in the design of antibiotics. The use of the penicillins that inhibit the synthesis of bacterial cell walls is an example of this principle. Of course, you should realize that the use of antibiotics also leads to a substantial loss of intestinal bacteria. It is reasonable to consider the use of dairy products containing bacteria (e.g., yogurt) or supplements of lactobacillus and other friendly intestinal bacteria during prolonged administrations of antibiotics. Parenthetically, another use of friendly bacteria is when you travel abroad. The spectre of diarrhea and other symptoms of gastrointestinal infections can loom over

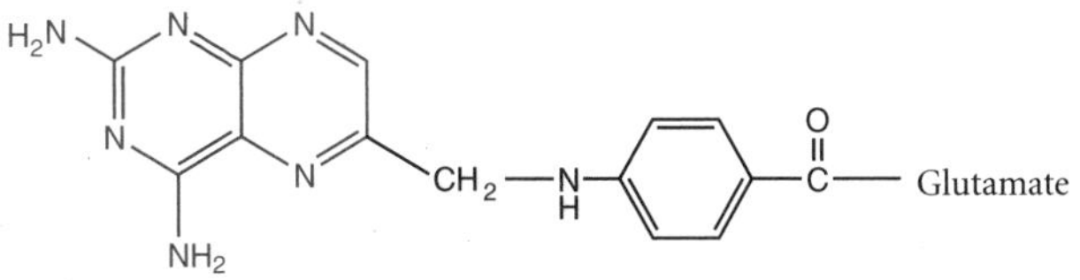

Aminopterin

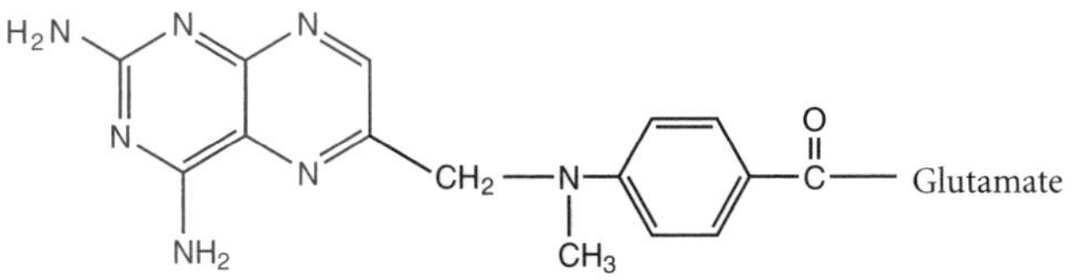

Amethopterin
(Methotrexate)

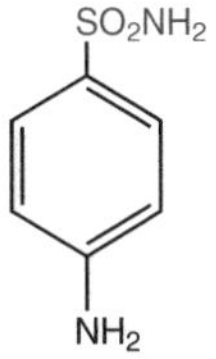

Sulfanilamide

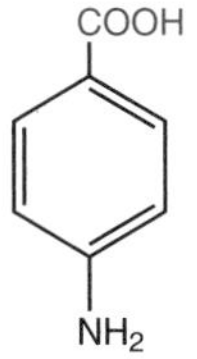

p-Aminobenzoic Acid
(PABA)

Figure 6–7 The structures of the antimetabolites methotrexate and amniopterin and of sulfanilamide and p-aminobenzoic acid. Methotrexate and aminopterin are analogues of folate that bind tightly to and inhibit DHFR. This limits DNA synthesis, a useful strategy in cancer chemotherapy and in the treatment of certain forms of arthritis. Sulfanilamide is an antimetabolite of p-aminobenzoic acid that arrests the synthesis of bacterial folic acid. Sulfanilamide is an antibiotic used to inhibit bacterial growth.

trips to exotic and otherwise desirable destinations. The daily use of friendly bacteria may potentially limit the spread of pathologic microorganisms.

The use of methotrexate was not as benign as that of sulfanilamide or penicillin, as methotrexate effectively slows down the growth of any rapidly growing cells in the body. Thus, cells of the intestinal mucosa and hair follicles can be disabled in these therapies. One more recent use of methotrexate is, interestingly, in the treatment of rheumatoid arthritis. This form of arthritis involves autoimmune, inflammatory responses centered at the joints. The use of carefully controlled quantities of methotrexate effectively decreases the production of white cells and decreases the immune response.

As women are more prone to rheumatoid arthritis than are men, care must be taken to stop the methotrexate therapy prior to pregnancy. However, if methotrexate is given before the disease produces permanent joint damage, the remission from this autoimmune disorder can be quite remarkable.

One further example of folate involvement in metabolism comes from the catabolism of the amino acid histidine. Histidine is an amino acid characterized by the presence of an imidazole ring in its R-group (Figure 6–8). During the catabolism of histidine, this ring is broken open, and a formimino group (-CH=NH) is created in the generation of the intermediate formiminoglutamic acid (FIGLU). This formimino group can be transferred to FH_4, forming N^5-formimino FH_4 (see Figure 6–5) and glutamic acid. If there is insufficient FH_4, FIGLU will accumulate. This is the basis of a test for folate deficiency, although it is not commonly used now. Histidine is given orally, and excretion of FIGLU in urine is an indication of the lack of the vitamin. It is possible that vitamin B_{12} deficiency, by lim-

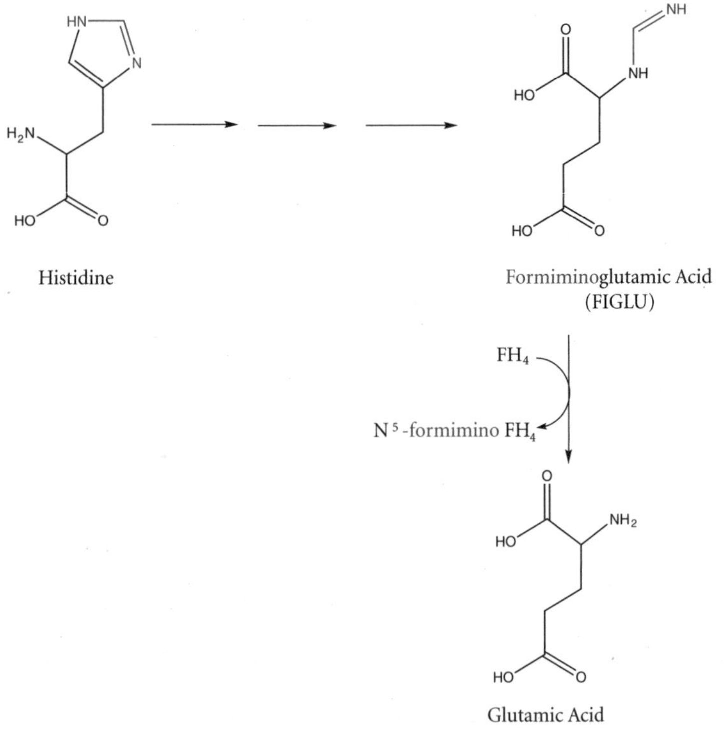

Figure 6–8 Histidine catabolism and FIGLU production. Histidine is broken down enzymatically to form formiminoglutamic acid (FIGLU), which possesses a formimino group (-CH=NH). This group can be transferred to FH_4 to form N^5-formimino FH_4 and glutamic acid. A test for folic acid deficiency involves an oral loading dose of histidine (20 g). If FIGLU is found in urine, a deficiency of folate is possible.

iting FH$_4$ production in cells (the folate trap), can also lead to elevated FIGLU excretion with a loading dose of oral histidine. However, experience with megaloblastic anemias has indicated that FIGLU excretion is not found in most cases of vitamin B$_{12}$ deficiency.

Besides its involvement in the synthesis of dTMP, the catabolism of histidine, the synthesis of methionine, and the catabolism of serine to glycine, folate is also important in the synthesis of purines, such as adenine and guanine.

Folate is absorbed within the intestine at the jejunum and requires the action of an enzyme (a peptidase called **conjugase**) that removes glutamate residues from the polyglutamate forms of the vitamin. The resulting F (or PteGlu) may be generated prior to folate uptake or possibly following uptake within the intestinal cells. F is converted to N^5-FH$_4$ by reduction and methylation. This monoglutamate form of FH$_4$ is the principal one found in the circulation, and there is evidence for transport by a specific plasma protein. Circulating folate is rapidly taken up by tissues.

Clinical Features of Folate Deficiency

Generally, both deficiencies in folate and vitamin B$_{12}$ will lead to megaloblastic anemia as shown by abnormal red cells, abnormal white cells, and elevated serum LDH (noted in Table 6–3). However, there are a number of important differences between the two conditions. Megaloblastic anemia due to folate deficiency is confirmed by finding low levels of plasma and red cell folate and responsiveness to folate therapy. Older and less used tests for folate deficiency are elevated excretion of FIGLU following histidine loading and abnormally fast clearance of intravenously administered folate. Suggestive features include a lack of neurologic symptoms and normal levels of methylmalonate in urine. Unlike the case of pernicious anemia (where there is little response to dietary cobalamin), individuals with folate deficiency respond very rapidly to therapeutic oral folate supplements (5 mg/d) or dietary folate (200 to 400 μg/d) unless there are general problems with intestinal absorption, as encountered in intestinal disease and alcoholism. You should make a specific diagnosis before initiating folate or vitamin B$_{12}$ therapy, as we have noted that folate can lessen some of the signs and symptoms of vitamin B$_{12}$ deficiency without remedying the important neuropathology associated with this deficiency. Megaloblastic anemias can also be found when there is no problem with dietary supply or absorption of the vitamins. This can occur in antimetabolite therapy (e.g., methotrexate) or in an inborn error of metabolism that compromises the use of folate or vitamin B$_{12}$.

You should pay special attention to the diets of elderly patients who live alone and manifest an anemia, as the incidence of dietary insufficiency among seniors is quite frequent.

Metabolism

In our efforts to introduce you gradually to certain topics in biochemistry, we have already shown how heme, found within hemoglobin and other heme proteins, is assembled and degraded by metabolic pathways consisting of enzymes working in sequence to produce a final product or products (Chapter 5). In Chapter 6, small enzyme pathways were described, featuring methylation reactions using cobalamin and folate. Now we wish to enter metabolism in some detail, in particular, featuring metabolic pathways that degrade compounds for the production of energy. This energy can be utilized in the synthesis of adenosine triphosphate (ATP) and phosphocreatine, for use in synthetic pathways. Medical students and those in related health-care fields may be relieved to know that metabolism, while important, is not the colossus it once was in biochemistry courses. Only some 10 to 15 years ago, metabolism was the chief biochemical diet fed to students, who were expected to memorize considerable strings of enzyme reactions, a little like putting to memory all the stops on each of the subway (metro/underground) lines within a large city like New York or London. The objectives for metabolism are now seen as more global—more an overall understanding of a pathway, including its purpose, its initial substrates and final products, and important points of regulation. Thus, while we present complete paths, we urge you to deal with forests and not trees and attempt to establish an overview that may be carried with you into future applications of biochemical theory in the practice of health care.

As well, a chain of reactions, by its very existence, relies on contributions from all its members. Thus, a genetic mutation that results in the deficiency of one enzyme can shut down a metabolic path, often resulting in a very profound and specific pathology. Enzyme paths can also be affected by drugs, and we will cover the basics of enzyme inhibition within this chapter. As well, the control of metabolism by insulin and its antagonists, adrenaline and glucagon, will be studied in the context of eating and fasting and with specific reference to that very prevalent disease, diabetes mellitus.

So what is metabolism? Well, you can see various wise heads being scratched and a safe global definition emerging. Metabolism is usually defined as all the enzymatic reactions taking place within the body. Many of these reactions are components of enzyme pathways, a concept we introduced in Chapter 3 and further expanded in Chapters 5 and 6 . Metabolism can be further subdivided into two major realms. As shown in Figure 7–1, anabolism comprises synthetic reactions that produce more complex molecules from simpler ones and requires energy, often supplied by ATP. In contrast, catabolism involves breakdown reactions that degrade more complex molecules into simpler ones, with energy being released in the process. This energy is in part conserved with the formation of ATP, or the reduced coenzymes nicotinamide-adenine dinucleotide (NADH) and nicotinamide-adenine dinucleotide phosphate (NADPH).

The complex molecules, which are of particular interest to us in this chapter, can be classified as proteins, polysaccharides, and fats (triglycerides). Nucleic acids, such as deoxyribonucleic acid (DNA) and ribonucleic acid (RNA), will be discussed in Chapter 8. Proteins have been described in Chapter 1, and in Chapter 3, we introduced glycogen, a polymer made up of glucose molecules. Glycogen is a very important polysaccharide, stored in granules, mainly within liver and muscle cells. Glycogen can effectively serve as a source of glucose, a molecule that we will see is commonly broken down in cells to provide energy. Glucose is, thus, a fuel

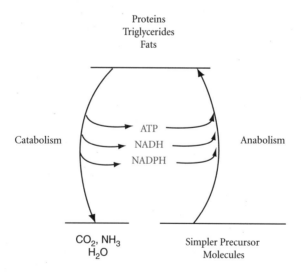

Figure 7–1 Pathways of catabolism and anabolism are compared. Generally, catabolic paths degrade larger molecules into simpler ones, with a release of energy, part of which is conserved in the formation of ATP and NADH. In contrast, anabolic paths convert simpler molecules or precursors into larger more complex molecules. This requires energy, often supplied by ATP or NADPH.

substrate for the body. Another form of stored fuel, more quantitatively important than glycogen, is fat or triglyceride (also known as triacylglycerol). Most of your fuel reserves are in the form of fat, which is contained within fat cells (adipose cells or adipocytes).

Each of these three classes of complex molecule can be broken down in catabolic pathways, as outlined in Figure 7–2. Glycogen is degraded to glucose-1-phosphate, a derivative of glucose, which is subsequently broken down in a pathway called **glycolysis**. Glycolysis yields energy that can be conserved, in part, by the formation of ATP. In glycolysis, glucose is converted to pyruvate, which is further metabolized to the molecule acetyl-CoA (acetyl-coenzyme A). This enters the Krebs or citric acid cycle (a circular enzyme pathway). The Krebs cycle releases carbon dioxide (which ultimately ends up in the air you expire from your lungs) and also produces the reduced coenzymes NADH and flavin adenine dinucleotide ($FADH_2$). These molecules have energies of reduction, and the passage of their electrons down a chain of carriers (called the **respiratory or electron transport chain**) releases energy. Oxygen is the final recipient of these electrons, and its reduction yields water. The respiratory chain is linked to a process known as **oxidative phosphorylation** that uses the energy released during the passage of electrons to drive the synthesis of ATP from adenosine diphosphate (ADP) and inorganic phosphate (Pi).

Proteins can be degraded by proteolytic enzymes (hydrolyzing peptide bonds) to yield amino acids. In turn, these can be stripped of their amino groups, and the carbon skeletons (in the form of pyruvate, acetyl-CoA, and oxaloacetate, to name a few) are further broken down within the Krebs cycle. Thus, proteins can be used to provide energy, but because of their diverse functional roles and importance in muscle, proteins are used as major fuel sources only in extreme circumstances (e.g., starvation).

Quantitatively, the most important stored molecules that act as fuel substrates are the fats (triglycerides). These are broken down to fatty acids, which can be degraded within a pathway known as β-oxidation. Acetyl-CoA is produced by β-oxidation and enters the Krebs cycle. You can see that the catabolic paths converge to a small number of simple molecules, of which acetyl-CoA is central to protein, glycogen, and fat breakdown.

Under normal circumstances, there is a balance between the catabolic and anabolic processes. Thus, while a protein, such as albumin, will be broken down after a certain length of time within the circulation, there is a balancing synthesis of albumin by the liver so that the concentration of this protein within blood remains reasonably constant. This is referred to as a steady state. Fat and glycogen build up in your body after eating, as you utilize glucose and fatty acids (coming from digestion) in the synthesis of these complex storage molecules. Between meals, you can draw on these reserves to provide fuel substrates for your daily activities. If you eat more food

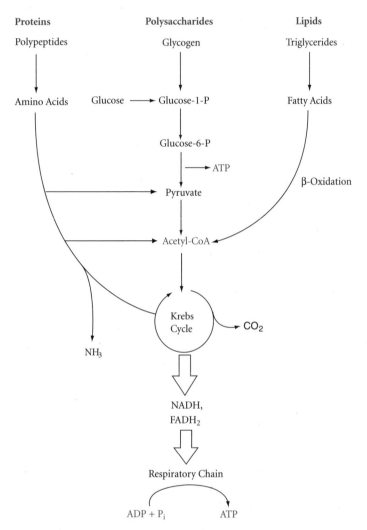

Figure 7–2 The major catabolic pathways. The breakdown of three major classes of macromolecules (proteins, polysaccharides, and lipids) is shown. The central path of glycolysis leads to a splitting of glucose into two molecules of pyruvate (three carbons), with a modest production of ATP. More ATP is generated following the conversion of pyruvate into acetyl-CoA and its entry into the Krebs cycle, with the subsequent production of reduced coenzymes NADH and $FADH_2$ supplying electrons for electron transport (via the respiratory chain). The energy released during electron transport drives oxidative phosphorylation and ATP production. Amino acids released during the breakdown of proteins can be stripped of their amino groups (released as ammonia) and the carbon skeletons, such as oxaloacetate, enter the Krebs cycle. Fatty acids are released in the catabolism of lipids (mainly triglycerides), and these are broken down by the process of β-oxidation to yield acetyl-CoA, which enters the Krebs cycle. Considerable energy in the form of ATP can be produced from fat catabolism. Adapted from Moran LA, Scrimgeour KG, Horton HR, et al. Biochemistry. 2nd ed. Englewood Cliffs (NJ): Neil Patterson-Prentice Hall; 1994.

(often measured in the form of Calories [with capital C] or kilocalories) than you utilize as fuel substrates, you put on weight in the form of fat. On the other hand, if you are fasting or dieting, you will begin to reduce the size of these stores (which, for the average North American, is usually a good thing!). Thus, there is a ledger of Calories taken in and Calories used, with the accounts explaining why that large-sized Hawaiian pizza, coupled with sitting at a desk for 8 hours studying your Biochemistry notes, results in a net weight gain. Not to mention what happens when you try to run for that number 52 bus that will take you downtown for the exam!

DIGESTION AND METABOLISM

Having mentioned eating in the paragraph above, it is important to draw a clear line between the enzymatic events taking place in the gastrointestinal tract and those events taking place within the cells of the body. In the stomach and intestine, enzymes are secreted to facilitate the breakdown of dietary components. Thus, proteolytic enzymes in the stomach and small intestine break down peptide bonds in proteins, ultimately to produce amino acids and a few dipeptides and tripeptides that are taken up by mucosal cells lining the small intestine. Similarly, starch (potatoes, pasta, bread) is degraded by amylase (secreted by the pancreas and entering the small intestine) and other glycosidases (that break the bonds between the simple sugar units) in the intestine to yield glucose. Glucose and other simple sugars, such as fructose and galactose, also come from the digestive breakdown of table sugar (sucrose) and milk sugar (lactose) by the enzymes sucrase and lactase, respectively. Thus, simple sugars are absorbed by the mucosal cells of the small intestine. Lactose intolerance is due to a deficiency in lactase. And milk sugar, in the large intestine, can be used by bacteria to produce a variety of gases, giving those with lactase deficiency a bloated feeling. Lactase deficiency is quite prevalent among adults (particularly among Asian adults) and can be treated by using a dietary supplement containing the deficient lactase enzyme (isolated from microorganisms). Dietary fat (triglyceride) is also broken down by lipases secreted principally by the pancreas. The liberated fatty acids and monoglyceride (one fatty acid attached by ester linkage to glycerol) products are taken up by the intestinal mucosal cells.

It is important to appreciate that the body uses the simple molecules that are absorbed following digestion to construct its own complex molecules. Thus, glucose and amino acids circulate within the blood and are used by various tissues in the synthesis of glycogen or proteins. Glucose can also be used by cells as a fuel substrate to generate ATP. Using dietary fatty acids and monoglycerides, triglycerides are usually synthesized within the intestinal mucosal cells and shipped out within lipoprotein particles (described in Chapter 2) to body tissues. At these locations, the triglycerides are broken down within the circulation and the simpler molecules taken up by nearby cells for use in triglyceride synthesis or for use as fuel substrates in the production of ATP.

Thus, it is not usually the case that large intact dietary molecules like proteins are taken into intestinal mucosal cells to become part of the body's repertoire of macromolecules. Rather, these molecules are first broken down and then the components are utilized to make complex molecules that are designed for the body. Many years ago, a set of dubious experiments that revolved around the biochemical basis of memory was performed. In these, rats were trained to climb, and then RNA was taken from the brains of these animals. The concept was that RNA was responsible for the synthesis of new proteins that were directly linked to the memory of this newly acquired skill. When this RNA was fed to a second set of rats (which did not have climbing in their basic training), sure enough, these animals were now quite competent climbers. Of course, these findings neglected the ability of the gastrointestinal tract of these animals to destroy the RNA. Keep this in mind when patients are hoping to change their lives by nutritional supplements that contain relatively large molecules. Unless the simpler components of these have therapeutic use, they will be wasting their money. Thus, it is important to recognize the power of digestion and the separate metabolic framework that takes place within the cells and tissues of the body.

ENZYMES AND DISEASE

We have talked about genetic mutations that lead to functional abnormalities in proteins, such as coagulation factors VIII and IX (causing the hemophilias), hemoglobin, or the enzymes of heme synthesis (causing the porphyrias). The section on porphyrias in Chapter 5 introduced you to the effects of enzyme deficiency within a pathway. Not only is there a decrease in the generation of the end product, there can also be deleterious effects associated with the build-up of the intermediates formed before the enzyme block within the pathway. These genetic defects result in what are called **inborn errors of metabolism**, many of which can be fatal. For example, an enzyme pathway that begins with A and produces G following a sequence of six enzymes can be represented as A→B→C→D→E→F→G.

A deficiency in the enzyme that converts C→D will reduce production of D, E, F, and ultimately G and increase levels of C and possibly A and B as well. If A, B, or C are toxic in high concentration or, if when they increase in concentration, they can be converted to toxic compounds by other pathways, then pathology can ensue. It's a little like the old adage that the devil (whose biochemistry is as yet an unknown quantity!) finds work for idle hands. If this is a little too retro, you may relate more closely to the fear, expressed by your parent(s), that hanging out in the local shopping mall would turn you into a moral degenerate—hence the need to keep you continuously occupied with school work, skating classes, hockey and football practices, music lessons, and so on. Isn't it interesting to see the number of quite respectable musicians in your class? When there is a slowdown in a pathway and an accumulation of intermediates, significant problems can ensue.

Phenylketonuria

This is an example of an inborn error of metabolism that occurs due to a defect in the enzymatic pathway responsible for the conversion of the amino acid phenylalanine into tyrosine, which serves as precursor in the synthesis of catecholamines, such as epinephrine (adrenaline). The latter is the hormone released into your circulation when you realize that there are approximately 100 pages of notes left to assimilate before an exam and you have, unfortunately, only 60 minutes to do this. The first step in this pathway is the conversion of phenylalanine into tyrosine by the enzyme phenylalanine hydroxylase (Figure 7–3). In this case, while tyrosine can be used to make epinephrine, it can also be used in protein synthesis. In classic or type I phenylketonuria, the enzyme phenylalanine hydroxylase is deficient. This occurs with a frequency of approximately 1 in 10,000 births. As a result, phenylalanine coming from the diet will accumulate in the body. The rising levels of phenylalanine can then be used as a substrate for an enzyme called **transaminase**,

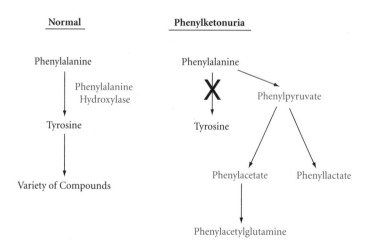

Figure 7–3 Phenylketonuria. A comparison of the normal pathway of phenylalanine metabolism through conversion into tyrosine and the paths that predominate in individuals with phenylketonuria (PKU), a condition usually due to a deficiency in the enzyme phenylalanine hydroxylase responsible for the conversion of phenylalanine → tyrosine. In PKU, phenylalanine is converted to phenylpyruvate, and then to phenyllactate, phenylacetate, and phenylacetylglutamine. These compounds can have deleterious effects in infants and children, leading to mental retardation.

which transfers the amino group from phenylalanine to the molecule pyruvate, forming phenylpyruvate and the amino acid alanine as products:

phenylalanine + pyruvate → phenylpyruvate + alanine

The molecules phenylacetate and phenyllactate can be formed from phenylpyruvate (see Figure 7–3). These compounds, phenylalanine and phenylacetylglutamine (formed from phenylacetate), can be found in the urine of individuals with this inborn error—hence the name phenylketonuria. Brain injury in babies and young children is associated with the build-up of these compounds in the body, and one way to treat the disease is dietary restriction in proteins containing phenylalanine (and enrichment in dietary proteins containing tyrosine). Phenylpyruvate can be detected in the urine or diapers of babies with phenylketonuria. This is a routine test for newborns in many parts of the world and is compulsory in North America and elsewhere.

There are many inborn errors, each the result of a specific genetic defect. It is more likely to find these enzyme deficiencies farther away from the central and more common pathways of metabolism (e.g., the enzymes of the Krebs cycle), as defects in these will inevitably be critical and will not be tolerated in embryonic and fetal development.

AN OVERVIEW OF METABOLIC PATHWAYS

Before we cover certain metabolic pathways in more detail, we shall attempt to present a big picture. This is shown in Figure 7–4. Again, don't be overwhelmed by the detail (and, believe us, this is a simplification of the entire metabolic route map). Rather, take highlighters of different colors and mark the different paths so that you can see the main routes. The image of intersecting subway lines is also useful here, as you will find that different pathways connect at specific points. The main "north-south" line is the catabolism of glucose, either absorbed from blood or generated following the breakdown of glycogen to the derivative glucose-1-phosphate (an ester of glucose linking carbon number 1 of this sugar to a phosphate molecule). Both glucose and glucose-1-phosphate can be converted by different enzymes into glucose-6-phosphate (with the ester situated now on carbon number 6 of glucose). Glucose-6-phosphate is part of the glycolytic pathway. **Glycolysis** simply means a splitting of sugar, for as the glucose-6-phosphate is further metabolized in glycolysis, this six-carbon sugar is broken into two three-carbon molecules. The three-carbon molecules are further metabolized, ultimately resulting in the formation of the three-carbon molecule pyruvate. 1,3-Bisphosphoglycerate is also formed during glycolysis. This compound can be converted by an enzyme reaction into 2,3-bisphosphoglycerate, the important allosteric modulator of the oxygen affin-

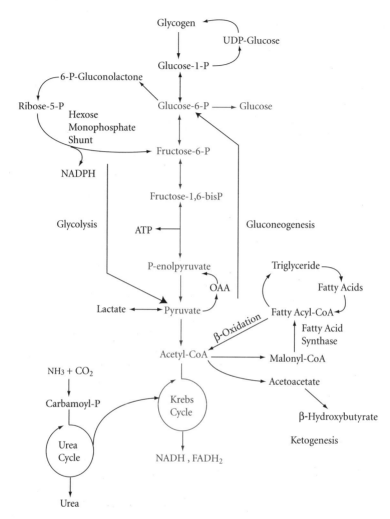

Figure 7–4 The major metabolic routes of intermediary metabolism. Again, it is important not to be overwhelmed by this flow chart but rather to concentrate on the start and end points. Think of it as a subway system, starting with glucose going into glycolysis and the Krebs cycle as the major north-south line. Glycogen synthesis utilizes glucose-6-phosphate, a member of the glycolytic path, while this same intermediate can be used by the hexose monophosphate shunt to produce ribose-5-phosphate, a precursor used in nucleic acid synthesis, and NADPH, used in fatty acid synthesis. To the east of glycolysis is the synthesis and breakdown of fatty acyl-CoA, formed using malonyl-CoA (derived from acetyl-CoA) or broken down following the hydrolysis of triglyceride in the process of β-oxidation. This path generates acetyl-CoA for the Krebs cycle or for ketone body (acetoacetate, β-hydroxybutyrate, and acetone) formation. To the west of the Krebs cycle, ammonia coming from the breakdown of amino acids is used by the urea cycle for the production of urea (which will be excreted by the kidneys). As well, it is possible to go from lactate or pyruvate to oxaloacetate (OAA) and then to phosphoenolpyruvate. Phospho-enolpyruvate can be converted to glucose, largely following a reversal of the enzymes of glycolysis, in the path called gluconeogenesis.

ity of hemoglobin (see Chapter 5). Along the glycolytic pathway, there is a small net production of ATP (two molecules per molecule of glucose entering the path). Within the mitochondria, pyruvate loses carbon dioxide, and the central intermediate acetyl-CoA is formed using CoA. Acetyl-CoA can enter the Krebs cycle, with the production of the reduced coenzymes NADH and $FADH_2$, which serve as sources of electrons for the respiratory chain that provides energy for the synthesis of ATP. The overall net output of ATP is 36 to 38 molecules per molecule of glucose. Basically, what is happening is that glucose is being broken down to carbon dioxide and water, and part of the energy released (about 40%) is conserved in ATP formation. This is the main glycolysis–Krebs cycle central line of catabolic metabolism.

We will also discuss, later in the chapter, the ability of certain tissues to make glucose in a pathway called **gluconeogenesis**. This can be highlighted with another marker and starts with the conversion of pyruvate to oxaloacetate (OAA), which is subsequently converted to phosphoenolpyruvate, followed by a reversal of glycolytic steps (with one exception) going northbound to form glucose-6-phosphate. The last step in gluconeogenesis is the conversion of glucose-6-phosphate to glucose. Gluconeogenesis occurs when levels of glucose are falling (say, during fasting) and glucose is needed for certain organs (principally, the brain).

If you have just eaten a meal, the glucose coming from dietary carbohydrates that is not needed for glycolysis is used to form glucose-6-phosphate, which is converted to glucose-1-phosphate, and this, in turn, is used to make the nucleotide-sugar uridine diphosphate (UDP)-glucose. UDP-glucose can donate glucose in the formation of the glucose polymer glycogen. This is the **glycogen synthesis pathway** and can be highlighted with another color.

Obviously, glucose-6-phosphate is a transfer station in our subway image because you can either go south to glycolysis, north to glycogen synthesis, or west in the **hexose monophosphate (HMP) pathway or shunt**. The major point of the HMP line is to produce five-carbon sugars (ribose-5-phosphate) from the six-carbon sugar glucose-6-phosphate, as well as the reduced coenzyme NADPH. Ribose-5-phosphate is important in the synthesis of nucleic acids, and NADPH is involved in a variety of reactions, including the synthesis of fatty acids. This HMP pathway is sometimes known as the **pentose phosphate shunt**. The term "shunt" comes from the return of the path to the level of fructose-6-phosphate, only one step south of glucose-6-phosphate in the glycolytic chain.

Another line (to the southeast of glucose-6-phosphate) is dedicated to **triglyceride** (triacylglycerol) **synthesis**. Fatty acyl-CoA (an activated form of fatty acid), along with a derivative of glycerol, can generate triglyceride. This fat synthesis pathway occurs in times of feasting. In contrast, the catabolic path begins with triglycerides and degrades these, liberating fatty acids, which are activated to form fatty acyl-CoA; these, in turn, can be degraded by **β-oxidation** to acetyl-CoA for use in the Krebs cycle. This complete breakdown of fatty acids (β-oxidation + Krebs cycle) produces considerably more ATP than that derived from glucose. Acetyl-CoA is a transfer station leading to the Krebs cycle, to fatty acid synthesis via malonyl-CoA, or to ketone bodies, such as acetoacetate. Acetyl-CoA can also be formed during the breakdown of carbon skeletons derived from various amino acids. The carbon skeletons of other amino acids can also enter the Krebs cycle via the production of pyruvate, fumarate, oxaloacetate, or succinyl-CoA. Lastly, in the southwest corner of our metabolic map is the **urea cycle**, which functions to convert relatively toxic ammonia derived from the amino groups of amino acids into the more benign urea, which is excreted in urine. There are intersections between the urea and Krebs cycles.

Again, this is an overview, which will be followed by more careful considerations of these paths; so, don't think we are abandoning you in a transit maze. More general points can be made looking at this metabolic map:

1. Anabolism and catabolism generally make use of different pathways because anabolic paths require energy for synthetic reactions, while catabolic paths involve steps that release energy. Usually, anabolism is not a simple reversal of catabolism. The one partial exception is gluconeogenesis, but we shall see that this is not a complete reversal of glycolysis. Often, catabolic pathways and anabolic ones are located in different cellular compartments. In this way, conditions may be optimized for each pathway (e.g., factors favoring oxidation reactions within the mitochondria and synthetic reactions within the cytosol). As well, the segregation of anabolic and catabolic pathways in this manner allows distinct control mechanisms for each. Thus, fatty acids are broken down to acetyl-CoA by β-oxidation in the mitochondria, while the synthesis of fatty acids using malonyl-CoA takes place in the cytoplasm.

2. Catabolic paths lead to the formation of ATP, NADH, or NADPH, molecules that can be used in a variety of situations, including anabolic pathways. For example, NADPH is required in the synthesis of fatty acids. Malonyl-CoA is the principal source of carbon for fatty acids, and malonyl-CoA is formed from acetyl-CoA in the cytoplasm in a reaction that utilizes ATP.

3. Levels of cofactors, particularly the ratios of oxidized/reduced cofactors, are important determinants in metabolism. Ratios of $NAD^+/NADH$ and $NADP^+/NADPH$ can determine the rates of catabolic pathways. If, for example, there is a relatively high concentration of NADH within a cell, this may slow the catabolism of glucose, as can relatively high concentrations of ATP. This allows the end products of carbohydrate catabolism to regulate catabolic rates. Reciprocal control of glycolysis and gluconeogenesis means simply that the two paths do not operate concurrently.

This makes sense, as it would be wasteful for the liver to make glucose and, at the same time, degrade this very molecule. Thus, a compound that stimulates glycolysis, such as adenosine monophosphate (AMP), which rises in concentration as levels of ATP fall, will inhibit gluconeogenesis simply because AMP serves as an indicator that cellular levels of ATP are low and, thus, glucose breakdown, not formation, is required.

4. Not all these metabolic routes are found in every cell or tissue. While glycolysis is universal in cells, the Krebs cycle is not found in red cells that lack mitochondria, and the cycle is not particularly active in white blood cells. The brain does not demonstrate a very active fatty acid β-oxidation pathway. Rather, the brain usually relies on glucose as its principal fuel substrate when an individual is not fasting. Similarly, the gluconeogenic pathway is found principally in the liver and kidney. You can also appreciate that tissues and organs can cooperate within metabolic schemes. For example, the molecule lactate, produced as an end product of glucose catabolism in red cells and in muscle undergoing strenuous activity (e.g., a 100-meter dash), is lost to the blood and can be picked up by the liver and converted to glucose by the gluconeogenic pathway.

5. The various catabolic paths do not usually function at the same time. For example, following a meal, there is likely sufficient glucose present to provide for cellular energy needs. Thus, triglycerides are not degraded; rather, fat reserves are built up through anabolism following a meal. Similarly, there is no need to use protein for energy under such conditions. In contrast, fasting or dieting will lead to a breakdown of triglycerides so that fatty acid breakdown provides ATP for most tissues, sparing glucose levels that can be augmented by gluconeogenesis in the liver, in an effort to keep the brain supplied with glucose. During fasting, the brain can also, with time, utilize small fuel compounds known as **ketone bodies**, which are formed as by-products of fatty acid oxidation.

REGULATION OF METABOLISM

The metabolic map looks like a subway system or, possibly, the major arteries of traffic running through a city. In this second image, you can appreciate that some control is needed, say, stop lights or traffic cops, to make sure that the streams of cars and trucks are running reasonably smoothly. In the morning, the inbound city traffic predominates, while in the late afternoon, the reverse flow out of the city is dominant—similar to metabolism, where anabolism and catabolism of glycogen or fat do not occur at the same time.

So, how can control be exerted by the biochemical mechanisms? One obvious way is the supply of substrates. An enzyme reaction may potentially have a high rate, but if substrate concentration is low, then the enzyme activity can be very effectively regulated by the supply of substrates. Thus, one metabolic pathway or enzyme providing a substrate for another can efficiently regulate the activity of the downstream enzyme or pathway.

Control can also be exerted through the use of inhibitors. We have mentioned these before, when discussing how aspirin inhibits cyclooxygenase, the key enzyme that converts arachidonic acid into eicosanoids (see Chapter 4). Aspirin is an example of an irreversible inhibitor, which acetylates cyclooxygenase and thus kills this enzyme. Of course, once this enzyme is dead, there is no going back, and more cyclooxygenase must be made by protein synthesis. Penicillin is another irreversible enzyme inhibitor that blocks bacterial wall synthesis. There are also poisons that are irreversible inhibitors. For example, a class of synthetic inhibitors known as the **organophosphates** (sarin, parathion, malathion, and diisopropylfluorophosphate) inhibit a variety of enzymes in two families, called **serine esterases** and **serine proteases**, that have serine as a catalytic amino acid residue at their active sites. Sarin is a nerve gas, but you may encounter parathion or malathion, which are used commercially as insecticides. These compounds effectively kill acetylcholinesterase, the enzyme that removes acetylcholine (the neurotransmitter, as we noted in Chapter 1, that is used in skeletal muscle contraction and in the central nervous system). These poisons can produce paralysis and are quite deadly. There are many examples of young children ingesting similar garden insecticides found in backyard sheds and garages.

Irreversible inhibition can result from the use of drugs, poisons, and toxins, but it is not usual to find irreversible inhibition as a part of normal metabolic control. This type of inhibition naturally limits your options (so, don't burn your biochemistry notes to heat your apartment in the winter, you may need them for other exams coming your way in the spring!).

Reversible inhibition, as its name indicates, is much more flexible and involves the natural products of metabolism. Simply stated, a reversible inhibitor (I) rising in concentration within a cell will bind to an enzyme (E), slow down or block its activity, and then disengage from the enzyme as the concentration of inhibitor falls, restoring enzyme activity. This can be shown as follows:

as I ↑   EI   as I↓   E
A--→B (reaction slowed)   A→B (reaction increases)

You might remember our turnstile–enzyme analogy from Chapter 3, where we showed substrate molecules, like commuters, streaming through subway turnstiles to enter transit stations, effectively being turned into product molecules. What would happen when a commuter approaches the turnstile and realizes that she or he does not have a ticket or a token? Naturally, she or he cannot proceed through. In other words, the reaction cannot take place. However, there is no mechanism whereby the enzyme can spit out this nonpaying commuter. Rather, she or he could sit within the turnstile, blocking turnstile traffic and slowing down the passage of commuters into the subway. This is known as **competitive inhibition**, where a molecule that looks like a substrate molecule (paying commuter) inhibits an enzyme by binding at the active site without a subsequent reaction taking place. Ultimately, this nonpaying commuter may be displaced from the turnstile by other paying commuters. However, if the subway station is flooded with nonpaying commuters (competitive inhibitors), prolonged enzyme inhibition will follow.

If you remember the velocity versus substrate concentration plots we showed in Chapter 3, the effect of a fixed concentration of competitive inhibitor in this reaction is shown in Figure 7-5. The curve is still hyperbolic but is shifted to the right. It simply means that you need an increased concentration of substrate molecules, relative to the inhibitor, before you can get up to the maximal enzyme velocity (Vmax). Remember that the concentration of substrate that gives one half of the Vmax is called the **Km** (Michaelis constant) for the reaction. You can see that the competitive inhibitor increases the value of Km for the enzyme, although the Vmax is not altered. It just takes a higher substrate concentration to get to the Vmax, a little like putting a piece of foam rubber under the accelerator in your car. You can get to the maximal speed; it just takes more pressure on the gas pedal. A specific biochemical example is the enzyme succinate dehydrogenase that converts succinate (within the Krebs cycle) to the product fumarate (Figure 7–6). It does this by introducing a double bond between the inner two carbons of succinate. Malonate is a competitive inhibitor for this reaction. Like succinate, which it resembles, malonate does have two -COO⁻ groups, but as it has only three carbons, it is impossible for the enzyme to create a double bond in this molecule (see Figure 7–6). Thus, malonate binds at the active site of the enzyme and cannot be processed. It prevents other molecules of succinate from immediately entering the active site of the enzyme, thus slowing the reaction rate.

An analogous situation arises when an enzyme has more than one substrate. For example, a phosphatase (E-1) may remove phosphate groups from two closely related molecules, A-P and B-P (using P to denote the phosphate group). If you are following the enzyme reaction using A-P as substrate, the addition of B-P will slow the reaction A-P → A + P. The effect of B-P will be similar to that of a competitive inhibitor. The one difference is that B-P does serve as a substrate for the enzyme, as B-P is converted to B + P. It is, thus, possible to slow down the hydrolysis of A-P by the production of B-P in another reaction sequence controlled by the enzyme E-2. Thus, a second reaction can control the hydrolysis of the original substrate A-P.

E-1

In the absence of B,   A-P → A + P (brisk reaction)

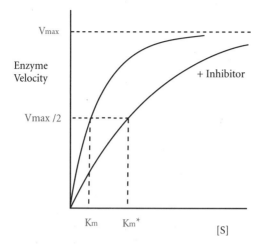

Figure 7–5 Michaelis-Menten enzyme kinetics showing the effects of a competitive inhibitor. The hyperbolic plot (enzyme velocity vs substrate concentration [S]) is shifted to the right, in the presence of the inhibitor, raising the Km value for the substrate to Km* while leaving the Vmax for the reaction unchanged.

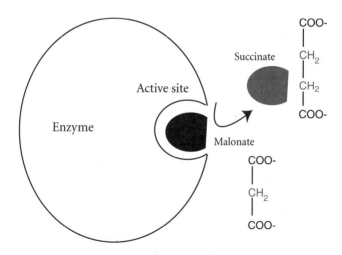

Figure 7–6 Competitive inhibition. Here the enzyme succinate dehydrogenase, which utilizes succinate as its substrate, can be very effectively inhibited by the molecule malonate. Malonate can bind at the active site of the enzyme but has only three carbons (in comparison with the four found in succinate), and thus, malonate cannot participate in the reaction. Malonate effectively blocks the active site of the enzyme and increases the Km value for the natural substrate succinate.

$$\text{In the presence of B,} \quad \begin{array}{c} \text{E-2} \\ \text{B} \rightarrow \text{B-P,} \end{array} \quad \begin{array}{c} \text{B-P} \rightarrow \text{B} + \text{P} \\ \text{E1} \\ \text{A-P} \dashrightarrow \text{A} + \text{P (slowed reaction)} \end{array}$$

You may find in other texts examples of a second kind of inhibition called noncompetitive inhibition. Here, the inhibitor binds not to the active site but at another locus on the enzyme. This inhibition does not affect the Km for a substrate, but it will lower the Vmax, as the binding of this inhibitor can cause a conformational change in the enzyme that will reduce the catalytic efficiency of the active site. It may be as simple as causing the catalytic amino acid residues involved in the reaction to move farther away from one another. While noncompetitive inhibition is a logical counterpoint to competitive inhibition, in actual fact, there are rather few examples of this within metabolism. What is more common is the next type of regulation of enzymes known as **allosteric modulation**.

Allosteric Enzymes

We have discussed allosteric effects in oxygen binding to the hemoglobin tetramer (see Chapter 5). You may recall that the binding of oxygen to one site in the tetramer increases oxygen affinity for a second heme site within a second subunit. "Allosteric" means other site; thus, binding oxygen at one subunit (polypeptide) can promote oxygen binding at a second subunit. Allostery can be seen in the cooperativity of a substrate binding to an enzyme (analogous to the cooperativity in oxygen binding by hemoglobin) and in the modulation of the enzyme activity. Allosteric effects are almost always seen with multisubunit enzymes. Thus, we must move into the realm of quaternary protein structure, namely, the association of separate polypeptides, that comprise a multisubunit enzyme.

Enzymes are often regulated by compounds that are neither substrates nor products of the enzyme. Thus, an enzyme (often the first in a metabolic path) may contribute to the synthesis of an end product; yet, the end product may have few structural similarities to the initial substrate. This end product can regulate the first enzyme by binding at a site that is removed from the active site. One example that we have mentioned in Chapter 5 is the synthesis of heme, the prosthetic group found in heme proteins, such as hemoglobin and myoglobin. You may recall that the first step in the pathway of heme synthesis is catalyzed by the enzyme ALA synthase, which converts the substrates succinyl-CoA and glycine into ALA (aminolevulinate). In subsequent steps, porphobilinogen, hydroxymethylbilane, and then a succession of complex porphyrinogens is formed until heme is produced, following the activity of last enzyme in the pathway ferrochetalase, which inserts an iron ion into the heme structure. Heme can regulate its synthesis by blocking the production of more ALA synthase molecules (a process called **repression**) and also by allosterically binding this enzyme. This allosteric regulation is an example of feedback inhibition, as rising concentrations of heme will slow down the first step in the synthetic pathway.

$$\text{E1} \leftarrow\text{---}$$
$$\text{Succinyl-CoA + glycine} \rightarrow \text{ALA} \rightarrow \text{Porphobilinogen} \rightarrow\rightarrow\rightarrow\rightarrow\rightarrow\rightarrow \text{Heme}$$

Heme is an allosteric inhibitor of ALA synthase (E-1). ALA synthase is considered to be the first committed step in the metabolic pathway that synthesizes heme. Regulating a path at this first committed step allows an economy of control for the pathway. If control were exerted at an enzyme farther along in the sequence of reactions, this would permit a loss of succinyl-CoA and glycine and an inefficient build-up of undesirable intermediates when heme is already present in optimal concentrations.

Another type of allosteric control is that exerted by a compound coming from another pathway or process that exerts an effect on an enzyme. There is usually a rationale for this type of control, as the allosteric modulator may effectively signal the increase or decrease in activity of the enzyme. For example, the enzyme that breaks down glycogen, producing glucose derivatives that enter glycolysis to initiate energy production, is glycogen phosphorylase. Glycogen phosphorylase exists as a dimer of identical subunits. This enzyme can exist in a relatively inactive form called **phosphorylase b**. If levels of adenosine monophosphate (AMP) begin to rise in the cell, it is usually a sign that levels of ATP are falling. AMP serves as an allosteric activator of phosphorylase b, since phosphorylase b becomes active and begins to degrade glycogen after the binding of AMP at the allosteric site. Thus, rates of glycolysis within the cell increase, and ultimately ATP can be made by the actions of the Krebs cycle, electron transport, and oxidative phosphorylation.

glycogen phosphorylase b (inactive)
$$\downarrow$$
glycogen phosphorylase b-AMP (active)
$$\downarrow$$
glycogen $\rightarrow$ glucose-1-phosphate $\rightarrow$ glycolysis $\rightarrow$ Krebs cycle $\rightarrow$ ATP

Allosteric multienzyme complexes typically show sigmoid kinetics. And allosteric inhibitors or activators (also known collectively as allosteric modulators) effectively shift the curve of enzyme velocity versus substrate concentration to the right or left, respectively (Figure 7–7).

Phosphorylation and Dephosphorylation in Regulation

Another mechanism in enzyme control is the covalent modification of the enzyme itself. We have noted this in the acetylation of cyclooxygenase by aspirin. However, this is not a reversible process, unlike phosphorylation/dephosphorylation. The phosphorylation of certain enzymes at amino acid residues that have -OH groups (e.g., serine, threonine, or tyrosine) will result in enzyme activation or inhibition. Thus, there are enzymes called **protein kinases**, which make use of ATP as a phosphate donor to generate a phosphate ester or esters at strategically located serines, threonines, or tyrosines within a substrate enzyme molecule. A protein kinase reaction for one serine residue (Ser) within an enzyme (E) is shown below:

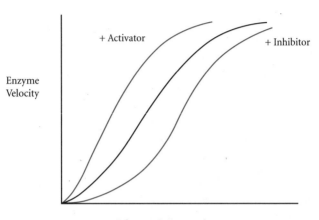

Figure 7–7 Allosteric kinetics. These enzyme kinetics are often shown by multisubunit enzymes that have distinct active sites and regulatory sites for the binding of allosteric inhibitors and activators. The shape of the enzyme rate versus substrate concentration curve is sigmoidal, as allosteric enzymes show cooperativity in the binding of substrate. An allosteric activator will shift the sigmoid curve to the left, while an allosteric inhibitor will displace the curve to the right.

$$\text{E-Ser-CH}_2\text{-OH} + \text{ATP} \rightarrow \text{E-Ser-CH}_2\text{-OPO}_3^{2-} + \text{ADP}$$

Protein kinases can be divided into two large groups: those that phosphorylate serine or threonine (serine/threonine kinases) and those that phosphorylate tyrosine (tyrosine kinases). Within each of these families are kinases that specifically phosphorylate individual proteins. We noted in Chapter 1 myosin light chain kinase (MLCK), cyclic AMP (cAMP)–dependent kinases (e.g., protein kinase A), and cyclic guanosine monophosphate (cGMP)–dependent kinases. As you may remember, these kinases were activated as a result of signalling pathways, each initiated by a stimulatory event (e.g., the action of a hormone or neurotransmitter at the cell surface). To allow a return to a nonphosphorylated form of an enzyme, phosphatase activities are employed.

$$\text{E-Ser-CH}_2\text{-OPO}_3^{2-} \rightarrow \text{E-Ser-CH}_2\text{-OH} + {}^-\text{OPO}_3^{2-} \text{ (inorganic phosphate)}$$

Thus, there can be enzyme regulation by a cycle of phosphorylation and dephosphorylation.

With respect to signalling and phosphorylation cycles, consider another route for the activation of glycogen phosphorylase b when glucose derivatives are needed for energy (Figure 7–8). The second messenger cAMP can activate protein kinase A, which, in turn, phosphorylates and activates an enzyme known as **phosphorylase kinase**. True to its name, this kinase will phosphorylate glycogen phosphorylase b converting it into an active form of the enzyme known as **glycogen phosphorylase a**. Glycogen breakdown then ensues.

It is not always the case that phosphorylation activates an enzyme. In some cases, phosphorylation will lead to enzyme inactivation. For example, while protein kinase A phosphorylates and activates glycogen phosphorylase, protein kinase A also phosphorylates glycogen synthase (the enzyme that assembles glycogen polymers using UDP-glucose) and inactivates this enzyme activity (Figure 7–9). This shows the regulatory balance between anabolic and catabolic processes, which ensures that both are not activated at the same time. In a corresponding manner, the same phosphatase that inactivates the phosphorylated glycogen phosphorylase will activate glycogen synthase by dephosphorylation.

Signal Transduction

As you can appreciate from the glycogen phosphorylase example above, phosphorylation and enzyme activation or inactivation are products of a

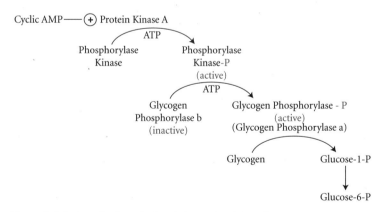

Figure 7–8 Pathway for the activation of glycogen breakdown. The second messenger cyclic AMP (itself generated from ATP following binding of adrenaline to the muscle cell) activates protein kinase A. This enzyme can covalently modify and activate the enzyme phosphorylase kinase by phosphorylation (addition of phosphate group[s]). The activated phosphorylase kinase, in turn, catalyzes the activation of the enzyme glycogen phosphorylase b by another phosphorylation reaction. This activated enzyme (known as glycogen phosphorylase a) catalyzes the degradation of glycogen to glucose-1-phosphate, which can be converted to glucose-6-phosphate.

chain of events initiated by cellular activation. We have used the example of adrenaline, which stimulates muscle cells, ultimately leading to the activation of glycogen breakdown. We described second messengers in Chapter 1, and these are important elements of this chain of activation. The initial step is the binding of a biologically active ligand (e.g., a hormone or neurotransmitter) to a specific receptor protein at the plasma membrane.

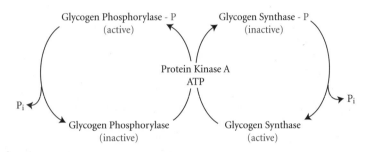

Figure 7–9 Phosphorylation and dephosphorylation. While the phosphorylated form of glycogen phosphorylase (glycogen phosphorylase a) is active, phosphorylation of glycogen synthase inactivates this enzyme. For both enzyme-phosphates, there is a phosphatase that removes this covalent modification, effectively deactivating glycogen phosphorylase (to produce glycogen phosphorylase b) while activating glycogen synthase. The differences in the response of the two enzymes to this cycle of covalent modification control the balance between the anabolic and catabolic reactions involving glycogen.

When adrenaline binds to its receptor on the muscle cell, there follows the activation of a **Gs-protein heterotrimer**, composed of α-, β-, and γ-subunits (Figure 7–10). G-proteins are so called because they can bind guanine nucleotides, which are relatives of the adenine nucleotides (see Chapter 8), at the α-subunit. During inactivity, this bound nucleotide is guanosine diphosphate (GDP). However, following binding of adrenaline to its receptor, the receptor (more specifically called the β-adrenergic receptor) interacts with the Gs-heterotrimer. As a result, GDP is exchanged for guanosine triphosphate (GTP), and the GTP–α-subunit complex dissociates from the βγ-subunits and interacts with the membrane-bound enzyme adenylate cyclase. This enzyme is activated and converts ATP into cAMP, the second messenger. We have noted how cAMP, through three additional enzymes in the signalling pathway, achieves the breakdown of glycogen. This is a signal transduction pathway, initiated with the binding of adrenaline, mediated by Gs-protein and cAMP and completed by the liberation of glucose derivatives for energy production.

This signalling event is transient because GTP attached to the α-subunit is readily hydrolyzed to GDP by a GTPase activity, and the α-subunit then rejoins the βγ-subunits in the resting αβγ conformation. Similarly, cAMP is readily destroyed by the action of cAMP phosphodiesterase and is, thus, short lived. This enzyme, interestingly enough, can be inhibited by caffeine, which prolongs the stimulatory effect of cAMP. Because the signalling cascade utilizes a series of enzyme activation events, there is a considerable amplification effect, as each enzyme can activate a large number of substrate enzyme molecules, which, in turn, will activate an even larger number of

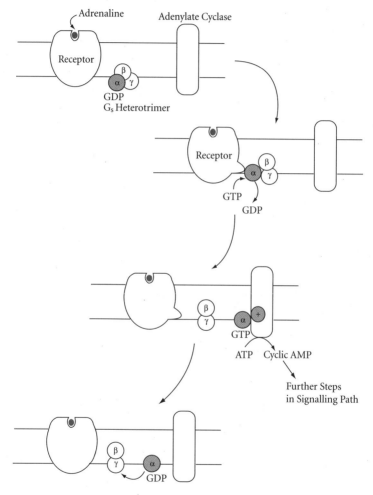

Figure 7–10 The activation of adenylate cyclase. When adrenaline binds to its receptor on the plasma membrane of a muscle cell, an activation of the Gs-protein heterotrimer occurs. This is accompanied by a release of GDP and an acquisition of GTP by the α-subunit of the trimer. This promotes a dissociation of the α-subunit, which can activate adenylate cyclase. This enzyme produces the second messenger cAMP, which initiates a signalling pathway. There is a GTPase activity within the α-subunit that degrades the bound GTP to GDP, leading to a return of the α-subunit and a reformation of the Gs-protein heterotrimer, with deactivation of adenylate cyclase.

their substrate enzymes. Because of this, a signalling pathway is often called a **cascade** (similar to the avalanche of protein events we described for coagulation in Chapter 4).

G-heterotrimers and adenylate cyclase/cAMP signalling are also involved following the binding of other hormones to their receptors in the plasma membrane. One example is glucagon, the starvation hormone, released from the pancreas during fasting. There are also hormones that will inhibit adenylate cyclase, following binding to their receptors and the activation of a different class of G-heterotrimers called **Gi** (Figure 7–11). Thus, it is the balance between the actions of stimulatory and inhibitory hormones that determines which signalling path is predominant. Interestingly, cholera toxin exerts its effects by entering intestinal cells and modifying the Gs-heterotrimer so that it remains in an activated state (GTP cannot be hydrolyzed to GDP). As cAMP switches on ion transporters in the intestinal cells, rapid and fatal dehydration can follow, as there is a continuous and massive loss of salts and water from these intestinal cells. In a similar manner, pertussis toxin (*Bordetella pertussis* infections cause whooping cough) modifies the Gi-heterotrimer so that inhibitory control cannot be exerted over adenylate cyclase.

Another signalling path described in Chapter 4 involves platelets and the phospholipid phosphatidylinositol 4,5-bisphosphate (PIP$_2$). Thrombin, on interaction with its receptor in the platelet plasma membrane, activates another class of heterotrimeric G-proteins referred to as **Gp** (Figure 7–12). The α-subunit–GTP complex of Gp can activate the enzyme phospholipase C, an enzyme that converts PIP$_2$ into membrane-bound diacylglycerol and water-soluble inositol trisphosphate (IP$_3$). IP$_3$ elevates the levels of cytosolic free calcium ions, and these, in concert with diacylglycerol, activate protein kinase C. This will lead to the shape changes of platelets, as noted in Chapter 4.

If calcium ion levels rise, another line of signalling can be activated by the association of calcium with calmodulin and the subsequent activation

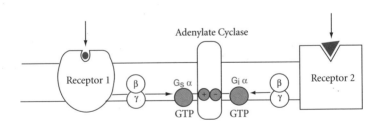

Figure 7–11 Balance of paths activated by stimulatory and inhibitory ligands. Just as there is a Gs-protein heterotrimer, whose Gsα-subunit can stimulate adenylate cyclase, there are also Gi protein heterotrimers, and here, the Giα-subunit (once activated) will inhibit adenylate cyclase. Thus, two different ligands or hormones can have opposing effects exerted through different G-proteins. Depending on which hormone predominates, there will be either a formation of cAMP or a block in the formation of this second messenger.

of calcium/calmodulin–dependent kinases, such as MLCK of smooth muscle (see Chapter 1). Rising levels of calcium can also activate phospholipase A_2, which, in turn, releases arachidonate from membrane phospholipids. Recall that arachidonate is the precursor for a variety of eicosanoids, including thromboxane A_2 in platelets (see Chapter 4).

Induction and Repression of Enzyme Synthesis

One final mechanism in the regulation of metabolism involves the synthesis of new enzyme molecules rather than the control of existing ones. In this situation, a specific signal given to cells, following signal transduction pathways, will result in the production or activation of transcription factors that promote the generation of messenger RNA (mRNA) from a particular genetic sequence within nuclear DNA. This sequence of events leads to increased synthesis of the encoded enzyme and is known as **enzyme induction**. Transcription is described in the next chapter in some detail. In Chapter 4, we noted the effects of corticosteroid anti-inflammatories on arachidonate release catalyzed by the enzyme phospholipase A_2. Corticosteroids promote the synthesis of mRNA encoding a protein called lipocortin 1. Thus, corticosteroids induce the synthesis of lipocortin 1, which inhibits phospholipase A_2 and thereby blocks the release of arachidonate and generation of eicosanoids. Corticosteroids also reduce the expression of cyclooxygenase 2 (COX-2), the enzyme that is usually upregulated in inflammatory

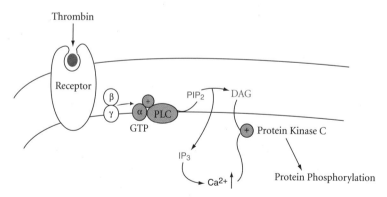

Figure 7–12 The inositide signalling pathway. In platelets, this pathway can be initiated by the binding of thrombin to its receptor, which activates a Gp-protein heterotrimer. In this case, the enzyme phospholipase C is activated and degrades the membrane phospholipid PIP_2. The inositol trisphosphate product (IP_3) of the enzyme triggers the release of calcium ions from the endoplasmic reticulum. The rising concentration of free calcium ions, together with the diacylglycerol product of phospholipase C, activates protein kinase C, leading to other protein phosphorylation events and cellular responses (such as platelet shape changes seen with platelet activation).

processes. Corticosteroids diminish the synthesis of mRNA for COX-2 and thus repress this key enzyme in eicosanoid synthesis. In a similar manner, as discussed in Chapter 5, phenobarbital can lead to the induction of the glucuronosyl transferases that are used in the liver to produce conjugated bilirubin. This drug can be used to treat neonatal jaundice, which may be caused, in part, by inadequate levels of these bilirubin-processing enzymes.

These induction and repression events are due to alterations of transcription (mRNA synthesis). It is also possible to regulate enzyme synthesis at the level of protein translation, the assembly of amino acids following the mRNA blueprint.

Generally, induction/repression events require a longer time span than the other regulatory mechanisms we have noted, as new protein has to be made, or else the synthesis of a protein associated with a distinct pathologic process has to be repressed and the existing protein degraded. In contrast, enzyme inhibitors and phosphorylation paths can exert their effects within seconds to minutes.

BIOENERGETICS

Many of the concepts of metabolism are focused on the production of energy and the formation of NADH (a coenzyme with energy associated with its reduced state) and ATP (the energy transferring molecule). ATP powers anabolism and is a vital component in muscle contraction and an important element in a number of membrane transport processes and kinase reactions. The basic concept underlying bioenergetics is the liberation of energy contained in various fuel molecules and the conservation of this energy in a useful chemical form. Thus, it is not enough to light a fire and produce heat from the combustion of wood or coal; some of the heat has to be saved for future use, somewhat like charging a car battery during the running of an internal combustion engine so that the battery can be used to run the starter motor and also the lights, air conditioning, and inboard audio system.

Molecules, such as ATP, ADP, AMP (the two less energetic relatives of ATP), NAD$^+$, and NADH are very important, as a cell can evaluate its energy levels by the concentrations of these molecules. The NAD$^+$/NADH, ADP/ATP, and AMP/ATP ratios are important in regulating catabolic events that lead to ATP and NADH production. This is similar to the operation of a thermostat that senses a drop in room or office temperature and signals the activation of a heating system to break down a fuel (natural gas or oil) to provide heat energy.

Without belaboring the principles of thermodynamics (likely not a favorite memory from previous courses in physical chemistry), there are usually changes in free energy when one or more substrates are converted into one or more products. The free energy change (ΔG) is given by the equation $\Delta G = \Delta H - T\Delta S$, where ΔH is the change in enthalpy (heat), T is the temperature in degrees Kelvin, and ΔS is the change in entropy (order or randomness). While enthalpy is pretty tangible, entropy is sometimes difficult to understand. As the degree of disorder increases in a system, there is a corresponding rise in entropy, and ΔS is a positive value. There is an inherent tendency toward disorder, as you may realize when you don't clean up your room/apartment/flat for a period of several weeks. In chemical terms, when you produce a number of smaller molecules from one substrate, there is an increase in entropy (i.e., an increase in disorder). Thus, any catabolic process will show an overall positive ΔS value. In this way, you can see that ΔG for a catabolic pathway (say, the conversion of glucose to two molecules of pyruvate) (see Figure 7–2) will be a negative value, as ΔH will be negative (as heat is lost) and ΔS will be positive (as a larger number of simpler molecules is produced). Generally, the magnitude of ΔG will depend on the extent of breakdown of a fuel substrate. Thus, the complete breakdown of glucose to CO_2 and H_2O (glycolysis and the Krebs cycle) will have a larger ΔG value than the less extensive conversion of glucose (six carbons) to pyruvate (three carbons) in glycolysis alone.

By a similar logic, when more complex molecules are constructed from a larger number of simpler molecules in an anabolic pathway, ΔG will be positive, and the reaction usually requires an energy input, often in the form of ATP. For example, the assembly of glucose molecules into the large polymer glycogen requires ATP.

As the cells of the body require a continuous supply of fuel substrates to maintain adequate levels of ATP, and as you are not continuously eating to supply these fuels, there is a need to store fuels (derived from digestion) in a convenient form. We have mentioned glycogen, and granules containing this polymer can be found in abundance both in the liver and in muscle (Table 7–1). We have noted that triglycerides are the most abundant form of stored fuel within the body, and fat does make up the bulk of your fuel reserves. Triglyceride is stored in adipose or fat cells, located at fairly obvious places throughout the male and female anatomies. The energy values for fat and glycogen are measured in kilocalories. Kilocalories are equivalent to Calories, although this second term is not terribly useful because it is easily confused with calories (with small "c"). When the media or your patients mention "calories," you can assume that they mean kilocalories. Perhaps because of this misunderstanding, there has, in recent years, been a move toward the use of the kilojoule (kJ) as a standardized unit of energy (1 kilocal = 4.18 kJ). As a professional within the health sciences, you are far more likely to encounter the terms kilocalorie (kcal) or Calorie; hence, we have used this unit in the following discussion.

You have more fat than glycogen stored in your body, and fat has several advantages compared with carbohydrate. Specifically, carbohydrate (glucose, glycogen, other sugars) will yield 4 kcal/g while fat yields 9 kcal/g.

Thus, Arctic and Antarctic explorers, who need foods high in caloric value, prefer to take foods rich in fat rather than carbohydrate. Another advantage of fat (triglyceride) is that it is hydrophobic and can be stored in an anhydrous condition, whereas the very polar glycogen must be stored in a hydrated form. Thus, glycogen (with all its associated water molecules) takes up more space. A useful image for this increased volume in hydrated carbohydrate is the considerable difference in volume between a cup of dry macaroni and that same sample of macaroni after it has been boiled (hydration). One advantage of glycogen is that glucose derivatives can be produced more quickly from this polymer, while fat is not as quickly mobilized as a stored fuel. In the adult male, on average some 135,000 kcal are stored in fat, with 900 kcal in glycogen and potentially 24,000 kcal in protein (see Table 7–1). The daily recommended food intakes (expressed in energy terms) for a 55-kg female and a 70-kg male are 2,200 kcal and 2,900 kcal, respectively. Thus, 1 kg of dietary fat (9,000 kcal) can sustain an adult for about 3 to 4 days. If our typical 70-kg male were stranded on a small desert island, with no coconuts or other food at hand, his fat reserves could sustain him for about 2 months. A similar time frame is available for the 50-kg female, although women are less likely to allow themselves to be marooned in this manner. It almost always seems to be males who needlessly place themselves in harm's way.

Of course, the number of kilocalories required on a daily basis will be a function of physical activity. Obviously, more kilocalories are required if our marooned male is running around, vainly attempting to attract the attention of a passing 747, instead of trying to improve his tan by languidly sunning himself on his exclusive beach. Another factor is the environmental temperature. Naturally, more kilocalories are required if you are shipwrecked in the Arctic, as opposed to a tropical island. Parenthetically, if you are stuck in a bus shelter in February and you begin to shiver, this is a sim-

Table 7–1
Compounds Used as Fuel within the Body*

Compound	Location	Grams	Kilocalories
Glucose	Blood, extra-cellular fluids	20	80
Glycogen	Muscle	150	600
Glycogen	Liver	75	300
Protein	Muscle	6,000	24,000
Fat (triglyceride)	Adipose tissue	15,000	135,000

*Values given are for a 70-kg male.

ple mechanism whereby skeletal muscular contraction produces heat to maintain body temperature.

If you consume more kilocalories than you need to, on a daily basis, your fat reserves will increase, and you will gain weight. This is part of a natural survival mechanism so that you will have fuel reserves to fall back on should food sources become scarce. The classic image is that of the bear that builds up considerable fat reserves in the fall and uses them up during hibernation in the long winter. While this mechanism was useful for our very distant ancestors, who might not have known where their next meal of woolly mammoth was coming from, it has distinct disadvantages for those without a food supply problem—hence the birth of the lucrative weight reduction industry. As a health professional, you will frequently encounter patients who have (or believe they have) a weight problem. It is incumbent on you to give them sound advice and guidance and to steer them away from deleterious dietary regimens that are centered on one or very few foods (i.e., the grapefruit, protein, or steak-and-eggs diet). Remember that dietitians are professionals who should be consulted in dietary matters. Often, medical practitioners have retained little or no knowledge of nutrition. Anorexia and bulimia similarly require the input of bona fide medical specialists.

CARBOHYDRATE METABOLISM

We have already mentioned glucose and its use as a fuel substrate in glycolysis and the Krebs cycle. Thus, glucose is an important fuel in the production of ATP by oxidative phosphorylation within the mitochondria. Glucose is the preferred compound used by the brain for energy production, and thus, it is critical to maintain a minimum blood glucose level. Naturally, blood glucose levels will increase following the consumption of sugars or more complex carbohydrates. However, fasting blood glucose levels are within a range of 4 to 5.5 mM (70 to 110 mg/dL). During a fast or starvation, fat will become the predominant fuel, but it is necessary to produce glucose to maintain the blood levels of this compound, predominantly for the brain.

Sources of Glucose

Many foods provide glucose. Sucrose or table sugar is made up of glucose and the simple sugar fructose; the milk sugar lactose is made up of glucose and galactose. Sucrose and lactose can be readily digested with a rapid production and absorption of glucose. A rapidly available source of glucose is grape juice, which is largely composed of this simple sugar. Complex dietary carbohydrates include starch (potatoes, bread, and pasta), which requires more extensive breakdown during digestion. Thus, these foods release glucose more slowly than sucrose or lactose. If you begin to fast, glucose can be quite readily supplied by the breakdown of glycogen found in the liver and muscle. We have noted how glycogen can be broken down by glycogen phosphorylase as a result of a signalling pathway initiated by the binding of adrenaline to a muscle cell surface. In a similar way, the starvation hormone glucagon, by binding at the liver cells, can facilitate the breakdown of liver glycogen. If the glycogen stores are depleted, which occurs in prolonged fasting or during a marathon race, the synthesis of glucose by gluconeogenesis in the liver takes place. The three-carbon compound lactate, produced by the muscles and red cells, can be used by the liver to generate glucose, with the use of energy provided by ATP.

Carbohydrate Oxidation and Energy Production

If glucose enters glycolysis and is broken down into the two molecules of pyruvate, there is a net production of two molecules of ATP as a result of the direct generation of ATP during two enzymatic reactions (Figure 7–13). Pyruvate is converted to acetyl-CoA, and this molecule enters the Krebs cycle, which subsequently generates the reduced coenzymes NADH and $FADH_2$. These coenzymes can donate electrons for the electron transport chain, and the loss of energy associated with the passage of these electrons down the chain accounts for the production of ATP in oxidative phosphorylation (ADP + phosphate $\rightarrow$ ATP + water).

Following the entry of each molecule of acetyl-CoA, 12 molecules of ATP are generated. Also taking into account the ATP produced in glycolysis, and the NADH produced during glycolysis and the conversion of pyruvate to acetyl-CoA, one glucose molecule will yield a grand total of 36 or 38 molecules of ATP. The total number of ATP molecules is tissue dependent because of different mechanisms whereby the reducing power of NADH produced in the cytoplasm (in glycolysis) is made available for electron transport within the mitochondria. The higher total yield of 38 molecules of ATP is found in the liver, while the muscles and brain show the smaller value of 36 ATP molecules.

Roles of Different Organs in Fuel Metabolism

You may appreciate by now that different organs and cells within the body have considerably different parts to play during fasting or feeding. The latter term is simply used to describe the well-fed state and is used likely because it has a certain alliterative appeal. The various organs can almost take on human personalities. The brain is the somewhat spoilt, favorite child, who prefers only one fuel, namely, glucose. Because of the importance of the central nervous system (in most humans!), sacrifices will be made in attempts to ensure that the brain is kept supplied with glucose. The liver is often described as the orchestra leader when it comes to nutrition and fuel metabolism, and, indeed, the liver is the parental figure struggling to keep everyone (particularly the brain) happy. Thus, if there is a decline in blood sugar, the liver will ultimately sacrifice its glycogen reserves in efforts to maintain the blood glucose level. The liver can also switch on its gluconeogenic pathway for the synthesis of glucose. Thus, the liver is a provider. Muscle, in our analogy, is a body-building sibling who is not particularly

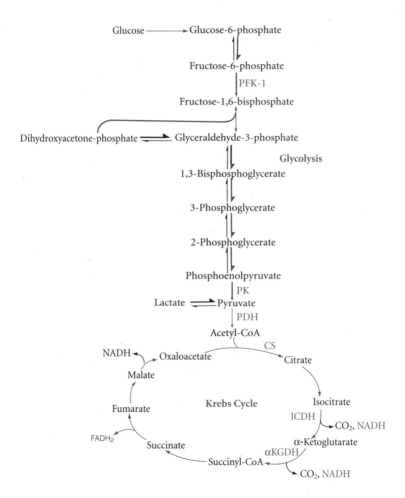

Figure 7–13 Glycolysis and the Krebs cycle. Key regulatory enzymes include phosphofructokinase-1 (PFK-1), pyruvate kinase (PK), and pyruvate dehydrogenase (PDH). Within the Krebs cycle, regulation is exerted at citrate synthase (CS), isocitrate dehydrogenase (ICDH), and α-ketoglutarate dehydrogenase (αKGDH).

interested in the fate of the family, as long as he or she is well fed. Thus, muscle (like the brain) is a consumer, but happily, muscle has a rather broader taste for fuel substrates and will consume either glucose or fatty acids derived from triglycerides. Naturally, if muscle degrades its own glycogen, the resulting molecules of glucose-1-phosphate will be used for its own glycolysis. Muscle, unlike liver, does not provide glucose for the blood. Adipose tissue is, of course, the couch potato, happily taking in whatever fuel substrates (glucose or fatty acids) that come its way, gaining weight and usually not exerting itself, unlike muscle, its more energetic sibling.

Diabetes Mellitus

Discussion of carbohydrate metabolism with health professionals inevitably brings us to a very common and very important metabolic disease. Diabetes mellitus (DM) affects about 4% of the population and is, thus, a highly prevalent disorder. You are much more likely to encounter diabetic patients than ones who have phenylketonuria. DM generally is due to a lack of the hormone insulin or a resistance to the effects of this hormone. The term "diabetes" (literally, a siphoning through) refers to the polyuria seen with the disease, and the term "mellitus" indicates that the urine of diabetics is actually sweet because of the presence of glucose. We leave it to your imagination to figure out how this latter finding was originally made. You may also encounter an entirely different condition (that does not involve carbohydrate metabolism) called **diabetes insipidus**, arising due to a deficiency of antidiuretic hormone and the attendant production of large volumes of urine that is not enriched in glucose.

DM can be classified into two broad categories. Type I DM generally has its onset before adulthood and is caused by a deficiency in insulin production. Insulin is made by the β-cells of the pancreatic islets of Langerhans. Pancreas has both an exocrine function (the production of catabolic enzymes for secretion and use in intestinal digestion) and an endocrine function (the production and secretion of hormones, such as insulin and glucagon, that enter the blood). In type I DM, it is likely that β-cells have been destroyed in an autoimmune reaction and, thus, there is a deficiency of this hormone. Autoimmune reactions involve the attack and destruction of body cells by the immune system. Type II DM is a more complex disease and usually affects adults who may have a tendency to be overweight. In this condition, there may be a resistance to the effects of insulin so that insulin cannot adequately modify the metabolism of cells that normally are insulin responsive. It is also possible in type II DM to detect impaired pancreatic function and deficits in insulin production and secretion. Of the two types of DM, type II is by far the more prevalent.

You may also see the terms insulin-dependent DM (IDDM) and non–insulin-dependent DM (NIDDM) used to describe type I and type II DM. The limitation in this older terminology is that some type II diabetics do show impaired insulin production. These type II diabetics can be treated with dietary restriction of simple sugars, drugs that increase insulin output, and ultimately insulin administration.

Under normal circumstances, insulin is made as a linear polypeptide known as **preproinsulin** (Figure 7–14), with a signal sequence at the N-terminus of this protein that facilitates its movement into the lumen of the endoplasmic reticulum. Remember, most plasma proteins are made in the liver by a similar mechanism, which we discussed in Chapter 2. Within the endoplasmic reticulum, the signal sequence is removed from this precursor polypeptide to generate the shorter proinsulin. In turn, disulfide (-S-S-) bridges are made between the side chains of amino acids, and the proinsulin is selectively cleaved by proteolytic enzymes to release C-peptide and produce mature insulin with its two distinct polypeptide chains linked by two of its three disulfide bridges.

When, following a meal, concentrations of glucose begin to rise in blood, glucose enters the β-cells of the islets of Langerhans and triggers a depolarization event, a rise in intracellular calcium, and a release of insulin from insulin granules within the β-cells (Figure 7–15). Thus, levels of insulin begin to rise in blood. Insulin is a hormone, and it can interact with insulin receptors found in the plasma membrane of striated muscle cells and adipose cells. The insulin receptor is composed of two α- and two β-sub-

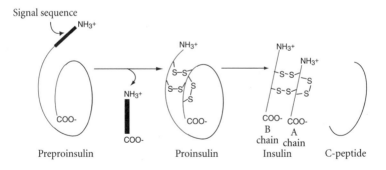

Figure 7–14 The production of insulin from its precursor proteins. Insulin is a hormone that is produced by the modification of a larger protein chain. Preproinsulin has a signal sequence at its N-terminus that facilitates the initial passage of this molecule into the endoplasmic reticulum (a path common to many secretory proteins; see Figure 2–2). The signal sequence peptide is removed by a signal peptidase to yield proinsulin. Three disulfide bridges are formed, and proteolytic cleavage reactions remove the large C-peptide, producing the two-chain structure of insulin, secured by disulfide bonds.

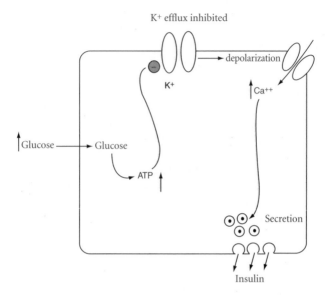

Figure 7–15 The release of insulin. As concentrations of glucose rise outside the β-cells of the islets of Langerhans following a meal, more glucose enters these, leading to a rise in cellular ATP. This is believed to inhibit the efflux of potassium ions, leading to depolarization of the plasma membrane and influx of calcium ions. This, in turn, triggers the release of insulin from insulin granules and ultimately the entry of insulin into the circulation.

units, and the binding of insulin triggers an activation of tyrosine kinase activity found in the β-subunits within the insulin-responsive cells (Figure 7–16). Muscle and adipose tissues generally show the most robust responses to insulin. Tyrosine kinase is a protein kinase that catalyzes the phosphorylation of tyrosine residues within proteins. The phosphorylation events mediated by tyrosine kinase initiate a signalling path for insulin. This type of signalling path, initially mediated by tyrosine kinase activities, is found for a variety of growth hormone receptors. The binding of insulin triggers principally anabolic responses within cells. However, a more immediately obvious result of insulin binding is the increased uptake of glucose shown by stimulated cells. Glucose normally enters cells making use of a glucose transporter that enables facilitated diffusion for this molecule. Insulin-responsive cells, such as muscle and adipocytes, have a type of glucose transporter called **GLUT 4** in the plasma membrane. Other glucose transporters, GLUT 1, 2, 3, and 5, can be found in other cells and tissues, but these are not sensitive to insulin stimulation. In the case of GLUT 4, there is also a population of these transporters held in membrane-bound vesicles just below the surface of the plasma membrane (Figure 7–17). Following the binding of insulin to its transporter, the insulin signalling path promotes the movement of these GLUT 4–bearing vesicles toward the plasma membrane and their fusion with it, dramatically increasing the density of GLUT 4 at the cell surface. This leads to a considerable increase in glucose uptake by these insulin-responsive cells. Diabetics quite frequently overdose themselves with insulin, which results in a precipitous drop in blood glucose because of the rapid sugar uptake by the muscle and adipose cells. This can result in insulin shock.

Insulin has other effects on the metabolism in these responsive cells. Again, this scenario is associated with eating and a plentiful supply of glucose and fatty acids coming from the diet. These metabolic responses to insulin include

1. Increased rates of glycolysis, as glucose is now the principal fuel available for energy metabolism;
2. Increased rates of glycogen synthesis, as any glucose in excess of the needs of glycolysis is stored as glycogen;
3. Decreased rates of glycogen breakdown, as there is no need to sacrifice glycogen stores when glucose is in abundance;
4. Decreased rates of gluconeogenesis, as there is no need to make glucose;

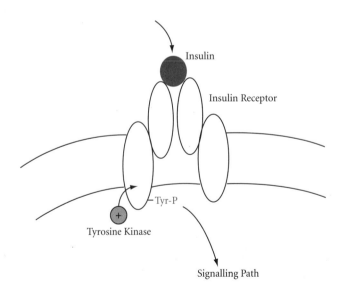

Figure 7–16 The insulin response. When insulin binds to its receptor (four subunits), there is an activation of a tyrosine kinase activity within the cytoplasmic domain of the insulin receptor. The active tyrosine kinase can autophosphorylate the receptor and lead to the binding and activation of various proteins that are involved in the insulin signalling pathway. This type of receptor tyrosine kinase is found for a variety of growth factors.

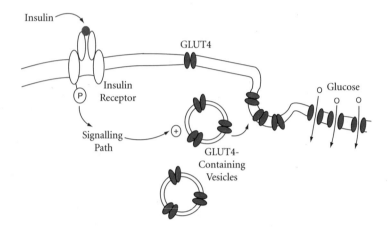

Figure 7–17 The recruitment of glucose transporters. Following insulin binding, one of the important physiologic responses is the recruitment of glucose transporters (specifically GLUT 4) to the plasma membrane. These proteins are found in vesicles lying just below the cell surface. With the rapid rise in numbers of glucose transporters on the cell surface, insulin-sensitive cells, such as muscle and fat, can rapidly internalize extracellular glucose.

5. Increased rates of fatty acid synthesis and triglyceride synthesis, as fat stores accumulate during this time of plenty;
6. Decreased rates of breakdown of triglyceride, as there is sufficient glucose to serve as fuel, and fat synthesis is the logical response; and
7. Increased rates of protein synthesis.

Generally, these metabolic responses are under the control of specific phosphorylation and dephosphorylation enzymatic events that control key enzymes in carbohydrate and fat metabolisms. The precise signalling mechanism, initiated by insulin binding and the associated regulation of enzymes by phosphorylation cycles, is still under active investigation and is not completely understood. It appears that the regulation of these enzymes, following insulin stimulation, is considerably more complex than the mechanisms established for adrenaline and glucagon, hormones that we will discuss shortly. Some of the effects of insulin at the enzyme level are noted in Table 7–2. Insulin is believed to increase glycogen synthase and decrease glycogen phosphorylase reactions by promoting dephosphorylation. Similarly, insulin is thought to elevate, by dephosphorylation, the activities of pyruvate kinase (PK), a key regulatory enzyme in glycolysis, and pyruvate dehydrogenase (PDH), a pivotal regulatory enzyme that produces acetyl-CoA for the Krebs cycle. Dephosphorylation is also believed responsible for the decreased activity of hormone-sensitive lipase, the enzyme responsible for triglyceride breakdown, and for the activation of acetyl-CoA carboxylase, a key enzyme regulating fatty acid synthesis.

Table 7–2
Enzyme Activities Controlled by Insulin and Glucagon

Enzyme	Effect of Insulin	Effect of Glucagon
Glycogen synthase	Increased (D)	Decreased (P)
Glycogen phosphorylase	Decreased (D)	Increased (P)
Pyruvate kinase (PK)	Increased (D)	Decreased (P)
Fructose 2,6-bisphosphatase	Decreased (D)	Increased (P)
Pyruvate dehydrogenase (PDH)	Increased (D)	
Acetyl-CoA carboxylase (ACC)	Increased (D)	Decreased (P)
Hormone-sensitive lipase	Decreased (D)	Increased (P)

D and P indicate that increased or decreased enzyme activities are associated with the dephosphorylated (D) or phosphorylated (P) forms of the enzymes.

The metabolic effects of insulin promote anabolism, while suppressing catabolism of glycogen and fat. Glucose is used as the predominant fuel in many tissues so that fat can be conserved and fat depots augmented by further synthesis of triglyceride. In the well-fed state, the effects of insulin and glucose availability predominate. Thus, glucose is used as the principal fuel substrate in the liver, skeletal muscle, brain, and adipose tissue. Muscle and the liver can use glucose to build up glycogen reserves, and the liver and adipose tissue can use glucose as a precursor for fat synthesis.

Hormones That Antagonize the Actions of Insulin

Insulin is a powerful hormone. Discovered by Canadian scientists Banting, Best, Collip, and Macleod, insulin, when administered to dogs, was found to be a potent hypoglycemic, promoting very rapid declines in blood glucose. When levels of blood glucose fall below 2 mM (40 mg/dL), coma and convulsions can ensue, as energy metabolism in the brain is compromised. If a diabetic has been administered an excess of insulin, glucose must be given quickly. Given its potency, insulin can be a very dangerous hormone. Thus, there is a need for other agents that can oppose insulin's action. The situation is comparable to the abilities of a very powerful receiver in American football. Whenever he is moving downfield, he will be accompanied by several opposing players in efforts to limit his potential actions.

There are, in fact, several hormones that oppose the actions of insulin. These hormones can gain the upper hand when levels of blood glucose begin to decline, between meals or in fasting or starvation. The first of these insulin antagonists is glucagon, a small polypeptide made by the α-cells of the islets of Langerhans. These cells release glucagon in response to falling levels of blood glucose. Glucagon exerts its actions by binding to a glucagon receptor in liver cells, initiating a signalling path that utilizes cAMP as a second messenger and the activation of protein kinase A. Stimulation of the liver by glucagon leads to the following effects on metabolic processes:

1. Rates of glycogenolysis increase so that the liver can release glucose into blood to help preserve blood glucose levels. The liver has a special enzyme known as glucose-6-phosphatase that allows it to generate glucose from glucose-6-phosphate formed during glycogenolysis.
2. Rates of glycogen synthesis decrease, as there is a need to mobilize glycogen reserves in the liver.
3. Rates of glycolysis are slowed in the liver in efforts to conserve glucose for other tissues, such as the brain.
4. Rates of gluconeogenesis are increased in the liver in order to generate glucose for release into the bloodstream.
5. Rates of fatty acid synthesis are slowed, as fat will now become a principal fuel in the production of energy, in efforts to preserve blood glucose.

The effects of glucagon are restricted to the liver, and given the central role that the liver plays in metabolism, the effects of glucagon are pivotal. Again, control is exerted at the level of protein phosphorylation. Thus, glucagon leads to the following special effects on the enzymes in the liver, mediated by phosphorylation (see Table 7–2):

1. Phosphorylation of glycogen phosphorylase to increase activity.
2. Phosphorylation of glycogen synthase to decrease activity.
3. Phosphorylation of pyruvate kinase (PK), a regulatory enzyme in glycolysis, to decrease glycolytic activity.
4. Phosphorylation and activation of fructose–2,6-bisphosphatase, an enzyme that removes fructose–2,6-bisphosphate, a simple sugar with two phosphate esters, which stimulates glycolysis by activating the glycolytic enzyme phosphofructokinase (PFK-1).

A second insulin antagonist is adrenaline. Adrenaline is released from the adrenal glands in response to signals from the brain initiated with falling blood glucose levels. Adrenaline has the following effects after binding to its receptors in different cells:

1. Muscle: The activation of glycogen phosphorylase occurs in a manner similar to that noted for glucagon in liver. Muscle does not have the enzyme glucose-6-phosphatase, and thus, glucose-6-phosphate produced from glycogen can be used in glycolysis for energy production in muscle. The absence of glucose-6-phosphatase means that muscle cannot contribute its glucose (derived from glycogen) directly to the bloodstream. This, again, underlines the consumer status of muscle.

2. Adipose tissue: Adrenaline can trigger the phosphorylation and activation of the enzyme hormone-sensitive lipase. This enzyme mobilizes fat stores in adipocytes by hydrolyzing triglycerides. We will discuss this more thoroughly later in this chapter in the section on lipid metabolism. This mobilization of fat is an important step, as it releases fatty acids for use as fuel substrates in order to conserve levels of blood glucose.

3. Liver: Binding of adrenaline to its receptor can lead to the breakdown of glycogen and the inhibition of fatty acid synthesis, thus shutting down fat anabolism, a logical prelude to the use of these compounds as fuels.

The glucocorticoids (e.g., cortisol, produced by the adrenal cortex) can also function as insulin antagonists, a feature of pharmacologic importance when these compounds are used as therapeutic agents.

Thus, type I DM, caused by low levels of circulating insulin, is associated with a hormonal imbalance in which insulin antagonists have the upper hand (Table 7–3). Although a diabetic may be well fed, with relatively high levels of blood glucose, the anabolic responses are muted. Levels of blood glucose remain high (hyperglycemia), as GLUT 4 glucose transporters are not recruited to the plasma membrane of fat and muscle cells. Glucose can enter urine (glucosuria) when blood glucose levels are beyond the kidneys' ability to reclaim glucose after glomerular filtration. Hyperglycemia can have

Table 7–3
Diabetes Mellitus: Metabolic and Clinical Findings

Metabolic signs	Increased glycogen breakdown
	Decreased glycogen synthesis
	Increased gluconeogenesis in the liver
	Decreased rates of glycolysis in the liver
	Increased fat mobilization
	Increased rates of fat β-oxidation and ketogenesis
Lab signs	Hyperglycemia
	Glucosuria
	Increased ketone bodies in urine (ketonuria)
	Increased fatty acids and ketone bodies in blood
Physical signs and symptoms	Polyuria, polydypsia
	Dehydration
	Kidney failure
	Coma

deleterious effects on cells. The mobilization of fat reserves by adrenaline cannot be blocked because of the absence of insulin. Thus, triglyceride breakdown predominates. In our discussion of fat metabolism, we shall see how the powerful mobilization of fat can cause problems for cells.

Type II DM can be caused by deficient production of insulin in adults. While these patients have β-cells, their function is impaired. Thus, drugs may be used in efforts to boost insulin production before the use of insulin therapy is initiated. These patients can have elevated plasma fatty acid levels as a result of fat mobilization triggered by adrenaline.

Type II DM can also be caused by insulin resistance. While insulin production and release are not impaired, there is a problem with cells that are normally insulin responsive. Likely, a defect lies in the insulin signalling pathway so that the binding of insulin cannot elicit the usual anabolic responses associated with this hormone or the rapid clearance of glucose from the blood. The suspected diabetic can be assessed using a glucose tolerance test, in which 100 g of glucose is given orally and blood glucose levels monitored with time. A prolonged elevation in blood glucose is often indicative of decreased glucose tolerance because of a defect in insulin production/secretion or insulin responsiveness. There are precise criteria to be followed for a glucose tolerance test, and certain drugs and aging can affect the response to glucose loading. Normally, blood glucose levels are maintained within a range of 4.5 to 5.5 mM, although levels down to 3.3 mM can be found in fasting and levels upward of 7 mM after eating carbohydrates.

Gluconeogenesis

This is rather an interesting pathway from the point of view of metabolic regulation and hormonal balance. It is found principally in the liver, although the kidney can make a contribution. Gluconeogenesis shares many of the enzymes of glycolysis, with a few critical exceptions (Figure 7–18). Gluconeogenesis functions to produce glucose, starting with simpler compounds. One major substrate is lactate, entering blood from muscle and the red cells. Gluconeogenesis can also utilize certain amino acids (such as alanine, supplied to the liver by muscle during starvation) or glycerol (liberated during the mobilization of triglycerides in adipose cells). The fatty acid components of triglycerides are broken down to form acetyl-CoA, which cannot serve as a substrate for gluconeogenesis.

Glycerol can be converted in two steps to the intermediate dihydroxyacetone phosphate, which is used for glucose synthesis. Alanine can be converted to pyruvate by the removal of its amino group. Lactate can be taken up by the liver and converted to pyruvate, which can be metabolized to phosphoenolpyruvate (PEP) using steps that lie outside the glycolytic path. This route to PEP is needed, simply because it is not feasible, from energy considerations, to directly reverse the glycolytic step that makes pyruvate from PEP. PEP can be converted to fructose-1,6-bisphosphate by a sequential reversal of glycolytic steps. The conversion of fructose-1,6-bisphosphate to fructose-6-phosphate again requires a different enzyme, fructose-1,6-bisphosphatase. Fructose-6-phosphate can be isomerized to glucose-6-phosphate, which, in turn, can be utilized to release free glucose into the circu-

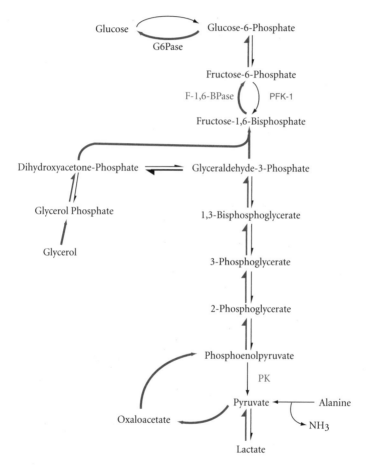

Figure 7–18 Gluconeogenesis. This pathway, principally found in the liver, uses many of the enzymes found in glycolysis and is rather unique, as these glycolytic enzyme reactions can be reversed. However, there is a need for a path to generate phosphoenolpyruvate from pyruvate, as well as a need for the enzymes fructose-1,6-bisphosphatase and glucose-6-phosphatase, which are not a part of glycolysis. These additional enzymes are required to detour around glycolytic enzymes whose reactions are not easily reversed. Gluconeogenesis does require energy (four ATP, two GTP, and two NADH molecules per glucose molecule) and yields glucose that can be released by the liver into the circulation in times of need.

lation via the action of hepatic glucose-6-phosphatase. Remember the role of the liver as the parental figure/provider in metabolism.

Glycolysis and gluconeogenesis are metabolic paths that have two opposite results: the degradation of glucose to pyruvate and the synthesis of glucose starting from pyruvate. Naturally, it would be wasteful to have both paths running at the same time (a little like a dog chasing its tail). Thus, there is **reciprocal regulation** of the two paths. Generally, this control is exerted at enzyme sites that are not shared between the two paths. For example, a rising level of AMP within cells is a sign that ATP and energy levels are falling. AMP serves as an allosteric activator for the enzyme phosphofructokinase-1 (PFK-1), the enzyme in glycolysis that converts fructose-6-phosphate to fructose-1,6-bisphosphate. At the same time, AMP is an allosteric inhibitor of fructose-1,6-bisphosphatase, an enzyme critical to gluconeogeneis. Thus, rising AMP (and falling ATP) stimulates glycolysis and shuts down gluconeogenesis.

While AMP is a signal arising within a cell for the control of its own cellular environment, hormones can bring signals that reflect the needs of other cells or tissues. Recall our image of the liver as the provider. Thus, when levels of blood glucose levels begin to fall, glucagon is secreted from the pancreas and interacts with its receptors in the liver. The liver responds through the production of cAMP, which affects a number of pathways. For glycolysis and gluconeogenesis, one step of particular interest is an activation of fructose-2,6-bisphosphatase (F2,6-BPase), which degrades the compound fructose-2,6-bisphosphate. This compound is an allosteric activator of PFK-1, a key regulatory enzyme in glycolysis and an allosteric inhibitor of fructose-1,6-bisphosphatase (F1,6-BP), a key enzyme in gluconeogenesis. Thus, the removal of fructose-2,6-bisphosphate slows glycolysis and removes the inhibition of gluconeogenesis. Cyclic AMP generated following the binding of glucagon to liver cells can also lead to the phosphorylation and inactivation of pyruvate kinase (PK), another key regulatory enzyme in glycolysis, thus slowing glycolysis in the liver.

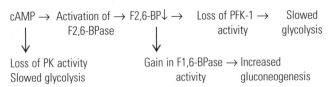

Insulin and glucagon, by their signalling pathways, can also regulate the synthesis of enzymes found within the glycolytic and gluconeogenic pathways. Thus, insulin acts as an inducer of the synthesis of phosphofructokinase-1 and pyruvate kinase, two key enzymes in glycolysis. This increases the number of the molecules of these enzymes, elevating rates of glycolysis. In contrast, glucagon acts as a repressor of the synthesis of these enzymes. Glucagon also plays the role of an inducer of enzymes of gluconeogenesis, including fructose-1,6-bisphosphatase and glucose-6-phosphatase. Thus, the numbers of molecules of these enzymes increase, as will rates of gluconeogenesis. In a corresponding manner, insulin serves as a repressor of the synthesis of these enzymes.

Glycolysis	Gluconeogenesis
Insulin: PFK-1↑ PK ↑	F1,6-BPase ↓ G-6-Pase ↓
Glucagon: PFK-1 ↓ PK ↓	F1,6-BPase ↑ G-6-Pase ↑

Recall, however, that the synthesis of new enzymes requires time, and thus, allosteric regulation and regulation by phosphorylation and dephosphorylation are speedier ways of controlling pathways.

A summary of regulatory enzymes in carbohydrate metabolism is shown in Table 7–4. We noted earlier that pyruvate dehydrogenase (PDH) is inactivated by phosphorylation and activated by dephosphorylation (following cellular stimulation by insulin). PDH converts pyruvate into acetyl-CoA and thus supplies the Krebs cycle with substrates. PDH is an important regulatory point for the Krebs cycle. PDH can be inhibited by its products (NADH and acetyl-CoA) and activated by its substrates (NAD^+ and CoA). Further, ATP is an allosteric inhibitor of the enzyme, and AMP is an allosteric activator. You can see that when the activity of the Krebs cycle slows, the NAD^+/NADH and AMP/ATP ratios may rise, prompting increased PDH activity to provide more acetyl-CoA substrate in efforts to increase the activity of the Krebs cycle.

The hexose monophosphate pathway (that produces the five-carbon ribose-5-phosphate and NADPH) is regulated at the enzyme glucose-6-phosphate dehydrogenase, the first step in this shunt. This enzyme is allosterically inhibited by rising levels of NADPH.

In general, the ADP/ATP ratio, AMP/ATP ratio, and the NAD^+/NADH ratio are critical in the control of glycolysis and the Krebs cycle, and rising

Table 7–4
Key Regulatory Enzymes in Carbohydrate Metabolism

Glycolysis	Phosphofructokinase-1 (PFK-1)
	Pyruvate kinase (PK)
Gluconeogenesis	Fructose-1,6-bisphosphatase (F1,6-BPase)
	Glucose-6-phosphatase
Glycogen metabolism	Glycogen phosphorylase
	Glycogen synthase

values for these ratios will trigger increased rates of glycolysis and Krebs cycle activity in efforts to restore levels of ATP and NADH within cells. A summary of the various means of regulating enzymes and metabolic pathways is shown in Table 7–5.

FAT METABOLISM

You will likely now appreciate that carbohydrate metabolism and the metabolism of fat are directly connected and are under hormonal control. Thus, many tissues will use glucose as a fuel substrate in a well-fed condition, while reserving the use of fat as a fuel for times of fasting and starvation and during prolonged exercise. And, as we shall see, in DM, fat is used as the principal fuel, with deleterious consequences for cells.

For nondiabetic individuals, fasting triggers a series of events that decreases the use of glucose as fuel and promotes the use of fat in many tissues and organs. As levels of glucagon and adrenaline rise in response to falling levels of blood glucose, cAMP is generated by adenylate cyclase within the adipose cells, and protein kinase A is activated (Figure 7–19). By phosphorylation, this kinase can activate hormone-sensitive lipase, the key enzyme regulating fat catabolism. It hydrolyzes the two outside ester links that attach the long-chain fatty acids to glycerol in storage triglycerides. The last fatty acid ester link (found in the intermediate monoglyceride) is hydrolyzed by the enzyme monoglyceride lipase. You should also note that rising levels of insulin will promote the dephosphorylation and inactivation of hormone-sensitive lipase. Insulin also promotes an inhibition of adenylate cyclase and a stimulation of the phosphodiesterase that inactivates cAMP.

The liberated free fatty acids (destined to be used as fuels in other cells) leave the adipose cells and are transported to various tissues of the body, bound to the plasma protein albumin. Thus, fasting will lead to an elevation of plasma free fatty acids. Fatty acids readily cross the plasma membrane of

Table 7–5
Methods of Metabolic Regulation

- Regulation of substrate supply
- Competitive and allosteric inhibition (competing substrates, end-product inhibition)
  Note: Reciprocal control of related pathways and control by $NAD^+/NADH$, ADP/ATP, AMP/ATP ratios
- Covalent enzyme modification (e.g., phosphorylation–dephosphorylation cycles under hormonal control)
- Induction or repression of enzyme synthesis

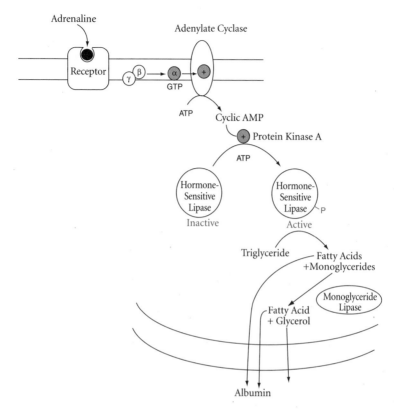

Figure 7–19 The mobilization of fat. Triglycerides in fat cells can be degraded by the action of the enzymes hormone-sensitive lipase and monoglyceride lipase. Hormone-sensitive lipase is activated in a phosphorylation reaction by protein kinase A, following the binding of adrenaline to a fat cell. Ultimately, fat mobilization yields one molecule of glycerol and three fatty acids, which are transported to other tissues bound hydrophobically to albumin. Rising levels of insulin in the circulation lead to dephosphorylation and deactivation of hormone-sensitive lipase.

cells and are then activated by enzymes known as fatty acyl-CoA synthetases (Figure 7–20). These reactions require ATP and CoA. CoA has an important sulfhydryl (-SH) group at the end of its structure. The fatty acyl-CoA synthetases create a chemical link between the -SH group of CoA and the carboxyl of the fatty acid, generating a thioester linkage. Because this bond has a relatively high free energy associated with it, fatty acids are activated by this process so that they can take part in other aspects of metabolism.

Fatty acyl-CoA molecules are generated outside the mitochondrial matrix. The mitochondria have two membranes, but the outer membrane has pores that allow relatively quick passage of smaller molecules (such as fatty acyl-CoA) into the intermembrane space (Figure 7–21). However, because of the large hydrophilic CoA part of the molecule, fatty acyl-CoA

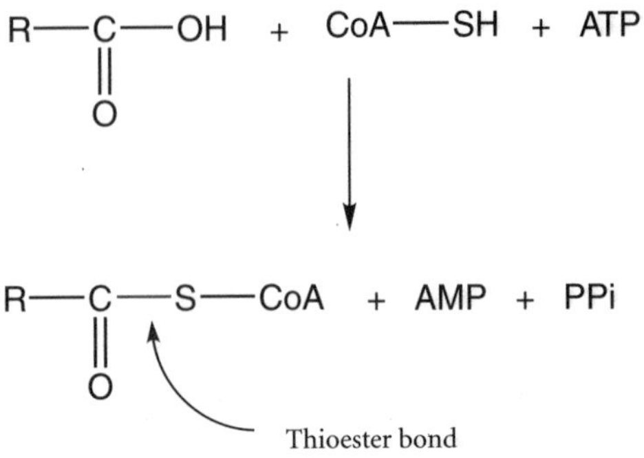

Figure 7–20 Fatty acyl-CoA synthetase. Fatty acids require an activation step before they enter into metabolism. This activation is catalyzed by enzymes known as fatty acyl-CoA synthetases that use the energy of ATP to create a thioester bond between the water-soluble CoA and the free fatty acid. Note that this reaction generates AMP and pyrophosphate (PPi), instead of the more usual ADP and Pi.

does not readily cross the inner mitochondrial membrane or enter the mitochondrial matrix. Yet, in fasting or starvation, these fatty acyl-CoA molecules will be used within the matrix as substrates for fatty acid oxidation and energy production. You might (quite reasonably) feel that this problem should have been "ironed out" during evolution. Synthesis of fatty acyl-CoA, thus, appears somewhat like building a boat in your basement, then realizing you can't take your new craft to the beach.

Of course, there is a rationale here. Simply stated, there is a specialized transport system within the inner mitochondrial membrane, and control of fatty acid oxidation can be exerted at the level of this transport mechanism. This mechanism is referred to as the **carnitine shuttle**, as carnitine plays a very central role in this process (see Figure 7–21). The enzyme carnitine acyltransferase I is located at the inner face of the outer mitochondrial membrane and converts fatty acyl-CoA to fatty acylcarnitine. Carnitine is much smaller than CoA, and this change in the molecule facilitates the passage of acylcarnitine through the inner membrane mediated by a transporter called a **translocase**. Once inside the matrix, the fatty acylcarnitine can be converted back to fatty acyl-CoA by carnitine acyltransferase II. The carnitine acyltransferases catalyze reactions that are readily reversible, allowing this initial shift to fatty acylcarnitine and the return to fatty acyl-CoA. During fasting, starvation, or prolonged exercise, this carnitine shuttle is very active but is shut down with rising levels of insulin in the blood following the ingestion of food.

The steps in the oxidation of palmitic acid (a fatty acid with 16 carbons) within the mitochondrial matrix are shown in Figure 7–22. This process is usually referred to as **β-oxidation**, simply because the process is centered on reactions at the carbon that is two carbons removed from the carboxyl

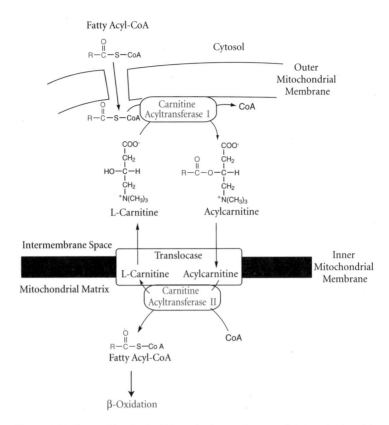

Figure 7–21 The carnitine shuttle. This mechanism employs two distinct molecules of the enzyme carnitine acyltransferase located in the outer mitochondrial membrane (CAT I) and the inner mitochondrial membrane (CAT II) and a translocase in the inner mitochondrial membrane. Initially, fatty acyl-CoA is converted into acylcarnitine, a molecule of much lower polarity that can be transported by the translocase into the mitochondrial matrix. Here the acylcarnitine is converted back into fatty acyl-CoA for use in mitochondrial β-oxidation. The carnitine shuttle is a very important control point for the generation of fatty acyl-CoA within the matrix and effectively controls rates of β-oxidation. Adapted from Moran LA, Scrimgeour KG, Horton HR, et al. Biochemistry. 2nd ed. Englewood Cliffs (NJ): Neil Patterson-Prentice Hall; 1994.

portion of the fatty acyl-CoA molecule. If the carbon next to the carboxyl carbon is referred to as the α-carbon, the next carbon along the chain is thus designated as the β-carbon. β-Oxidation of fatty acyl-CoA molecules effectively removes a two-carbon piece from the carboxyl end of the fatty acid chain. This is accomplished in four steps that produce one molecule each of the reduced coenzymes $FADH_2$ and NADH (in two dehydrogenase reactions) and require one molecule of water (the hydratase reaction) and a new molecule of CoA (the thiolase or acyl-CoA–acyltransferase reaction). Thus, after one β-oxidation sequence, one molecule of acetyl-CoA (two carbons)

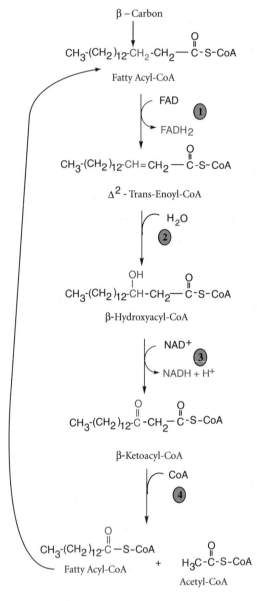

Figure 7–22 β-Oxidation of palmitoyl-CoA. In this mitochondrial catabolic path, there are four steps that work in sequence, ultimately to facilitate the removal of a two-carbon fragment (as acetyl-CoA) from this 16-carbon fatty acyl-CoA chain. The steps are (1) dehydrogenation, (2) hydration, (3) dehydrogenation, and (4) release of acetyl-CoA. This sequence of steps can be repeated until all the fatty acyl chain is converted into eight acetyl-CoA molecules. During each sequence of β-oxidation, there is also the generation of NADH and FADH$_2$, which can be used for ATP production via the electron transport chain and oxidative phosphorylation.

is produced as well as a fatty acyl-CoA molecule with a fatty acid chain two carbons shorter (14 carbons) (see Figure 7–22).

By repeating the process with the shorter fatty acyl-CoA, another molecule of acetyl-CoA is produced. Thus seven β-oxidation sequences will completely convert the 16-carbon fatty acyl-CoA to eight acetyl-CoA molecules. It's a little like cutting a log into eight equal pieces; you need only cut seven times to produce the eight end products.

After the seven β-oxidation sequences, seven molecules each of $FADH_2$ and NADH will be generated. These can be used by the electron transport chain and oxidative phosphorylation to generate 14 and 21 molecules of ATP, respectively, on the basis of the energies of reduction associated with these two reduced cofactors. Of course, the eight acetyl-CoA molecules can enter the Krebs cycle, and more energy can be released and conserved in the form of ATP. Each turn of the Krebs cycle (following the entry of one acetyl-CoA) yields 12 ATP, on the basis of the generation of NADH and $FADH_2$ during the cycle and the operation of electron transport and oxidative phosphorylation.

Thus, one molecule of palmitoyl-CoA can yield 131 molecules of ATP, following β-oxidation, the Krebs cycle, and electron transfer/oxidative phosphorylation. The corresponding values for glucose are 36 or 38. Accordingly, fat can produce considerably more energy than can carbohydrate. As well, another advantage to fatty acid breakdown in mitochondria is the large production of water molecules. With 131 molecules of ATP are generated 146 molecules of water. Camels are reputed to require very little water, largely because they make use of their fat deposits (in their humps) on long journeys as sources of energy.

Ketone Bodies, Alternative Fuels, and Diabetes Mellitus

The complete oxidation of fatty acids does have one potential drawback. The problem arises because overall rates of β-oxidation of fatty acids can exceed the ability of the Krebs cycle to handle the intermediate product acetyl-CoA. The potential result is a build-up of acetyl-CoA within the mitochondria (a little like the result with a fast-running faucet or tap bringing water into a sink that has a relatively small drain). If acetyl-CoA molecules rise in concentration within the mitochondria, they can be used in a second pathway (independent of the Krebs cycle) that generates compounds known as **ketone bodies**. The production of ketone bodies (ketogenesis) occurs primarily within the liver mitochondria. The path for ketone body synthesis is shown in Figure 7–23. The three ketone bodies are acetoacetate, β-hydroxybutyrate (made by the reduction of acetoacetate), and acetone (from the spontaneous decarboxylation of acetoacetate).

The ketone bodies, acetoacetate, and β-hydroxybutyrate, when supplied in reasonable quantities, can be very useful. They are water-soluble fuel sub-

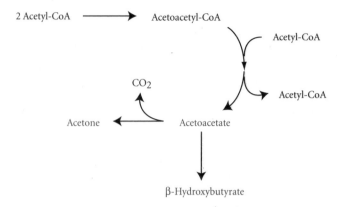

Figure 7–23 Ketone body formation. In this pathway, two molecules of acetyl-CoA can be used to form the four-carbon acetoacetyl-CoA. In turn, this molecule is used to generate the ketone body acetoacetate. This molecule can be reduced enzymatically to form β-hydroxybutyrate or decarboxylated chemically to form acetone, the two other ketone bodies. Acetoacetate and β-hydroxybutyrate are largely formed by the liver and released into the circulation as fuel compounds for other tissues.

strates that are released from the liver and travel in blood to other tissues. Here, the ketone bodies can be broken down to acetyl-CoA, which can feed the Krebs cycle. A number of tissues can make use of ketone bodies when glucose supplies are limited. In our analogy of provider and consumers in the family, you can picture the liver as the anxious single parent attempting to keep everyone reasonably well fed and happy when times are tough (i.e., during fasting or starvation). Thus, the liver produces ketone bodies as fuel substrates that may serve as substitutes for glucose. Even the brain, with time, can make use of ketone bodies as fuel.

If you study an individual who is fasting, you will, indeed, find evidence of fat mobilization, rising fatty acid levels in cells and in blood, increased rates of β-oxidation, and rising levels of circulating ketone bodies. However, the nondiabetic, fasting patient has one very important control over this whole process. While insulin levels are depressed during fasting, there is always some insulin present. Insulin is a powerful inhibitor of fat mobilization, and even low levels of insulin can thus act as a brake on the overall rate of β-oxidation. If there is no insulin present, as in type I DM and some cases of type II DM, this braking mechanism is not present, and a truly remarkable quantity of storage triglyceride can be broken down in adipose cells as a result of adrenaline stimulation. This will lead to very high rates of β-oxidation (also assisted by the absence of insulin) and spectacular rates of ketone body synthesis. The quantities of ketone bodies produced by the diabetic liver can be staggering. This is shown by the very high levels of ketone bodies in blood (ketonemia) and the spillover of ketone bodies into urine (ketonuria). This will be accompanied by hyperglycemia and glucosuria. The presence of ketone bodies in urine can be detected using Dip-Stix or other simple chemical procedures.

The high concentrations of ketone bodies in blood lead to metabolic acidosis and a drop in tissue pH. In addition, the glucose and ketone bodies in blood and extracellular fluids serve to dehydrate cells, leading to a loss of tissue electrolytes and water, polyuria, a lowering of blood pressure, and ultimately diabetic coma. The hypotension can also result in anuria and kidney failure.

The administration of insulin to insulin-responsive diabetics very rapidly changes this picture. Insulin blocks both triglyceride mobilization (by inhibiting hormone-sensitive lipase) and β-oxidation (by inhibiting the action of carnitine acyltransferase I, an enzyme of the carnitine shuttle, as noted in Figure 7–21) and thus eliminates ketone body production, shutting down the use of fat as fuel. As well, insulin promotes the entry of glucose into muscle and fat cells and clears the blood of excess glucose. Insulin stimulates fat production, a process we will discuss next. You can perhaps appreciate the almost god-like status that Frederick Banting acquired when he became the sole dispenser of insulin back in the early 1920s. Virtually overnight, there were spectacular reverses in the progression of the disease, and juvenile diabetics were rapidly pulled back from the edge of death. The very generous participation of Eli Lilly & Co. in the commercial production of pure insulin, making considerable quantities of the hormone available to Banting and, thus, to child and teenage diabetics at this time, cannot be overlooked.

Fatty Acid Synthesis

As soon as levels of insulin begin to rise, usually following a meal in non-diabetic patients, there is a stimulus to synthesize fatty acids and augment the triglyceride reserves within the fat cells. The synthesis of fatty acids basically involves the addition of two carbon units to each other to make a long fatty acid chain. Although the process is approximately the reverse of fatty acid β-oxidation, the synthesis of fatty acids takes place in the cytosol of cells and utilizes quite a different metabolic machinery from that used for fatty acid breakdown inside the mitochondrial matrix.

The initial steps require the use of acetyl-CoA (as a source of two-carbon units) in the cytosol. As acetyl-CoA is largely made within the mitochondria via the action of pyruvate dehydrogenase (in a well-fed state, when insulin levels are relatively high), a mechanism is needed to remove acetyl-CoA from the matrix and regenerate this molecule in the cytosol. Acetyl-CoA is highly hydrophilic and will not readily pass through the inner mitochondrial membrane. Instead, acetyl-CoA reacts inside the matrix with a molecule of oxaloacetate in a step catalyzed by citrate synthase, the first step in the Krebs cycle. Citrate can be transported to the cytosol by a transporter in the inner membrane (Figure 7–24). Once in the cytosol, an enzyme called citrate lyase uses citrate, ATP, and CoA to regenerate acetyl-CoA and oxaloacetate. Thus, the initial conversion of acetyl-CoA into citrate within the mitochondrial matrix simply facilitates the generation of acetyl-CoA outside the mitochondria.

In the cytosol, acetyl-CoA is carboxylated by an important enzyme, known appropriately enough as **acetyl-CoA carboxylase** (sometimes abbreviated as ACC, but be careful, as three-letter abbreviations for enzymes can often show redundancy within biochemistry). ACC is a complex enzyme that has biotin as a prosthetic group and the ability to both transfer carbon dioxide to biotin and then transfer that bound carbon dioxide to acetyl-CoA. Thus, ACC can both carry and transfer carbon dioxide. The overall reaction is noted below:

$$CH_3\text{-}C\text{-}S\text{-}CoA + ATP + HCO_3^- \rightarrow \ ^-OOC\text{-}CH_2\text{-}C\text{-}S\text{-}CoA + ADP + Pi$$
$$\underset{\text{Acetyl-CoA}}{O} \qquad\qquad\qquad \underset{\text{Malonyl-CoA}}{O}$$

Here, bicarbonate (HCO_3^-) serves as the source of carbon dioxide, and ATP provides energy for the carboxylation. The product (with the extra carboxyl group) is known as malonyl-CoA. Acetyl-CoA carboxylase is important, as malonyl-CoA provides most of the carbons for fatty acid synthesis. You will soon see that the extra carboxyl group is added to acetyl-CoA so that the decarboxylation of malonyl-CoA provides an energy kick that helps to drive the assembly of two-carbon units in fatty acid synthesis. ACC is the major point of regulation for fatty acid synthesis. Thus, when ACC is phos-

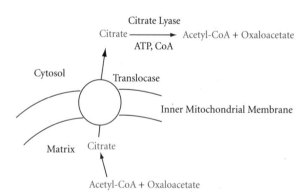

Figure 7–24 Citrate and the production of acetyl-CoA in cytosol. To supply acetyl-CoA for the cytosolic acetyl-CoA carboxylase and for fatty acid synthase, acetyl-CoA is converted into citrate by the action of mitochondrial citrate synthase, an enzyme of the Krebs cycle. Citrate can be transported from the mitochondrial matrix to cytosol, where it is converted to acetyl-CoA and the molecule oxaloacetate by the action of citrate lyase.

phorylated, its activity is greatly decreased, and this phosphorylation is a result of signalling pathways initiated by the insulin antagonists glucagon and adrenaline. In contrast, when insulin levels are rising, dephosphorylation and activation of ACC predominate.

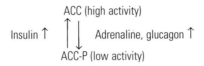

Fatty acid synthesis is carried out by **fatty acid synthase** within the cytosol. This synthase is one large polypeptide, but it carries seven separate active sites, which carry out seven reactions. This is quite possibly the most complex enzyme that we have studied to date. The fatty acid synthase reactions are shown in Figure 7–25. While this mechanism appears complex, try to get an overview of the whole reaction. Essentially, each sequence of reactions in fatty acid synthesis adds a two-carbon unit to a growing acyl chain. The enzyme reactions involve the addition of two carbons from malonyl-CoA (the original carbons of acetyl-CoA used to make the malonyl-CoA), with subsequent steps needed to convert these two carbons into $-CH_2-CH_2-$. One interesting feature of fatty acid synthase is that the complex has an acyl carrier protein (ACP) component with a terminal -SH group. It is this ACP that carries the growing fatty acyl chain bound in thioester linkage during the reactions of fatty acid synthase.

Initially, one molecule of acetyl-CoA is used to prime the reaction sequence. (After this, all the incoming carbons are supplied by malonyl-CoA.) This first reaction transfers the acetyl group to the ACP arm. In turn, this acetyl group is donated to the first enzyme of the fatty acid synthase sequence. Malonyl-CoA then enters the picture, and the malonyl group is transferred to ACP. These two molecules now come together as the acetyl group is transferred to the malonyl group in a condensation reaction. This is driven by the decarboxylation of the malonyl group. The loss of carbon dioxide liberates energy that is used, in part, to link the two-carbon units to form a four-carbon unit attached to the ACP arm. There is, then, a sequence of reactions as the four-carbon unit is taken by the ACP arm to the different active sites of fatty acid synthase. At each site, a different chemical reaction takes place: reduction of the keto group to form $-CO-CH_2-$ $CHOH-CH_3$, dehydration to liberate water and to form $-CO-CH=CH-CH_3$, and finally reduction of this double bond intermediate to form $-CO-CH_2-$ CH_2-CH_3. Thus, the end product of the first enzyme sequence is a butyryl group bound to ACP ($ACP-S-CO-CH_2-CH_2-CH_3$). This four-carbon unit is then transferred to the active site of the first enzyme of the sequence, and a second molecule of malonyl-CoA reacts with the ACP arm. In turn, the malonyl group is again decarboxylated in a second condensation reaction,

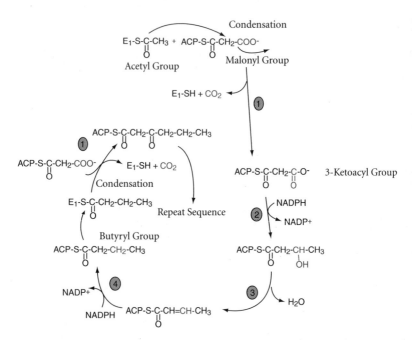

Figure 7–25 Fatty acid synthase. This is a large complex enzyme with seven active sites and an ACP arm to hold the growing fatty acid chain. Initially, an acetyl group is transferred to the active site of the first enzyme, while a malonyl group is attached to the ACP arm. The acetyl group condenses with the malonyl group in a reaction driven by the release of carbon dioxide. The condensation step is reaction 1: the resulting four-carbon compound (3-ketoacyl-ACP) then enters a sequence of reactions that ultimately yields a saturated four-carbon chain attached to ACP. Step 2 is reduction utilizing NADPH; step 3 is dehydration; and step 4 is an additional reduction reaction. This four-step sequence is repeated with another malonyl group and a condensation reaction with the saturated four-carbon chain. After seven sequences of the operation of the synthase, a 16-carbon fatty acid (palmitate) is released from the ACP arm.

as the four-carbon chain is transferred, forming a six-carbon chain attached to ACP. Again, the sequence of reactions ultimately forms $ACP\text{-}S\text{-}CO\text{-}CH_2\text{-}CH_2\text{-}CH_2\text{-}CH_2\text{-}CH_3$.

During each sequence of reactions catalyzed by fatty acid synthase, the two reductions utilize one molecule each of NADPH. Remember that this reduced coenzyme is supplied primarily by the hexose monophosphate pathway. After seven sequences (the first one generated the four-carbon acyl group, and each of the six following sequences added two carbons each), a 16-carbon fatty acyl chain, attached to ACP, is formed. The thioesterase activity within the synthase complex utilizes a molecule of water to release the new 16-carbon fatty acid (also known as **palmitic acid**).

Overall, considering the necessary preliminary formation of malonyl-CoA from acetyl-CoA by ACC and the seven sequences of fatty acid synthase, the generation of one molecule of palmitic acid requires eight molecules of acetyl-CoA, seven molecules of ATP, and 14 molecules of NADPH.

Once palmitic acid is released, it can be activated by fatty acyl-CoA synthetase to form palmitoyl-CoA. This activated form of fatty acid can be used to generate triglycerides by the transfer of fatty acid to form ester linkages on the glycerol backbone of triglycerides. Triglycerides can be formed within the adipose cells and also within the liver and intestinal mucosal cells for the assembly of lipoproteins (as we outlined in Chapter 2). The predominance of insulin in the circulation will maintain relatively high rates of fatty acid synthesis and triglyceride synthesis (while blocking the mobilization of fat reserves and inhibiting β-oxidation).

A summary of biochemical reactions involving fat and carbohydrate that are favored by insulin (times of feeding) on the one hand and by the insulin antagonists adrenaline and glucagon (times of fasting, starvation) on the other is given in Table 7–6.

PROTEIN METABOLISM

Having discussed carbohydrates and fat, it is important not to ignore proteins, which are another major food component and are found throughout the body as structural components (e.g., collagen) and as functional components, such as enzymes, receptors, transporters, and contractile elements in muscle. We have briefly noted the steps in the synthesis of proteins, notably plasma proteins, in Chapter 2 and of globins in Chapter 5. As well,

Table 7–6
Metabolic Pathways Affected by Insulin and Insulin Antagonists (Glucagon, Adrenaline)

Pathway	Insulin	Insulin Antagonist
Glycolysis	+	–
Gluconeogenesis	–	+
Glycogen synthesis	+	–
Glycogen breakdown	–	+
Fat mobilization	–	+
Fatty acid β-oxidation	–	+
Ketogenesis	–	+
Fatty acid synthesis	+	–
Triglyceride synthesis	+	–
Protein synthesis	+	–

in Chapter 8, we will consider the genetic code that directs the assembly of amino acids into proteins. In this last section of metabolism, we wish to mainly consider how proteins are broken down, the reactions that remove nitrogen from amino acids to form urea, and how the remaining carbon skeletons can be degraded or recycled.

Only in prolonged fasting and starvation (and in DM) is there a net loss of proteins, as these are used to provide fuel or carbon sources for gluconeogenesis. Under normal conditions of dietary food intake and insulin availability, there is a dynamic balance between protein breakdown and synthesis so that individual protein levels are maintained. Thus, there is a turnover of proteins, as old molecules are destroyed and new ones made to take their place. This emphasizes the functional importance of proteins in the body. The half-life of albumin is approximately 20 days, while some enzymes may have a half-life of only a few hours or even less. The synthesis of protein relies on the availability of the 20 amino acids, and these can be derived from dietary proteins or are contributed by the breakdown of existing proteins within the body. Certain amino acids can be made from other available amino acids or from intermediates formed in glycolysis, the Krebs cycle, and the hexose monophosphate pathway. The amino acids that can be made in the body are termed nonessential, while those that must be supplied in dietary protein are called essential amino acids. A deficiency in just one essential amino acid can retard growth; thus, children are particularly at risk if they have poor or restricted dietary sources of protein.

Proteolysis

The hydrolysis of a protein within the body is carried out by enzymes known as **proteases**. These utilize water to break the peptide bonds between amino acids, and they have a specificity for certain amino acids found within a protein sequence. For example, the protease trypsin, active in the intestinal digestion of dietary protein, recognizes the amino acids lysine and arginine and hydrolyzes the peptide bonds on the carboxyl side of these amino acid residues. Inside the cells and tissues of the body, proteolysis takes place within two compartments. The first is the lysosome, a small cellular particle that contains many different hydrolases that break a variety of chemical bonds found within proteins, carbohydrates, lipids, and other low-molecular-weight molecules (Figure 7–26). The interior of the lysosome is acidic, favoring these hydrolytic reactions. Cellular compounds can be brought inside the lysosomes to accelerate their breakdown. As well, materials internalized by cells in the process of phagocytosis can also be broken down in the lysosomes. Thus, lysosomes act somewhat like "garburettors" inside the cell, degrading larger molecules and releasing their smaller components for recycling. For example, cathepsins are lysosomal proteases that

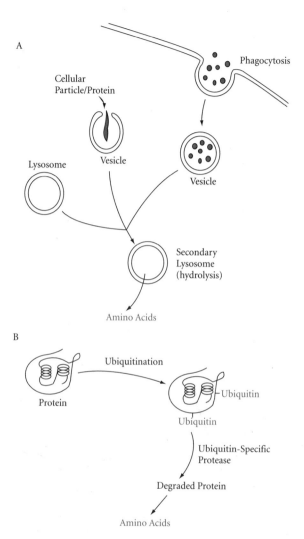

Figure 7–26 Intracellular proteolysis. *A,* Proteins can be degraded inside subcellular organelles called lysosomes that contain a battery of hydrolytic enzymes. The protein substrates may come from cellular components or from proteins brought into the cell by phagocytosis. The amino acid products of lysosomal proteolysis can emerge from the lysosomes and be recycled in protein synthetic events. *B,* Proteins can also be degraded within the cytosol after tagging with a small protein called ubiquitin. This ubiquitination serves as a signal for the actions of ubiquitin-specific proteases found in large multimolecular protein complexes, known as proteasomes.

degrade incoming proteins. The lysosomal digestion of proteins releases amino acids that can be used for the synthesis of new proteins.

Another locus for protein degradation is cytosol. Here, proteases known as **calpains** can be activated by rising levels of intracellular calcium ions. Protease activities are also found in proteasomes, which degrade specific proteins that have been marked for degradation. Proteasomes are giant complexes containing different types of proteases and other protein factors. Proteins may be tagged by receiving a specific biochemical marker, called **ubiquitin**, that earmarks them for hydrolysis. Ubiquitin is a small protein that can form chemical bonds with the side chains of lysine amino acid residues in target proteins. This process is called **ubiquitination** and requires ATP. Proteasomes (with ubiquitin-specific protease activities) recognize the ubiquitin tag and begin to degrade the marked proteins.

Short-lived proteins have sequences that are enriched in the amino acids proline, glutamate, serine, and threonine. By the one-letter abbreviations for these four amino acids, these amino acid regions are sometimes referred to as PEST sequences. These sequences appear to mark these proteins for degradation, possibly by promoting ubiquination reactions.

Transamination and Transdeamination Reactions

Once amino acids have been liberated following proteolytic reactions, they can be recycled in the synthesis of new proteins. However, there are paths for the disposal of amino acids that involve the transfer of amino groups. One such reaction is transamination. The example in Figure 7–27 shows the

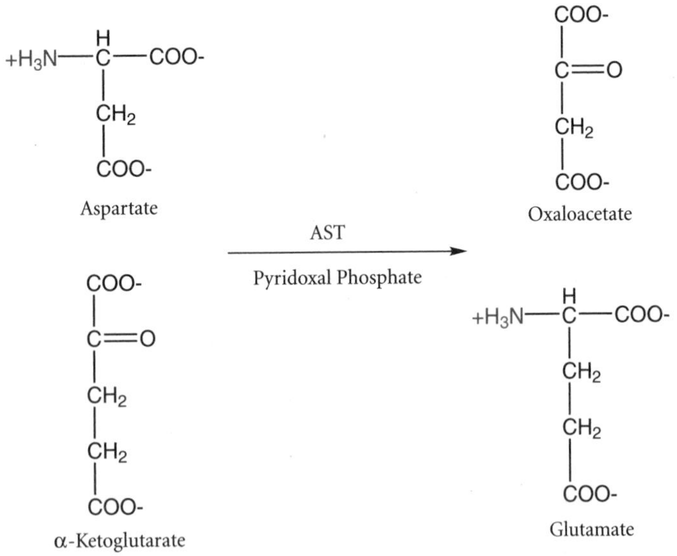

Figure 7–27 Transamination. Aspartate transaminase (AST) transfers the amino group from aspartate to α-ketoglutarate, forming glutamate and oxaloacetate (the carbon skeleton of aspartate).

removal of an amino group from the amino acid aspartate and its transfer to α-ketoglutarate, an intermediate of the Krebs cycle. This forms the amino acid glutamate, leaving behind the compound oxaloacetate, the carbon skeleton derived from aspartate. The enzyme catalyzing this reaction is aspartate aminotransferase (AST), a serum enzyme marker that we discussed in Chapter 3. Another aminotransferase and serum enzyme marker, known as alanine aminotransferase (ALT), transfers an amino group from the amino acid alanine to α-ketoglutarate, generating glutamate and pyruvate (the carbon skeleton of alanine). For the transaminases, the cofactor pyridoxal phosphate (vitamin B_6) is essential for the reaction mechanism. A number of amino acids can be used as substrates in similar reactions that form glutamate from α-ketoglutarate. Thus, the removal of amino groups from a variety of amino acids will generate glutamate as a common product. This is useful because the enzyme glutamate dehydrogenase catalyzes a deamination reaction:

$$\text{Glutamate} + H_2O + NAD(P)^+ \Longleftrightarrow \alpha\text{-ketoglutarate} + NH_3^+ + NAD(P)H + 2H^+$$

The combination of specific transaminases with glutamate dehydrogenase allows an efficient processing of the various amino acids through the common intermediate glutamate, whose amino group can be removed in the formation of ammonia (Figure 7–28). The combination of a transaminase with glutamate dehydrogenase results in a process referred to as **transdeamination**. As ammonia is toxic, a special route is necessary for its removal from the body. This is the function of the urea cycle, which takes incoming ammonia and uses it in the formation of urea. Urea is removed

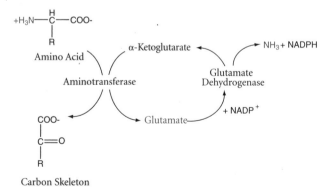

Figure 7–28 Transamination coupled to glutamate dehydrogenase. A variety of aminotransferases transfer the amino groups of the 20 amino acids to α-ketoglutarate with the formation of the amino acid glutamate. In turn, glutamate is converted to α-ketoglutarate with the release of ammonia by the action of glutamate dehydrogenase. The combination of these two reactions is called transdeamination.

from the blood by the kidneys and represents the principal excreted form of nitrogen coming from amino acid breakdown.

The ammonia liberated in transdeamination and in other reactions can also be used in the synthesis of the amino acids glutamine and asparagine. Glutamine itself can be used as an amino group donor in the synthesis of the purine bases that are found in nucleic acids (see Chapter 8).

Urea Cycle

This is shown in Figure 7–29. Again, try to get an overview of the process rather than getting bogged down in the details of the specific intermediates. The urea cycle (Figure 7–29) takes place in the liver and involves two cellular compartments, the mitochondria and cytosol. Initially in the mitochondria, ammonia and carbon dioxide are used along with ATP to form carbamoyl phosphate. Remember how carbamates can be formed by a reaction of carbon dioxide with the N-terminal amino groups of the subunits of hemoglobin (see Chapter 5). The carbamoyl group is transferred to a rather unusual amino acid called **ornithine** to form another amino acid known as **citrulline**. Try to focus on the fate of the carbamoyl group as we proceed through the subsequent reactions in the cycle that occur within the cytosol. What follows is the combination of citrulline and a molecule of the amino acid aspartate to form argininosuccinate. Note how the carbamoyl group is involved in a reaction with the amino group of aspartate. Energy (in the form of ATP) is required for the reaction, and the interesting guanido group (-NH-C (=NH)-NH-) links the two parts of this larger molecule. In the next step, the smaller portion of the argininosuccinate is removed in the loss of the molecule fumarate. This yields the amino acid arginine (which maintains possession of the guanido group). The last step of the cycle is a hydrolysis reaction, where water is utilized to facilitate the loss of urea from arginine, regenerating ornithine that can be used in the cycle as it begins again in the mitochondria. The whole purpose of the urea cycle is the production of harmless urea from the rather toxic ammonia made by glutamate dehydrogenase. Mutations that lead to defective enzymes in the urea cycle or liver damage (e.g., cirrhosis) can lead to elevated levels of blood ammonia (hyperammonemia). Ammonia, in sufficient concentrations, is toxic and can produce blurred vision, tremor, coma, and death. Normally, the liver is an organ that is involved in a variety of detoxification reactions, including the conversion of ammonia into urea. Urea is the major solute found in human urine.

Regulation of the urea cycle is found at the first step catalyzed by carbamoylphosphate synthase. The molecule N-acetylglutamate can allosterically activate this enzyme. If the activity of the urea cycle is too slow, there is a build-up of the intermediate arginine (see Figure 7–29), a molecule that

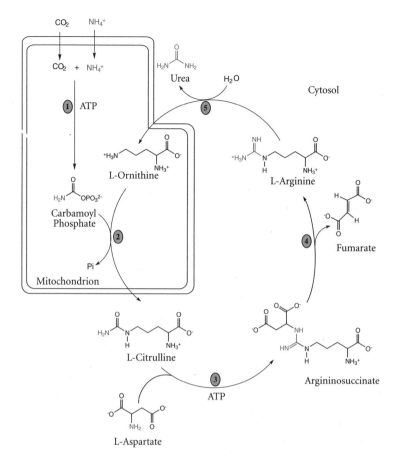

Figure 7–29 The urea cycle. Ammonia is converted to carbamoyl phosphate in the presence of carbon dioxide and ATP. The cycle begins within the mitochondria and transfers the carbamoyl group to the amino acid ornithine. The citrulline product enters the cytosol, where it is joined with a molecule of aspartate. The argininosuccinate product is converted to arginine and urea is liberated from this molecule in a hydrolytic step. The enzymes involved are (1) carbamoylphosphate synthase, (2) ornithine transcarbamoylase, (3) argininosuccinate synthase, (4) argininosuccinase, and (5) arginase. Adapted from Murray RK, Granner DK, Mayes PA, Rodwell VW. Harper's biochemistry. 25th ed. Stamford (CT): Appleton and Lange; 2000.

activates the synthesis of N-acetylglutamate and, thus, increases the activity of the urea cycle.

Fate of Carbon Skeletons Derived from Amino Acids

During transamination reactions and that catalyzed by glutamate dehydrogenase, carbon skeletons are released from amino acids. Figure 7–30 shows a number of carbon skeletons that are derived from amino acids and how these enter into metabolism. The carbon skeletons can be used for energy production, either as components of the Krebs cycle or as intermediates that enter the cycle. Note the generation of α-ketoglutarate, succinyl-CoA, fumarate, oxaloacetate, and citrate. Another possible fate of these compounds is their use in gluconeogenesis in the production of glucose. It is also possible for acetyl-CoA and pyruvate (two other products derived from certain amino acids) to be used in energy production, ketogenesis (the formation of ketone bodies), or fatty acid synthesis. The fate of these carbon skeletons will be guided by nutritional status and the balance of insulin and its antagonists. Thus, carbon skeletons derived from amino acids may be used as energy sources and as sources of glucose in prolonged fasting and starvation. In contrast, the skeletons coming from a variety of amino acids (such as leucine, isoleucine, alanine, aspartate, lysine, and glycine), supplied by the diet in excess of the needs of protein synthesis (well-fed condition), may be used in the formation of fat and glycogen.

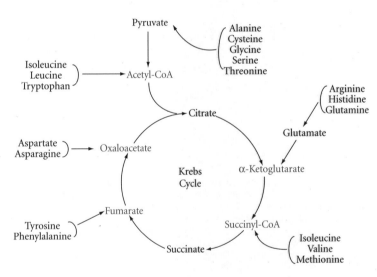

Figure 7–30 The fate of carbon skeletons produced from amino acids. In transamination and transdeamination reactions, carbon skeletons from the 20 amino acids are converted into various metabolites, including pyruvate, acetyl-CoA, and various Krebs cycle intermediates. These compounds can be used in energy generation or for ketone body synthesis or gluconeogenesis.

Recombinant DNA Technology and Its Application to Medicine

Throughout the chapters of this book, we have made many references to diseases and mentioned the genetic basis for specific biochemical defects. As noted in Chapter 1, within deoxyribonucleic acid (DNA), there are many different genetic sequences (genes), each containing a code for the amino acid sequence of a specific protein. The specific sequence of amino acids in a protein dictates the folding and, ultimately, the three-dimensional shape of that protein, and shape is vitally important to protein function.

There can be variations in the identity of individual amino acids at certain points within a protein so that one protein from two unrelated individuals may not be precisely the same. However, many of these amino acid variations do not compromise the function of proteins. Unfortunately, there are also changes or mutations within genetic codes that do lead to serious changes in protein structure and loss or alteration of protein function. These molecular changes are inheritable and can lead to disease. One of the greatest challenges facing medicine in the third millennium is the identification of these genetic flaws and the development of technologies to facilitate the correction of these mutations or the introduction of normal genetic sequences to permit the biosynthesis of functional proteins within the cells of the body. It is no exaggeration to say that the greatest advances in medicine that you are likely to see within your professional lifetime will be within the realm of genetic technology. Indeed, over the past 25 years, there has been a remarkable explosion in the development of DNA-based techniques. Many genetic flaws tied to genetic disease have already been discovered, including the genetic basis for sickle cell anemia and cystic fibrosis. Probes have been designed to identify genetic defects, and these are the tools used for the genetic diagnosis of disease. The year 2000 marked the first complete "draft" sequencing of human DNA in the Human Genome Project, and this DNA sequence will ultimately serve as a genetic roadmap for molecular biologists hunting down the genetic mutations that are the causes for a wide variety of genetic diseases. In this chapter, we hope to provide you with information that describes the use of recombinant DNA (rDNA) technology, the techniques that are the basis of genetic engineering.

STRUCTURE OF DNA

Before we enter the realm of rDNA, it is necessary to provide a background on DNA structure so that you have a working knowledge of this important macromolecule. You should appreciate that one molecule of human DNA is very much larger than any of the proteins that we have discussed. Comparing proteins and DNA by size is rather like comparing a car with a very long freight train. And any motorist who has had to wait for a freight train to pass at a level crossing is only too aware of this enormous difference in size.

One of the greatest accomplishments within the past century was the elucidation of the double-helical structure of DNA by James Watson and Francis Crick in 1953. This discovery explained many observations in genetics and was the key to understanding the precise mechanisms for the inheritance of genetic traits and genetic diseases. The discovery of the double helix held within it enough power to propel the emerging science of molecular biology (commonly identified as the biochemistry of DNA and genetics) for more than 25 years.

The double-helical structure of DNA indicates that DNA has two strands. Each is made up of building blocks, referred to as **nucleotides**, linked by phosphodiester bonds connecting the 3′ and 5′ carbons of adjacent nucleotides (Figure 8–1). Besides the linking phosphate group, each nucleotide has a sugar molecule called **deoxyribose**. The term "deoxy" simply indicates that at carbon 2 in the sugar ring, there is no oxygen, in contrast to ribose, a related sugar that does contain an -OH group at this carbon. Each nucleotide also has a cyclic structure, a nitrogen-containing base. In DNA, you find four bases, called adenine (A), guanine (G), cytosine (C), and thymine (T). You will note that A and G are larger than C and T, and A and G are called **purine bases**, while C and T are designated **pyrimidine bases**. The term "nucleoside" is used to refer to the sugar-base unit, while nucleotide designates the full base-sugar-phosphate structure.

The backbone of each chain or strand of DNA is a series of hydrophilic deoxyribose-phosphate units, with a hydrophobic base attached to each sugar. Remember, when we discussed amino acid structure in Chapter 1, we noted that if amino acids had only single amino and carboxyl groups, pro-

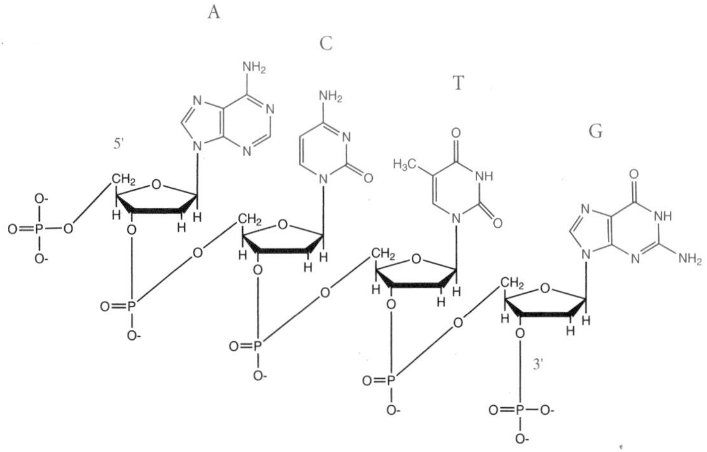

Figure 8–1 Structure of one strand of DNA, consisting of nucleotides linked by phosphodiester bonds between 3′ and 5′ carbons found on the deoxyribose component. Nucleotides consist of phosphate and deoxyribose, as well as one of four bases: adenine (A), guanine (G), cytosine (C), and thymine (T). Note that the DNA strand has a distinct polarity shown by the 5′→3′ orientation of the phosphodiester bonds.

teins would be very monotonous polymers, incapable of performing the wide variety of tasks that they do. However, the R-groups attached to amino acids confer on each protein an individuality in structure and in function.

So too, the deoxyribose-phosphate backbone of DNA is repetitious and cannot form the basis of a code that directs the assembly of amino acids into proteins. Instead, the genetic code is founded on the sequence of bases occurring within the nucleotide subunits of DNA. Each of the bases—A, G, C, and T—can be likened to a different musical note so that different meaningful tunes are composed using the base sequences found within the genes (or genetic sequences) of DNA. A gene is a specific sequence within the DNA that contains the code (or melody in our analogy) for a specific polypeptide.

The two strands of the DNA double helix come together so that the sugar-phosphate backbone is on the outside of the double helix, while the bases on the opposite strands interact at the center of the helix. Just as proteins have a specific orientation with an amino or N-terminus and a carboxyl or C-terminus, each strand of DNA has a specific orientation based on the phosphate connections between the 3′ and 5′ carbons of deoxyribose. Thus, each DNA strand has a 5′ end and a 3′ end. You can see that the two strands of DNA in the double helix run in opposite directions (based on the 5′→3′ orientation) (Figure 8–2). This is called an **antiparallel configuration**.

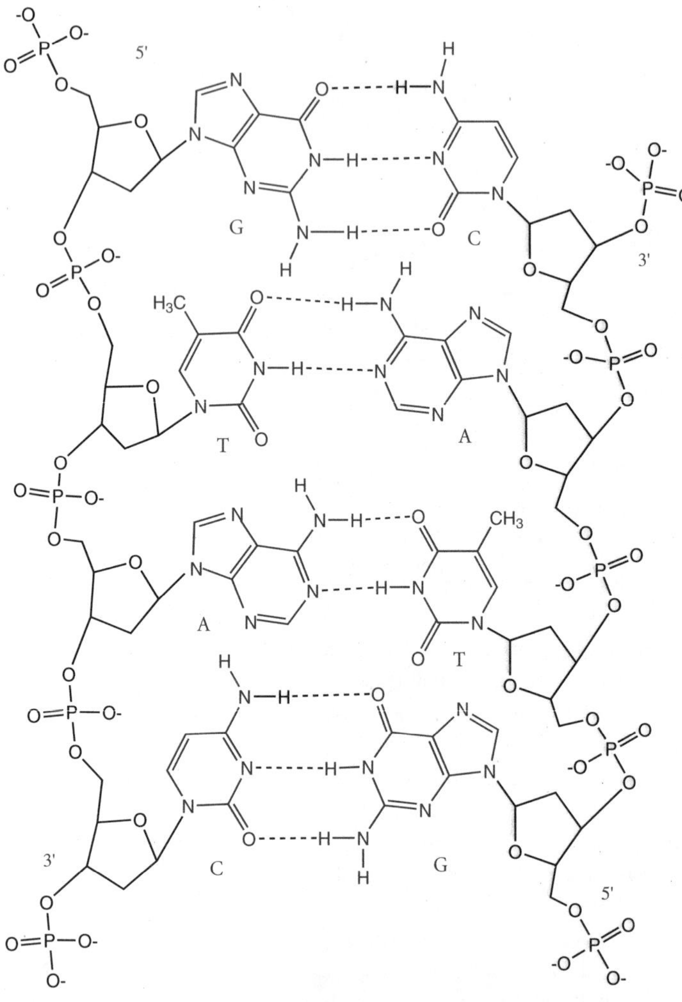

Figure 8–2 Base pairing between two strands of the DNA is an important force supporting the double-helix structure. Note that the base pairs are found within the center of the helix and that the larger purine bases (A, G) interact with the smaller pyrimidine bases (T, C), giving specific A-T and G-C pairs, on the basis of H-bonding between the bases. Also note the opposite polarity of the two strands, based on the orientation of each strand (5'→3' matches 3'→5'). The dotted lines indictate H-bonding. Adapted from Moran LA, Scrimgeour KG, Horton HR, et al. Biochemistry. 2nd ed. Englewood Cliffs (NJ): Neil Patterson-Prentice Hall; 1994.

When you look inside the double helix, you will find very specific pairing between the bases of nucleotide subunits in the two strands. A pairs with T, while G pairs with C. Thus, each purine base pairs with a specific pyrimidine base. These characteristic base pairs of DNA are held together by noncovalent bonds called hydrogen (H) bonds. In these bonds, one H found in an N-H structure of one base is shared with an O or N on the opposite base. We also saw this type of bond between amino acids within the α-helical and β-sheet structures of proteins (see Figure 1–3). In the DNA double helix, there are two H bonds between A and T and three H bonds between G and C. This base pairing between opposite strands in DNA is very critical for the formation of the double helix

The double helix has been compared to a ladder, with the long sides formed by the two sugar-phosphate backbones, while the base pairs represent the rungs or steps in the ladder. DNA is helical; thus, if you twist the opposite ends of this molecular ladder you can get an idea of the shape of the double helix. This is shown in Figure 8–3, which indicates a diameter of 2 nm for the double helix. It takes 10 nucleotide subunits to travel once around the helical structure (i.e., make one complete rotation around the spiral). You can also see that there are two types of grooves on the outside of the double helix, a larger (major) groove and a smaller (minor) groove. These grooves are important as they allow access to the base sequences. Thus, specific proteins can find specific base sequences within DNA and control the expression of certain genetic sequences within the double helix.

The **base pairing** between nucleotides in opposite strands of the DNA helix means that the sequences of bases within the two strands are complementary. Thus, for every A and C within one strand, there is a matching T and G within the other strand, forming the base pairs A-T and G-C (Figure 8–4). This specific interaction can be disrupted by heat; thus, subjecting the DNA double helix to elevated temperatures leads to denaturation, in which there is a separation of the double helix to form two single strands. However, the complementary nature of the base pairs of these two strands will allow a re-formation or **hybridization** of these two strands, once again forming the double helix when the two strands are cooled. Hybridization has been compared to the joining together of two parts of a zipper. Hybridization of two complementary DNA strands may occur either in solution or on a support surface, such as nitrocellulose filter paper. Hybridization, driven by **base complementarity**, is a very important technique used in recombinant DNA technology.

Hybridization can be carried out under different conditions and for different purposes. High-stringency conditions usually involve elevated temperature and low ionic strength (low salt concentration) and permit the hybridization of two DNA strands that have an exact complementarity in their bases. Only exact base pairing would allow the joining of the two DNA strands under these conditions. In other circumstances, you may wish hybridization to occur when there is not a perfect base-pair match. For example, you may have a short sequence of nucleotide subunits that matches, by complementarity, part of the DNA code for a murine (mouse) protein, and you wish to identify a human DNA strand that has a very sim-

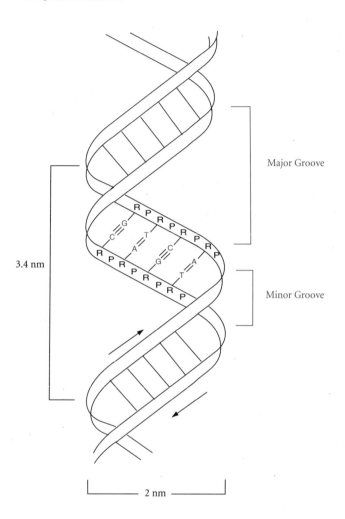

Figure 8–3 Dimensions and structure of the double helix indicate the presence of major and minor grooves along the outside of the helix that are important for proteins accessing the base sequences inside. One complete turn of the helix is found within 3.4 nm of vertical displacement. Adapted from Murray RK, Granner DK, Mayes PA, Rodwell VW. Harper's biochemistry. 25th ed. Stamford (CT): Appleton and Lange; 2000.

ilar code. The human DNA sequence does not precisely match the murine code; thus, hybridization may occur under conditions of low stringency, which allows base pairing but will tolerate some mismatches of base pairs. This procedure would help you identify the human DNA that contains a code for the human protein that is similar in structure to the murine protein.

5' - AGCGTCA - 3'
3' - TCGCAGT - 5'

Figure 8–4 The complementary nature of base pairing is shown by this common abbreviated notation for a segment of duplex DNA structure. The nucleotides are represented by single letters corresponding to each of the four bases so that the A-T and C-G interactions can be seen.

A relatively short sequence of nucleotides that has complementarity to a specific sequence of bases within a longer DNA strand is known as a **probe**. The probe is usually labeled, either by radioactivity or by a fluorescent group, which allows you to visualize the interaction between a probe and the specific DNA sequence. We will discuss the use of probes in greater detail later in this chapter, but you should remember that hybridization allows the use of probes in specific sequence identification.

MORE COMPLEX CONFIGURATIONS OF DNA

When earlier we used the image of a freight train to convey the enormous length of DNA, we were hardly doing justice to DNA's tremendous length. It has been estimated that if you could link the DNA molecules from one nucleus end to end, the resulting double helix would stretch right around your waist. This, of course, presumes that you could see and hold this hypothetical DNA chain and also makes some suppositions about the size of your waist (a potentially delicate subject). The point is that DNA molecules are very long, and they must be packed with some care to fit into the nucleus of a cell. It is somewhat like your first trip to summer camp when your father or mother, by the use of highly developed life management skills, were able to fit into your duffel bag or suitcase everything you needed for 2 weeks. Only as you struggled to repack these articles for your return home did you realize how much packing skill had been involved. (Likely the acquisition of various forms of wildlife during your stay did not help this process.)

To return to DNA, your cells must fold these long DNA chains into tightly packed structures called **chromosomes**. This is accomplished by a number of folding and coiling events (Figure 8–5). First, the double helix is wrapped around proteins called **histones** and is organized into structures called **nucleosomes**. The nucleosomes are further wound into **solenoids**, which are, in turn, folded into the chromosomal structure. Chromosomes do occur in pairs, and each is a continuous DNA double helix inherited from your mother or your father. When you look inside the nucleus of a human cell that is not dividing, you will be unable to distinguish the 23 chromosome pairs. Rather, the chromosomes are part of a mass of DNA double helices and proteins that is called **chromatin**. The chromosomes are visible in metaphase, during mitosis, and are often shown in textbooks as the classic linked pairs. However, each chromosome in metaphase has repli-

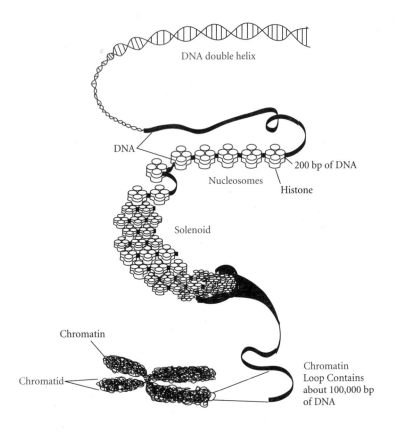

Figure 8–5 The DNA double helix is folded first into nucleosomes with the aid of histones, then into the larger solenoids, and ultimately into loops of chromatin that make up a chromosome. Note that the two chromatids shown have just been produced in mitosis, and each of these chromatids is identical. Appreciate that this pair of chromatids has been generated from one parent chromosome. Adapted from Jorde LB, Carey JC, White RL. Medical genetics. St. Louis (MO): Mosby-Year Book Inc.; 1995.

cated and appears as a pair of identical daughter **chromatids** linked at a point on each chromatid called the **centromere**. These linked pairs of metaphase daughter chromatids should be distinguished from the parent chromosome. In nondividing cells, you have pairs of these parent chromosomes (that are not linked), and each chromosome of the pair, one from your mother and one from your father, is different.

Besides histones, a number of proteins can interact with DNA. Regulatory proteins with specialized structural domains can access and interact with specific base sequences within the double helix. Thus, individual genes within DNA can be regulated by proteins. Transcription factors are proteins that bind to DNA sequences near a gene and even at DNA sites far away from a gene and facilitate the transcription of a genetic sequence by the enzyme ribonucleic acid (RNA) polymerase II. This enzyme effectively reads the code held in the DNA genetic sequence and transcribes it into messenger RNA (mRNA), the blueprint that is used in the assembly of amino acids into proteins. We shall discuss transcription in greater detail later in this chapter.

STRUCTURAL ELEMENTS FOUND WITHIN DNA

We have discussed the nucleotide subunits of DNA structure and also the folding and overall organization of this double-helical macromolecular structure into chromosomes. What are also important are structures that you will encounter as you proceed along the very long highway that is DNA, rather like the cities and towns that you will encounter while traveling across the country.

Genes

As we have noted, these are the genetic sequences that hold the codes for specific polypeptides within the human body. Thus, you can select a specific chromosome and point to a specific spot or locus as a gene that codes for the protein albumin. Your nuclear DNA contains about 32,000 genes (at latest estimate), and the total DNA in a complete set of 23 chromosomes coming from each parent accounts for about 3×10^9 base pairs. Remember that you have a complete set of genes from each parent. The DNA that actually codes for proteins represents only about 1.1 to 1.5% of the total genome (the total nuclear DNA). Among the remainder can be found noncoding sequences that are located within genes, important regulatory sites that control the expression of the genes and also sites involved in DNA duplication (replication) and the division and segregation of chromosomes. However, this still leaves a considerable proportion of human DNA that is not involved in transcription, replication, or chromosome division, and this has been termed "junk DNA."

Before we cast out this apparently nonfunctional DNA, we should take a closer look at the elements within it. When last you cleaned your room or office and discarded, in a massive purge, all those elements that you felt you did not need, it took only 24 hours before you found that many discarded items were important or had come into importance within this brief interval of time. (Please treat your old biochemistry notes and handouts with the requisite care owing them. The notes you have today could easily be needed for some comprehensive exam that looms in your future!)

Pseudogenes

Once you step outside the domain of those genetic sequences that code for proteins, or regulatory regions, you will encounter other types of structures within DNA. Pseudogenes may appear to be genetic sequences within DNA, but they cannot be used in the production of proteins. This can be caused by problems in the formation of mRNA from these sequences by transcription. Pseudogenes can lack regulatory regions that allow RNA polymerase II to recognize the pseudogene as a genetic sequence. There are many pseudogenes found within human DNA. We have not as yet talked about the synthesis of mRNA from DNA, and mRNA is the mature blueprint genetic code that directs the synthesis of a particular protein. It is believed that pseudogenes may arise when mRNA molecules are used to make DNA, a rather unusual process controlled by a viral enzyme called reverse transcriptase. This enzyme is of particular importance in the rDNA techniques, which we will be discussing in the latter part of this chapter.

Repetitive DNA

These are sequences of bases that are not genetic sequences but can be repeated up to thousands or millions of times within nuclear DNA. Repetitive sequences can make up 40 to 48% of the total DNA. Dispersed repetitive DNA can be divided into short interspersed elements (SINES, 90 to 500 bp) and long interspersed elements (LINES, 6 to 7 kb). These repeated elements do not occur with the frequency of the smaller sized satellite DNA, as noted below (Figure 8–6). Prominent among the SINES is the Alu family of repeats that are about 300 bp in length. The Alu repeats make up 2.88×10^8 base pairs, about 10% of the total DNA. Alu repeats can be found with high frequency in gene-rich areas of DNA.

Satellite DNA

These are also repetitive DNA sequences but are smaller in size and tend to be clustered at certain areas within chromosomes. Alpha-satellite DNA is made of tandem repeats of 171-bp sequences that can go on for several millions of base pairs in total length. These repeats are found close to centromeres in the chromosome structure. Minisatellites are composed of 20 to 120 bp and can extend for many thousands of base pairs in total, while microsatellites are tandem repeats of 2 to 5 bp that extend over a 100 base pairs in total. The best described microsatellites are dinucleotide repeats. Microsatellites are useful because they can be used in chromosome mapping. You can appreciate that the bulk of DNA is not composed of genes. Thus, finding a gene within a chromosome can be a "needle in a haystack"

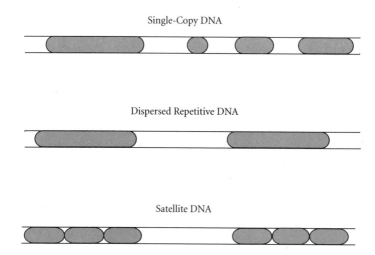

Figure 8–6 Single and repetitive DNA can be found within DNA sequences. Single-copy DNA may represent genes or pseudogenes, while repetitive DNA can be dispersed throughout the DNA molecule or present as satellite repeats that are in tandem and can run on for long stretches within the DNA sequence. Adapted from Jorde LB, Carey JC, White RL. Medical genetics. St. Louis (MO): Mosby-Year Book Inc.; 1995.

proposition. We will talk further about the hunt for disease genes; microsatellite markers can be particularly useful in these searches, particularly when researchers may have little or no idea of the nature of the protein or the gene that is the cause of the pathology in question.

MITOCHONDRIAL DNA

There is some DNA that is associated with the mitochondria, although it is usually less than 0.1% of the size of the total nuclear DNA. Mitochondrial DNA has genetic sequences coding for a limited number of mitochondrial proteins. There are genetic diseases that result from mutations in mitochondrial DNA, and the frequency of occurrence of mitochondrial mutations is rather high, quite possibly because of the oxidative nature of the mitochondrial matrix and a lack of DNA repair mechanisms that are found within the nucleus. Mitochondrial DNA is of interest because it is maternally inherited. In the fusion of the egg and sperm during fertilization, there is an equal contribution of nuclear DNA from both maternal and paternal cells, but it is the mitochondria in the egg that are progenitors for the mitochondria in the developing embryo and fetus. Although some of the sperm mitochondria may enter the egg during the fusion process, these are destroyed following fertilization. Thus, it is believed that the mitochondria in the cells of women and men can be traced back to a first mother (Eve, if you will).

RIBONUCLEIC ACID

RNA is a relative of DNA but has a number of distinctive features. RNA is made up of nucleotide subunits, but these nucleotides have the sugar ribose, instead of deoxyribose. RNA contains the bases A, G, C, and U, where U is the pyrimidine uracil (found instead of thymine, which is characteristic of DNA). Modified bases and unique bases can also be found in RNA, in contrast to DNA, where modified bases occur less frequently. RNA is single stranded and, thus, does not exist in a double-helical form, although the single strand of RNA can loop back on itself, forming a helical-like interaction (e.g., the "hairpin" structure). There is also a variety of different classes of RNA, including ribosomal RNAs, messenger RNAs (mRNA) that carry the genetic coding blueprint for the assembly of proteins, and transfer RNAs (tRNA), a number of species that bind to specific amino acids and facilitate the precise assembly of amino acids into proteins.

EUKARYOTIC GENES, mRNA, AND TRANSCRIPTION

While we have introduced the gene as a concept, we have not noted the specific elements of gene structure. A gene is a sequence of bases that contains a code used in the production of a specific protein. However, in a human gene, the code is actually interrupted and is not continuous. The gene is made up of coding sequences or segments called **exons**, but these are usually separated by noncoding sequences called **introns** (Figure 8–7). There are also regions that are not coding elements in front of the first exon and following the last exon. As you can imagine, it is particularly important to locate a particular DNA gene sequence within the vast lengths of DNA so that the DNA genetic code can be effectively reproduced within mRNA in the process of transcription. On the 5′ side of the eukaryotic gene are found regulatory regions. **Promoters**, which contain the sequences TATA and CAAT and are known as the TATA box and CAAT box, are the sites of transcription initiation. Promoters are sites where transcription factors come together to position RNA polymerase II in front of the gene sequence (Figure 8–8). Mutations within promoter sequences can significantly reduce gene transcription. RNA polymerase II proceeds along the DNA gene sequence and synthesizes mRNA. Farther upstream from the promoter regions or downstream from the genetic sequence are found other regulatory elements called **enhancers**. These can also facilitate transcription by interacting with promoter regions, likely by DNA looping to allow contact with RNA polymerase II. Enhancers may be involved in the tissue-specific

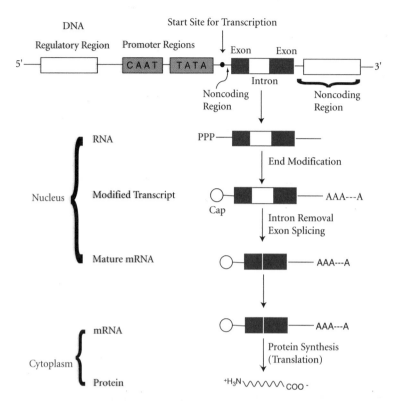

Figure 8–7 The eukaryotic gene and transcription are pictured. Note that a gene consists of both exon sequences that contain the genetic code and intervening intron sequences. Thus, transcription initially produces a primary RNA transcript with both exon and intron sequences. This transcript is capped and also is given a poly-A tail to protect the mRNA from degradation. As well, the intron sequences are removed to produce the mature mRNA that can enter the cytoplasm and direct protein synthesis. Adapted from Murray RK, Granner DK, Mayes PA, Rodwell VW. Harper's biochemistry. 25th ed. Stamford (CT): Appleton and Lange; 2000.

expression of certain proteins, as enhancers are active only in certain cell types. While each cell has a complete complement of chromosomes and of genes, you should appreciate that only certain genes are expressed in each cell type. Thus, enhancers may take part in allowing the production of hemoglobin in reticulocytes and albumin in hepatocytes while permitting the synthesis of enzymes of glycolysis in all cell types (as these enzymes are important in cellular energy production). Regulation of transcription is of particular importance within individual cell types.

Other regulatory elements include chromatin openers that facilitate the exposure of a gene to RNA polymerase II and response elements, which are DNA sequences that bind other regulatory molecules, for example, cyclic

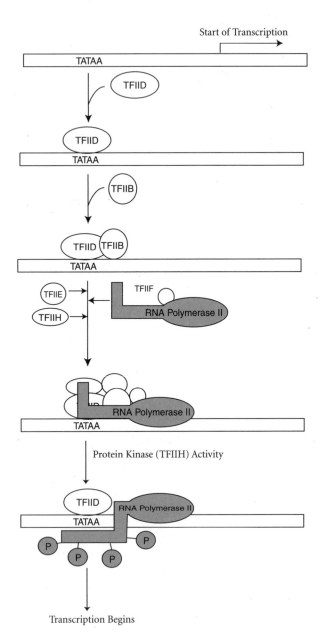

Figure 8–8 The transcription of a gene requires the assembly of transcription factors at a promoter sequence (such as a TATA box). The transcription factors allow RNA polymerase II to be positioned near the initiation site and phosphorylated so that the polymerase can proceed with transcription. Adapted from Alberts B, Bray D, Lewis J, et al. Molecular biology of the cell. 3rd ed. New York: Garland Publishing; 1994.

AMP (cAMP) (as noted in Chapter 7), retinoic acid, and steroid hormone-receptor complexes. Silencers are DNA sequences that decrease the transcription of genes. Within these regulatory events, you may hear of cis and trans acting effects. A **cis locus** is a DNA sequence that is relatively close to the gene and controls transcription. A **trans acting element** indicates regulation of transcription by a gene distinct from that being transcribed (and quite possibly on another chromosome) and involves the synthesis of a protein that will play a role in transcription.

Part of the complication in the understanding of DNA in general and transcription in particular is the double-stranded nature of the DNA helix. While the two strands of DNA are complementary, only one strand has the actual genetic or coding sequence, while the other DNA strand holds a complementary (template or antisense) sequence (Figure 8–9). In transcription, the RNA polymerase recognizes a sequence of bases in one strand of DNA and uses ribonucleotides containing A, G, C, and U to assemble a complementary sequence in the product mRNA. Because of this complementarity during assembly, the actual coding strand of DNA cannot be used, simply because the resulting mRNA would have the antisense base sequence. Thus, it is the antisense or template strand of DNA that is used in transcription to generate mRNA with the true code that matches the DNA coding sequence.

Transcription proceeds in a 5′→3′ direction, generating a primary RNA transcript that has the complete sequence of exons and introns found within the gene. This primary transcript is modified by a structural cap made at the 5′ end and by the addition of many adenine-containing ribonucleotide subunits at the 3′ end (the so-called poly-A tail). These modifications serve to protect the RNA transcript from enzyme attack and degradation. However, this modified transcript still contains sequences that cannot be used as a blueprint for protein synthesis, simply because many of the regions of the modified transcript are based on intron sequences.

DNA Strands

Coding   ⟶ 5′-T G G A A T T T C G C G G A T T A C A A T G T C A C A C A G G A A C A G C T A T G A C C A T C -3′
Template ⟶ 3′-A C C T T A A A G C G C C T A A T G T T A C A G T G T G T C C T T G T C G A T A C T G G T A G -5′
mRNA   ⟶   5′- A U U U C G C G G A U U A C A A U G U C A C A C A G G A A C A G C U A U G A C C A U C -3′

Figure 8–9 The double-helical nature of DNA is based on complementary base pairing between the two DNA strands. Thus, one strand contains the relevant genetic or coding sequence (oriented in a 5′→3′ direction), while the opposite strand has the antisense or template sequence (oriented in a 3′→5′ direction). It is the template strand that is used in transcription to direct the synthesis of mRNA, which by base complementarity will have the coding sequence.

Production of Mature mRNA

To achieve the true coding sequence in mRNA, the intron sequences must be removed, and there can be a large number of these. Often, the mature mRNA can be less than 20% of the size of the primary transcript. The gene for the muscle protein dystrophin, for example, has 70 introns. The removal of introns is carried out by spliceosomes, composed of a number of proteins and small nuclear RNA molecules. Intron sequences are marked by the bases G and U on the 5′ side of the intron and A and G on its 3′ side (Figure 8–10). The spliceosome promotes the formation of a lariat based on this GU....AG boundary. The intron sequence is removed, and the abutting exon sequences are bonded together. Thus, the mature mRNA is composed of the 5′→3′ sequence of exons found within the gene. This mRNA base sequence holds the code for the assembly of amino acids, and the mRNA sequence is read at the ribosome, while tRNA molecules bring specific amino acids for sequential assembly into protein, following the instructions of the mRNA code. The conversion of the mRNA code into protein is known as **translation**.

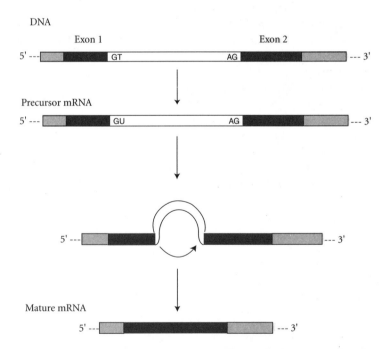

Figure 8–10 Introns are removed from primary mRNA transcripts by the action of spliceosomes. These large particles remove the intron sequences, which are demarcated by the 5′ GU.......AG 3′ nucleotide dimers. A lariat is formed using the intron sequence to facilitate the excision of the intron and the bonding of the adjacent exon sequences. Adapted from Brock DJH. Molecular genetics for the clinician. Cambridge (UK): Cambridge University Press; 1993.

RECOMBINANT DNA (rDNA) TECHNIQUES

What we have discussed so far represents, in a very abbreviated manner, the major discoveries that followed the proposal in 1953 that established the double-helix structure of DNA. These were very significant findings, but by the mid- to late 1970s, there was a feeling that molecular biology had come as far as it could, with the techniques that were available. What then happened was another remarkably important series of discoveries that propelled molecular biology by another quantum leap. The word "recombinant" refers to DNA molecules from different sources that have been combined to form a new hybrid DNA molecule. It was this ability to specifically modify and graft together DNA molecules that was the heart of the new initiative and brought scientists closer to the goal of genetic engineering.

At this point, a list and short description of these technologies and tools will outline the areas that we will be discussing from now on in this chapter:

1. Restriction enzymes: These enzymes, isolated from bacteria, cut duplex (double-stranded) DNA at very specific sites. These enzymes recognize specific base sequences in DNA and produce fragments that can be incorporated into other molecules of duplex DNA cut by the same enzyme. These fragments can be used to generate recombinant DNA.

2. Cloning of recombinant DNA: In this procedure, DNA fragments produced by restriction enzymes can be introduced into DNA vector molecules. The vectors can be incorporated into bacteria (or other cells), which then make large numbers of copies of the vector. A clone can refer to these identical DNA molecules produced by the bacterial cell.

3. DNA sequencing: There are different techniques for DNA sequencing, but the one of major interest is the dideoxy method developed by Fred Sanger. In this procedure, a single-stranded DNA molecule of unknown base sequence is used as a substrate in a DNA polymerase reaction (Figure 8–11). This enzyme will use the unknown DNA strand as a guide and assemble deoxynucleotides into a new strand of DNA that is complementary to the unknown. A primer that matches the first few nucleotides at the 3′ end of the unknown is required, and the polymerase reaction synthesizes the new DNA strand in a 5′→3′ manner.

The interesting feature of this technique is the use of dideoxynucleotides, each containing one of the four DNA bases. In these dideoxynucleotides, there is no -OH group at carbon 3 of the deoxyribose; thus, phosphodiester bridges cannot be constructed when this dideoxynucleotide is used by the DNA polymerase. Four tubes can be set up, each with the unknown DNA strand, the short primer, DNA polymerase, the four normal deoxynucleotides containing the bases A, G, C, and T, and also a small quantity of one of the dideoxynucleotides

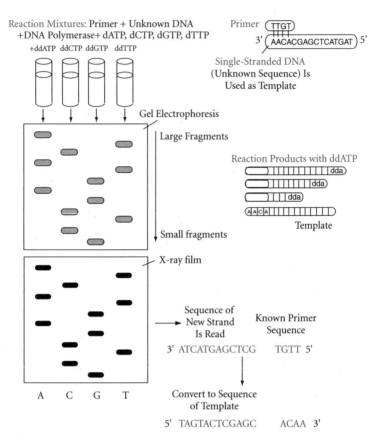

Figure 8–11 Sequencing of unknown DNA strands by the Sanger method involves the use of dideoxynucleotides. Here, a small primer is constructed to match the 3′ end sequence of the unknown DNA; then, DNA polymerase and nucleotides are used to synthesize a matching strand of DNA, following base pairing. Four incubations are used, each with the unknown DNA, primer, polymerase, nucleotides, and a small quantity of one of the four dideoxynucleotides. These artificial nucleotides, when selected for use by the DNA polymerase, terminate the enzyme reaction. Thus, if the products of each incubation are separated by electrophoresis, a sequence of bases in the new DNA strand can be read, and from this, the unknown DNA sequence deduced by base-pairing rules. Adapted from Brock DJH. Molecular genetics for the clinician. Cambridge (UK): Cambridge University Press; 1993.

(ddATP, ddGTP, ddCTP, or ddTTP). When the DNA polymerase chooses one of the dideoxynucleotide substrates, the polymerization stops.

Thus, incubation with ddATP, for example, will lead to the production of a number of incomplete DNA fragments, each ending with ddA where an A nucleotide is found in the sequence. These fragments can be separated by gel electrophoresis on the basis of their size, with the smallest fragments running the quickest. If a radioactive form of the primer is used, these bands can be localized on the gel using an overlaying x-ray film. The use of each of the four dideoxy nucleotides will produce a different set of DNA fragments, each ending in a specific base found within the unknown sequence. By reading the bands from the shortest to the longest, the actual sequence of the bases in the newly made DNA strand can be read, and from this, by complementarity, the sequence in the original unknown DNA strand can be constructed.

4. Hybridization: This complementary binding of DNA molecules, or of DNA and complementary deoxynucleotide probes, is a vital part of many of the new technologies. It is also possible for hybridization to occur between mRNA and a complementary strand of DNA, a feature central to the functioning of reverse transcriptase, which we describe below.

5. Reverse transcriptase: One of the central ideas arising from the Watson and Crick discovery was that there was a definite direction in the flow of genetic information, proceeding from DNA to mRNA and finally from mRNA to protein. However, a viral enzyme, reverse transcriptase, which uses mRNA to construct a complementary DNA sequence, thus reversing the sequence of information transfer, was identified (and made available).

6. Blotting techniques: In these electrophoretic procedures, fragments of DNA or RNA or intact proteins can be separated on gels and the bands transferred by blotting onto nitrocellulose sheets. The sheets can then be exposed to antibodies to allow the identification of specific proteins or exposed to labeled probes for the identification of DNA or RNA fragments with complementary sequences.

7. Synthesis of deoxynucleotide probes: This involves the chemical synthesis of specific oligodeoxynucleotide sequences that can be used to identify longer DNA fragments with sequences complementary to the probe.

8. Site-directed mutagenesis: This technique allows the replacement of a single amino acid in a protein with another amino acid to evaluate the importance of single amino acids in protein function.

9. Knock-out genes: In this procedure, animals that lack a specific functional gene can be reared. This can allow an assessment of the importance of a particular protein.

RESTRICTION ENZYMES

This was the discovery and technological breakthrough that revitalized molecular biology. The restriction enzymes are powerful because they cut duplex DNA by the recognition of a specific base sequence. They were isolated from a number of bacteria, and now hundreds are available. The enzymes have abbreviated names for the bacteria from which they were isolated. Thus, *EcoRI* indicates an *Escherichia coli* source, R represents the strain of bacteria (RY13), and the Roman numeral I allows a distinction to be made, as more than one enzyme comes from this source. (There is an *EcoRII*.)

The restriction enzymes are endonucleases because they can cut the phosphodiester bonds within a DNA strand, while exonucleases restrict their activity to the ends of DNA molecules. The restriction enzymes were novel because they recognized a specific sequence in the two DNA strands. This sequence is between 4 and 8 bp in length. The restriction enzymes that recognized 7 or 8 bp were called rare cutters because these sequences would occur less frequently in DNA, and fewer (and larger) DNA fragments would be produced by the action of these enzymes. Restriction enzymes occur as dimers and, thus, can recognize sequences within the two strands of duplex DNA. Specifically, these are called **palindromic sequences** because they have the same base sequence in either direction for the two strands (recalling that the two strands run in an antiparallel direction). One example of a palindrome often given: rats live on no evil star. Most word palindromes are rather uninformative and do not emphasize that the reading in two different directions takes place on the two DNA strands. A better representation (although not perfect) would be:

5′ rats live 3′
3′ evil star 5′

Restriction enzymes can produce fragments with sticky ends or with blunt ends. This is shown below for the enzymes *EcoRI* and *HpaI* (from *Haemophilus parainfluenzae*).

EcoRI:	5′ G ↓AATTC 3′ 3′ CTTAA↑G 5′	Gives sticky ends after attack
HpaI	5′ GTT ↓AAC 3′ 3′ CAA↑ TTG 5′	Gives blunt ends after attack

The meaning of the term "blunt ends" is hopefully obvious, but "sticky ends" indicates that after hydrolysis, it is possible (because of the complementary base pairs) to realign the overlapping (sticky ends) and re-establish the connections between the severed nucleotide sequences. This latter step can be carried out by DNA ligase. It's a little like having Velcro at the cut ends that allows the strands to reassociate. The beauty of the specific hydrolysis of duplex DNA sequences is this: when two different DNA molecules are cut by the same restriction enzyme, it is possible to take one fragment from one DNA molecule and hybridize it with a fragment produced from the second DNA molecule (Figure 8–12). We will speak of this in greater detail when we come to molecular cloning techniques.

Because of the specificity of the restriction enzymes, it is possible to produce a reproducible and characteristic population of DNA fragments from one DNA molecule. These can be separated from one another, by electrophoresis, to produce a banding pattern. This can be called a **fingerprint** and is based on the specific sites for restriction enzyme hydrolysis within

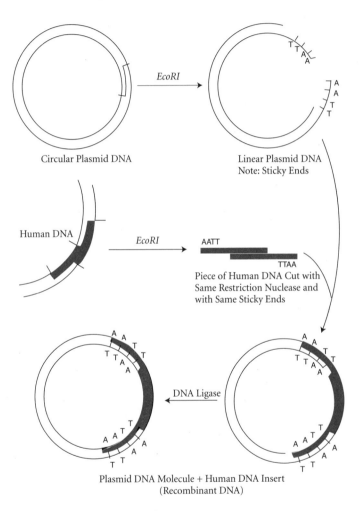

Figure 8–12 The restriction endonuclease *EcoR1* attacks specific sequences found in duplex DNA. Thus, "sticky ends" can be produced at a restriction site within a circular bacterial DNA plasmid. A DNA fragment produced from human DNA by the same enzyme will have complementary "sticky ends" and will be able to hybridize with the opened bacterial plasmid. DNA ligase will seal the new human fragment into the bacterial plasmid vector. Adapted from Murray RK, Granner DK, Mayes PA, Rodwell VW. Harper's biochemistry. 25th ed. Stamford (CT): Appleton and Lange; 2000.

DNA. This fingerprinting is particularly effective for smaller DNA molecules, as the number of fragments produced from the total human DNA could be very large and difficult to separate from one another. For example, the DNA molecule in the simian virus 40 (SV40, 5.1 kb) when hydrolyzed by *HindIII* (*H. influenzae* Rd) gives 12 characteristic fragments seen on electrophoresis.

MOLECULAR CLONING

In this technique, duplex DNA fragments produced by restriction enzyme hydrolysis are incorporated into DNA vectors that will carry the incorporated fragments into bacteria (or other cells), where both the vector and newly incorporated DNA can be produced in relatively large amounts. Thus, the DNA is cloned, or reproduced, in large numbers.

There are a number of different types of vectors that can be used. The smallest are the plasmids, which are small circular duplex DNA molecules from bacteria that can hold DNA inserts up to about 10 kb. Plasmids are extrachromosomal DNA, and they can be duplicated within bacteria to high copy numbers; for example, within *E. coli,* this number can be as high as 1,000 per cell. Phage (bacteriophage) vectors are usually linear duplex DNA molecules from these bacterial viruses that can accommodate duplex DNA inserts up to about 20 kb. Vectors for larger DNA inserts are cosmids (hybrids of plasmids and phage), which can take up to 40 kb of DNA, yeast artificial chromosomes (YACs), which are constructed using yeast centromeres, telomere sequences (DNA sequences found at the ends of chromosomes), and the DNA insert, which can be quite large (up to 1,200 kb). The YACs containing DNA inserts are inserted into yeast rather than bacteria.

The steps in cloning can be illustrated using a plasmid called **pBR322**. This plasmid has genes for tetracycline resistance (Tet^r) and for ampicillin resistance (AMP^r) (Figure 8–13). In other words, the bacteria have in these plasmids genes that can be used to direct the synthesis of enzymes that will inactivate the antibiotics. This certainly emphasizes the potential for bacteria to adapt to, and deal with, poisons directed against themselves.

The Cutting Step

Within the AMP^r gene, there is a DNA sequence that is a site for the restriction enzyme *PstI* (*Providencia stuartii*). Thus, hydrolysis of pBR322 with *PstI* will disrupt the AMP^r gene, while leaving the Tet^r gene intact. If human DNA is also incubated with *PstI*, many fragments will be produced, which will have complementary sticky ends to the sticky ends in the hydrolyzed plasmid (see Figure 8–13).

The Incorporation Step

When the human DNA fragments are mixed with the *PstI*-digested pBR322, base complementarity will lead to the hybridization of the human DNA

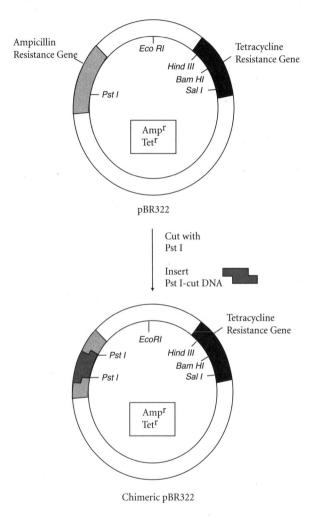

pBR322

Chimeric pBR322

Figure 8–13 The plasmid pBR322 contains both AMP^r and Tet^r genes. As well, there is a restriction site for *Pst1* within the AMP^r gene. Thus, the cutting of pBR322 at this site and the insertion of a human DNA fragment will lead to the formation of chimeric pBR322. The infection of bacteria with the chimeric plasmid will be shown by bacterial progeny that are resistant to tetracycline but sensitive to ampicillin. Thus, when plated on agar, bacteria that have taken up the chimeric plasmid vector can be identified. The nature of the human DNA fragment within individual transformed bacterial colonies can be identified by the use of appropriate oligonucleotide probes. Adapted from Murray RK, Granner DK, Mayes PA, Rodwell VW. Harper's biochemistry. 25th ed. Stamford (CT): Appleton and Lange; 2000.

fragments with the plasmid. The enzyme DNA ligase can now be used to covalently seal these new fragments into the plasmid vector. You should appreciate that you have produced a large population of different recombinant DNA molecules, as individual plasmids will carry different human DNA fragments.

The Transformation Step

Adding these vectors with their human DNA components to *E. coli* will result in the infection of these bacterial cells with this recombinant DNA. Usually, the multiplicity (frequency) of infection is arranged to be approximately one plasmid vector per cell.

The Cloning Step

One good thing about using bacteria in molecular cloning (which is not so good if you have a "strep" throat or an infected finger) is that bacteria multiply very rapidly. Thus, overnight, each transformed *E. coli* cell can produce many identical daughter cells, and there will be a replication of the circular plasmids within the bacterial cells as well. As the infectivity is approximately one plasmid per cell, each transformed cell will have one of the human fragments contained in the plasmid vector. The transformed bacterial culture may now be analyzed by "plating" the cells on petri dishes with agar containing either ampicillin or tetracycline. The plating technique allows a small sample of the culture to be spread quickly with a needle over the agar surface, leaving single cells on the agar. The cells will grow, each producing a colony of identical cells. Be aware that these cells are also called **clones**, and this term can describe identical cells or identical recombinant DNA.

The usefulness of having these antibiotic-resistance genes becomes apparent. Transformed bacterial cells will be able to grow on the tetracycline-agar, but not on the ampicillin-agar, as the incorporation of human DNA into the vector disrupted (and thus inactivated) the AMP^r gene. Any *E. coli* cells that have been transformed will have the Tet^r gene and will grow, forming colonies on the tetracycline-agar. It is possible to place a circular filter gently on top of the tetracycline-agar so that cells from the agar are transferred onto the filter. The filter can then be carefully placed on an ampicillin-containing plate so that the pattern of colonies found on the tetracycline plate is reproduced on the ampicillin plate (or replicate plate). Not all the transferred colonies will grow because those with disrupted AMP^r genes will die on the ampicillin plate. Those colonies from the tetracycline plate that do not grow on the ampicillin-agar will be those that have been transformed. Each of the transformed colonies will contain one of the human DNA fragments within the vector.

The Selection Step

It is likely that you are interested in one fragment of the human DNA that has a specific sequence (e.g., a sequence containing a gene). At this stage, it is necessary to select those colonies that contain a specific DNA fragment. If part of this sequence is known, it is possible to synthesize a complementary, labeled oligonucleotide probe. By transferring colonies from the tetracycline plate to a nitrocellulose filter and lysing the colonies with sodium hydroxide (NaOH), the denatured DNA may be exposed to the single-stranded probe. Hybridization with the probe will indicate those colonies that have the DNA fragment of interest. As you can see, it is useful to have a number of replicate tetracycline plates so that the original colonies can be used in subsequent steps. The plasmid vectors with the human DNA insert of interest can be recovered from the colonies, and by the use of *PstI*, the human DNA fragment (now in much larger quantity) can be recovered from the vector. Thus, by the use of a bacterial host, you have selected and amplified the quantity of a particular human DNA fragment or fragments.

Libraries

You can see that there are potential commercial applications in molecular cloning. Companies can produce a population of fragments from the DNA of individual organisms, insert these into an appropriate vector, clone them, and sell the vector-DNA populations to scientists. This preparation could then be used in the cloning of a large variety of different fragments, depending on the genetic sequence of interest. These populations—collections of cloned rDNA (recombinant DNA) fragments—are called libraries.

A genomic library is made by incubating DNA from a particular cell or tissue with a restriction enzyme. This incubation is not taken to completion (i.e., all possible sites for enzyme activity are not hydrolyzed). Rather, an incomplete digestion generates a smaller population of larger DNA fragments. The rationale is the larger the fragment, the more likely it is to find an intact gene. If 3×10^9 bp are found within the human genome, then considering an average fragment size of 20 kb, about 1.5×10^5 DNA fragments will be produced. Phage or yeast artificial chromosomes (YACs) are used as vectors to accommodate the size of fragments generated. Thus, a genomic library represents all the DNA sequences, including genetic sequences and sequences that do not code for proteins.

A cDNA library is a different type of DNA collection and, as you will appreciate, is more practical in many aspects than the genomic library. The "c" in cDNA stands for complementary. The cDNA library is produced using that rather valuable and nonconformist enzyme reverse transcriptase. If you select one cell type and isolate the mRNA pool from that cell, reverse transcriptase allows you to generate DNA sequences that match the blueprint sequences found in mRNA (Figure 8–14). The enzyme uses mRNA as a template to generate a complementary strand of DNA. The mRNA strand is then degraded, and the enzyme can further produce a new strand of DNA to match the single DNA strand made from mRNA. These DNA sequences match the sequence of exons found in the genes within the genome. These duplex DNA molecules can be inserted into vectors (it's a little more involved than the genomic library procedure), and these can be cloned. You can purchase a cDNA library that contains DNA sequences coding for each protein expressed within a particular cell or tissue. The size of the DNA molecules within the cDNA library is considerably smaller than those DNA fragments found in a genomic library. It is estimated that there are about 10^4 different mRNA species (and thus 10^4 proteins expressed) within one cell type. If you are interested in a particular protein, you must select a cDNA library from a cell or tissue that produces that protein. For example, reticulocytes are a good choice for the study of globins. cDNA libraries can thus differ considerably from cell to cell and tissue to tissue. As well, it is pos-

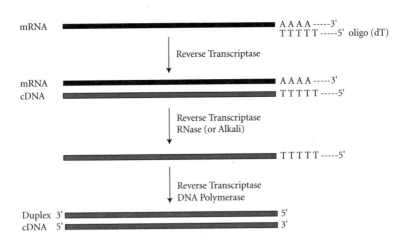

Figure 8–14 The action of reverse transcriptase (of viral origin) takes mRNA and produces a complementary DNA strand. This hybrid mRNA–DNA can be attacked by RNase activity within the transcriptase to eliminate the original mRNA template. Following this, the new DNA strand can be used to generate a complementary DNA strand that contains the original mRNA coding sequence. Thus, cDNA that has a complete genetic sequence without introns is produced and is considerably smaller than the gene sequences found in genomic DNA. Adapted from Brock DJH. Molecular genetics for the clinician. Cambridge (UK): Cambridge University Press; 1993.

sible that a specific protein may be expressed at a certain stage of development; thus, timing is important in the selection of a cDNA library.

A cDNA library can be used in a similar manner to a genomic library but with the assurance that complete coding sequences are present within duplex DNA molecules. cDNA libraries are used in bacterial transformation, and individual transformed colonies will contain a single coding sequence. Colonies can be selected using oligonucleotide probes and the appropriate cDNA recovered. Probes may be constructed, if part of the sequence of the protein of interest is known. The recovery of the cDNA will allow sequencing of the component bases, and this, in turn, will allow you to determine the complete sequence of amino acids in the protein. Another application using cDNA is the commercial production of proteins that may be difficult or possibly dangerous to isolate from animal sources. For example, growth hormone can be isolated from the pituitaries of cows, but given the possibility of contracting encephalopathies or other virus-based neurologic diseases from bovine tissues, it is preferable to transform bacteria with the human cDNA for this protein and allow the bacteria to produce the protein. The protein can be made in considerable quantity and can be purified from the bacterial source.

PROBES IN rDNA TECHNOLOGY

We have mentioned probes in several applications, and it would be wise to explain the different kinds of probes that can be used and how they can be constructed. A cDNA probe can be made by the action of reverse transcriptase with a specific mRNA. A single-stranded DNA probe may be generated from the duplex DNA product. The cDNA probe may allow the selection of a genomic DNA fragment carrying the complete sequence of exons and introns.

More usually, probes are oligonucleotide sequences of at least 18 nucleotides. If a characteristic mutated sequence of nucleotides is known for a specific disease gene, a probe that is complementary to the DNA sequence containing the specific mutation can be constructed. For example, cystic fibrosis (CF) is caused by the lack of a functional chloride ion channel in cellular membranes. This defect results in the production of thick mucus in the digestive tract and lungs (as well as other locations), leading to gastrointestinal and respiratory problems. A common mutation associated with CF is the loss of three nucleotides from the normal genetic sequence, resulting in the loss of one amino acid, phenylalanine, at position 508 in the amino acid sequence of the chloride channel (Figure 8–15). Using the sequence that includes the mutation, a probe that can be used to identify this mutated sequence in other samples of human DNA can be made. Thus, the probe can be used to screen for CF caused by this particular mutation.

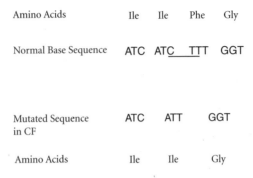

Amino Acids	Ile	Ile	Phe	Gly
Normal Base Sequence	ATC	ATC	<u>TTT</u>	GGT

Mutated Sequence in CF	ATC	ATT	GGT
Amino Acids	Ile	Ile	Gly

Figure 8–15 The sequence of DNA found in the CF gene has one particularly common mutation. This consists of a lack (deletion) of a sequence of three nucleotides (underlined) found in the control DNA resulting in the loss of a phenylalanine residue at position 508 in the chloride channel encoded by the CF gene. This loss leads to improper folding of the CF chloride channel (CFTR), and this mutant protein is destroyed by the cell. The F508 mutation is found with high frequency in Denmark and northern Europe but is less common in southern Europe and the Middle East. In total, some 800 mutations have been detected in the CF gene.

A third route to probe construction lies in the knowledge of a specific amino acid sequence within a protein. The genetic code found in DNA and mRNA consists of triplets of bases, with each triplet coding for one amino acid (Figure 8–16). Thus, it is possible to generate the coding sequence if the amino acid sequence is known. Unfortunately, there is one problem: for certain amino acids, it is possible to have more than one triplet code. For example, in the sequence

-Tryptophan-Tyrosine-Methionine-Isoleucine-Tyrosine-Tryptophan-

tryptophan and methionine have only one triplet code each, while tyrosine has two, and isoleucine has three codons. Thus, a number of probes are needed to adequately test the different possibilities in the genetic sequence. The number of probes corresponds to the number of coding choices for each amino acid: (1) (2) (1) (3) (2) (1). Thus, there are 12 possible genetic sequences that could produce the above sequence of amino acids, and 12 possible probes are required. This requirement for multiple probes is known as **probe degeneracy**. If you have a knowledge of odds in selecting lottery tickets, you may see this more clearly, but the total number of possibilities is equal to the product of the choices at each position. One of the 12 possible mRNA sequences for the amino acid sequence is shown below, as is the corresponding complementary probe sequence that will be used to bind to coding sequences in DNA.

5'-UGG-UAC-AUG-AUA-UAC-UGG-3' mRNA

3'-ACC-ATG- TAC- TAT- ATG-ACC-5' probe

RNA Codons	Amino Acid
GGA, GGC, GGG, GGU	Glycine
GCA, GCC, GCG, GCU	Alanine
UUA, UUG, CUA, CUC, CUG, CUU	Leucine
AUA, AUC, AUU	Isoleucine
GUA, GUC, GUG, GUU	Valine
UUC, UUU	Phenylalanine
UAC, UAU	Tyrosine
UGG	Tryptophan
UGC, UGU	Cysteine
AUG	Methionine
AGC, AGU, UCA, UCC, UCG, UCU	Serine
ACA, ACC, ACG, ACU	Threonine
GAC, GAU	Aspartic acid
GAA, GAG	Glutamic acid
AAC, AAU	Asparagine
CAA, CAG	Glutamine
AAA, AAG	Lysine
AGA, AGG, CGA, CGC, CGG, CGU	Arginine
CAC, CAU	Histidine
CCA, CCC, CCG, CCU	Proline
UAA, UAG, UGA	Stop

Figure 8–16 The genetic code shows how mRNA base triplets are translated into specific amino acids. Note that there is no duplication of mRNA codes among amino acids, that is, one code, such as GCA, only specifies one amino acid (alanine). However, there can be more than one mRNA code for one amino acid (degeneracy), that is, alanine has the codes GCA, GCC, GCG, and GCU. This can complicate the construction of oligonucleotide probes on the basis of amino acid sequences in proteins.

Usually, probes should be a minimum of 18 nucleotides in length, corresponding to a sequence of six amino acids.

A fourth type of probe is based not on DNA sequences but on protein. Antibodies (immunoglobulins) are proteins that can be made by the immune system in response to a foreign protein entering the body. For example, if a human protein is purified and injected into a rabbit, the animal may respond by producing antibodies that will specifically bind to the human protein. These are called **polyclonal antibodies** and can be used to identify the human protein. Thus, the molecular cloning procedure outlined earlier in this chapter can be extended so that the bacterial cells may use the new human cDNA to generate a human protein. In turn, this protein, produced by a particular bacterial colony, may be identified by the binding of the polyclonal antibody. As you might expect, there can be a few potential glitches in this procedure (rather like an inventor proceeding from the bicycle to the motorbike). First, it would be necessary to have not only the genetic sequence within the bacteria but also a good promoter within the vector to ensure that the bacteria would transcribe human cDNA into mRNA.

The next hurdle may be thought of as the modifications that some proteins require in human cells, following translation (protein synthesis). For example, glycosylation reactions add sugar (oligosaccharide) chains to specific amino acids in some human proteins. Bacteria do not carry out such modifications. However, the oligosaccharide chains in the human protein may be very important to the binding of polyclonal antibodies. If this is the case, the bacteria may synthesize the protein without sugar chains, and this protein would be undetectable using the antibody to the human protein.

It's a little like an automotive plant producing the basic car, while the dealership adds extras, such as racing stripes or an advanced, full-surround, 200 decibel stereo system. If you are waiting at the automotive plant trying to recognize "your" car by hearing the heavy duty sounds of Metallica, you may be waiting a long time. Nonetheless, if you are fortunate and the antibody, indeed, recognizes a human protein made in bacteria, you may label the antibody with radioactivity and use it to identify the colony that is making the human protein. Such bacteria that can successfully make human proteins are called **expression vectors**.

BLOTTING TECHNIQUES AND THE POINTS OF THE COMPASS

An important technique in rDNA technology is the ability to separate DNA and RNA molecules or their fragments as well as proteins and to identify these using probes. Electrophoresis, using a polyacrylamide or agarose gel medium, is used to separate these macromolecules. These polymerized gels have a consistency somewhat like that of a fruit roll-up (although the taste is definitely different and not recommended). Electrophoretic separations are done generally with respect to the size of molecules so that smaller molecules run more quickly within the gel. One difficulty is that gels are not an ideal medium for the binding of probes to DNA, RNA, or protein. Thus, blotting techniques were developed to transfer the separated bands to a different medium. For example, different bands of DNA separated within the gels are denatured using mild alkali, and the single strands of DNA from individual bands are transferred by blotting onto sheets of nitrocellulose (Figure 8–17). The nitrocellulose is then dried and exposed at an elevated temperature to a labeled probe so that hybridization can occur under stringent conditions. The labeled bands are then visualized using x-ray film and the specific DNA bands with complementary sequences to the probe identified. DNA separations were the first to be carried out with the blotting procedure and are named Southern after their originator.

The usefulness of the Southern blotting procedure can be outlined by the following applications. Point mutations in DNA may either eliminate or create sites for restriction enzyme hydrolysis, changing the nature of the fragments produced by the enzyme, and this may be shown by a change in banding patterns seen in Southern blotting, using a probe to a large sequence of bases in DNA (Figure 8–18). A mutation that removes part of a genetic sequence may also be identified by a reduction in the size of the DNA fragments generated by enzyme hydrolysis. Similarly, a translocation of DNA into a particular restriction sequence may be identified by a larger fragment produced by restriction enzymes. Southern blotting may also be used to assist in the selection of cloned rDNA that is identified by probe

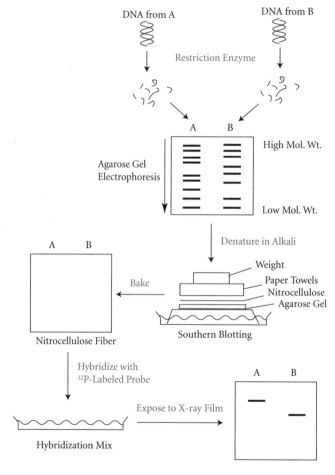

Figure 8–17 Southern blotting is used in the identification of DNA fragments, separated in agarose gels by electrophoresis. The DNA bands on the gel are denatured using alkali and blotted onto nitrocellulose. On nitrocellulose, the DNA can be exposed to radioactively labeled probes and DNA bands with sequences complementary to the probe identified using x-ray film. Adapted from Brock DJH. Molecular genetics for the clinician. Cambridge (UK): Cambridge University Press; 1993.

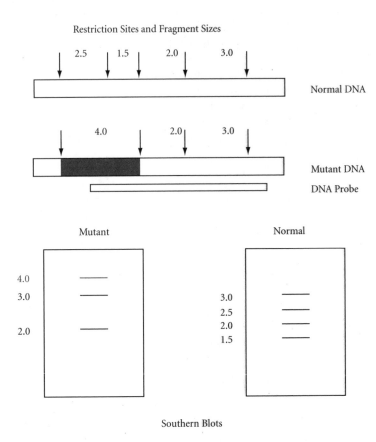

Figure 8–18 The loss of a restriction site within a DNA fragment will lead to a loss of smaller DNA products of the enzyme digestion, as well as the emergence of a larger fragment. This can be detected by Southern blotting, using a probe that will bind to all relevant areas.

hybridization in several transformed bacterial colonies. If the human genomic DNA fragment is recovered from each of the colonies, Southern blotting would show which of the human DNA fragments is the largest. In the search for an intact gene, the largest cloned DNA fragment may be the best starting point.

Northern blotting is a similar technique, developed to identify RNA molecules. No scientist conveniently named Northern invented the procedure; rather, the name simply emerged from a blossoming inventiveness based on associated compass direction headings. Northern blotting allows detection of the presence or absence of specific mRNA species, increased levels of mRNA (which could indicate increased transcription of a gene or genes, say, following treatment of cells with hormones or drugs), and size changes in mRNA leading to the production of mature mRNA from larger primary transcripts. Again, probes would allow the identification of specific mRNA species within a population.

Western blotting is designed to identify specific proteins. After separation of a variety of proteins by gel electrophoresis (usually, polyacrylamide gel electrophoresis, run in the presence of the detergent sodium dodecyl sulfate, hence SDS-PAGE) the protein bands can be transferred by blotting and specific proteins identified using labeled antibodies. Western blotting is sometimes called an **immunoblot**. The specificity of antibody detection of proteins is a very useful technology and can, for example, be used to detect chorionic gonadotrophin in urine in a pregnancy test.

Dot Blotting

The pregnancy test noted above would not require separation of the hormone from other proteins but simply relies on the specificity of the antibody to detect the protein within a mixture of compounds. So, too, can DNA sequences be identified within a mixture, using a specific probe. For example, if there is a specific mutated sequence within a gene that is the basis of a genetic disease, a very specific oligonucleotide probe for the mutated sequence can be produced. The probe in this case is termed an **alelle-specific oligonucleotide** (ASO) and is usually 18 to 20 bp in length. In dot blotting, the DNA fragments are delivered as a single spot onto nitrocellulose and the binding of the ASO to the denatured DNA determined under conditions of high stringency. If a probe for the normal gene sequence is also used, it is possible to identify the presence of only the mutated sequence (homozygous for the disease gene) or of both the mutated and the normal sequence, which could indicate a carrier of the mutation (heterozygous for the disease gene) (Figure 8–19). This technique can be used in the molecular diagnosis of a specific disease mutation.

POLYMERASE CHAIN REACTION

This is a very useful technique employed in the amplification of DNA fragments. Thus, a very small quantity of DNA can be used to produce a much larger quantity of the same DNA sequence. This could be done using bacterial hosts and transformation, but the polymerase chain reaction (PCR) is a purely chemical technique that is much simpler if you have identified a specific DNA fragment that you wish to reproduce. In a way, PCR is the photocopier technique within rDNA technology.

In PCR, the duplex DNA fragment is denatured by heat to two single strands. Using the single strands, you wish to make complementary DNA

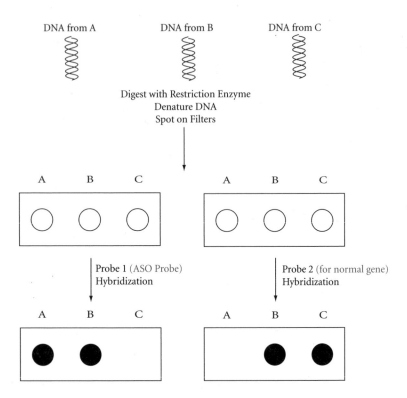

A = homozygous for mutation; B = heterozygous for mutation (carrier); C = normal control.

Figure 8–19 Allele-specific oligonucleotide probes complementary to specific mutated sequences within genes can be used in the dot blotting technique to identify the presence of the mutation, which may cause disease. Probe 1 is the ASO probe to the mutation, while probe 2 will bind to the normal genetic sequence. Thus, probe 1 will bind to DNA fragments from patients homozygous for the mutated gene, while both probes 1 and 2 can bind to DNA fragments from an individual who is a carrier for the defect (i.e., one chromosome bears the mutated gene, while the second chromosome of the pair bears the normal gene). Be aware that the probe will detect the mutation but not necessarily the disease, which is dependent on the manifestation of signs and symptoms. Adapted from Brock DJH. Molecular genetics for the clinician. Cambridge (UK): Cambridge University Press; 1993.

copies (Figure 8–20). However, the DNA polymerase that accomplishes this reproduction needs to have a short primer sequence complementary to the 3′ ends of the two single strands before it can proceed. It's a little like starting a car engine by using a starter motor. Thus, a knowledge of the base sequence close to the 3′ ends of the DNA single strands is important, as it allows you to construct primers that will facilitate the DNA polymerase activity. Recall that the dideoxynucleotide DNA sequencing technique also used a primer sequence before the polymerase was engaged. If you have the

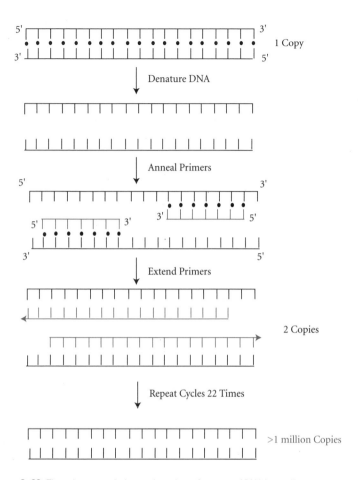

Figure 8–20 The polymerase chain reaction takes a fragment of DNA in small quantity, denatures the DNA to two strands at elevated temperature, and uses primers to the 3' ends of each strand to construct complementary strands to each, effectively duplicating the original duplex DNA fragment. This cycle can be repeated over and over again, in each case duplicating the quantity of duplex DNA present. This can magnify the duplex DNA by a factor in excess of 1 million after 22 cycles. Adapted from Brock DJH. Molecular genetics for the clinician. Cambridge (UK): Cambridge University Press; 1993.

primers and the enzyme, polymerization will proceed in a 5′→3′ direction, and at the end of one cycle, the original duplex DNA fragment will now have a duplex copy. One problem that was encountered initially was the heat stability of the DNA polymerase because the second cycle of PCR requires the heat-denaturation of these two identical duplex DNA fragments. This was solved by employing heat-stable DNA polymerase. An early example was Taq polymerase that could work at 65 to 75°C. Thus, the cycling in the presence of primers and enzyme could go on for hours as each cycle doubled the original quantity of duplex DNA. Over a million copies of the duplex DNA can be made after 22 cycles of PCR. So, remember, if some kind soul (whose name might be Regis) offers you either $100 or the proceeds from the serial doubling of a penny over 25 cycles, you definitely should go for the penny option. (Don't say this book doesn't give you practical advice!)

You can appreciate the advantages of PCR. It is relatively quick and can be used to give you large quantities of a specific DNA fragment that can then be sequenced if you are hunting for a disease gene. Similarly, the amplification factor of the technique allows the identification of criminals on the basis of small amounts of blood, hair, or semen, the identification of fathers in paternity suits, or the identification of viral or bacterial infections. (You may be hoping to create a prehistoric world over the weekend, like certain film directors who consider it possible to clone a dinosaur using DNA trapped in amber from times long past. This could have been the origin of the movie entitled "Forever Amber." Mind you, students have noted that even finding a piece of amber is a challenge, let alone one with an insect that had just gorged itself on dinosaur blood. Not to mention problems with DNA degradation after thousands of years.)

The other potential difficulty with PCR is that of contamination. If you have a technique that can transform a penny into a hundred thousand dollars, you should be careful of what exactly goes into the machine. For example, before you can claim that you have discovered DNA on the meteorite from Mars (nicely amplified by PCR), it is important to ensure that this "extraterrestrial" DNA does not look a lot like your DNA, which may have inadvertently come from your hands while examining this interesting piece of Martian real estate.

SOMATIC CELL HYBRIDIZATION, IN SITU HYBRIDIZATION, AND FLUORESCENCE IN SITU HYBRIDIZATION

Chemistry does take you quite a long way within the reaches of rDNA technology, but the "bio" in front of biochemistry certainly has significance within molecular biology. Thus, a question that came to the forefront in the search for disease genes was simply on which chromosome can I find this gene? This is indeed a good question because a knowledge of the chromosomal location of the disease gene can simplify the search for a precise gene locus.

Somatic cell hybridization attempted to answer the chromosomal locus question. In this procedure, human cells and tumor cells from another species, such as mouse, are hybridized to form a cell (heterokaryon) with the chromosome complements of both species (for human and mouse: 43 pairs in total). This cellular hybridization is promoted by the presence of Sendai virus or by the use of the chemical polyethylene glycol. As the hybrid cells undergo division, there is, with time, a tendency to lose chromosomes. Stable hybrid cells that have only a few of the human chromosomes remaining after these divisions could be found. A number of different hybrid cell lines, each containing a small number of human chromosomes, can be isolated and exposed to a radioactive probe complementary to a specific human DNA gene sequence. By checking which of the hybrid cells bound the probe, it was possible to figure out which chromosome was the likely locus for the gene in question. For example, positive probe results with hybrids 1 (human chromosomes 1, 7, 19), 2 (human chromosomes 3, 7, 22), and 3 (human chromosomes 7, 14, 16) would indicate human chromosome 7 as the location of the gene in question.

In situ hybridization utilizes the fact that at metaphase within mitotic division, chromosomes can be both seen and identified on the basis of their size and characteristic banding patterns. Thus, the metaphase chromosomes could be exposed to a radioactive probe to a particular DNA sequence, and with an overlaying x-ray film, the chromosome and area within the chromosome hybridizing the probe could be identified. This is a form of **karyotyping**. In situ hybridization certainly had some drawbacks, including relatively low resolution (the exact area of the chromosome was fuzzy at best), the procedure did take time, and there was the possibility of hybridization to more than one chromosome or one chromosome area.

Fluorescence in situ hybridization (FISH) is an improved version of the in situ technique described above. In this procedure, fluorescent labeled probes are used to hybridize with the separated metaphase chromosomes, and the fluorescence can be seen by employing a fluorescence microscope. This technique is quicker (you don't have to wait to have the x-ray film developed), has better resolution (often to within 1 million base pairs of the gene locus on the chromosome), and avoids the use of radioactivity. It is also possible to use several fluorescent probes at one time and distinguish binding areas for several chromosomes, on the basis of the fluorescent color for each probe. Individual chromosomes can be isolated and used in the generation of **chromosomal libraries**. Knowledge of the chromosomal location for the gene within the human genome and the corresponding use of a chromosomal library can greatly simplify the search for a disease gene.

THE HUNT FOR DISEASE GENES

One principal application of recombinant DNA technology is in the localization of genes that cause disease. From this localization can come the identification of the mutation in the genetic sequence (and in the amino acid sequence of the corresponding protein) and the possibility of generating a probe specific for the mutated sequence that can serve as a molecular diagnostic. There is a variety of possible approaches in the hunt for the gene, depending on how much is known about the biochemistry of the disease.

To go back to the history of biochemistry, before the discovery of the DNA double helix (molecular biologists may date these years as BWC, or Before Watson and Crick), Linus Pauling categorized sickle cell anemia as a molecular disease. This disease is characterized by fragile, elongated, sickle (or banana, if you prefer) -shaped red cells that can hamper the circulation through blood capillaries and lead to anemia. This is caused by a mutation in the β-globin gene that effectively replaces the amino acid glutamic acid at position 6 in the β-subunit of hemoglobin (whose structure we cover in greater depth in Chapter 5) with the amino acid valine. This can lead to a polymerization of hemoglobin at low oxygen pressure, and these long polymers can actually distort the shape of the red cell (a little like a child putting a whole candy bar in his or her mouth). Interestingly, this amino acid change leads to a change in charge on hemoglobin S (for sickle cell) so that it is less negative than normal hemoglobin. Thus, the electrophoretic migration for hemoglobin S was distinct from that of normal hemoglobin and led to the elucidation of the amino acid mutation in this protein. This effectively linked a mutated protein to the disease, and this led to the discovery of the disease gene. This approach may be called a **functional approach**, as sickle cell anemia was first linked to a dysfunctional hemoglobin within the red cells. Once the protein was characterized, the gene was readily identifiable. Thus, if the symptoms of a particular disease point readily to a problem in the function of a specific protein, the study of that protein and the use of probes based on the protein sequence can lead directly to the disease gene.

If the disease is not linked to a specific protein mutation (and a corresponding defined loss of function), it may still be possible to narrow the area of investigation by proposing a likely protein whose potential dysfunction may be a cause for a disease. This can be called the **candidate gene approach**. For example, the disease retinitis pigmentosa (RP) affects vision and leads to blindness. Rhodopsin, a protein involved in light absorption at the retina, was a potential candidate. Locating and studying the rhodopsin gene helped identify the involvement of this gene in RP.

As you might expect, the identification of a protein/gene candidate for a disease is not always possible. Disease symptoms may not point to a specific cellular function, much less to a specific protein. For example, CF is a disease marked by thick mucus secretions that cause chronic difficulties in respiration and digestion, among other serious problems. A specific protein dysfunction is not apparent from the symptoms. Without a protein, how can research proceed? It's a little like trying to find someone's telephone number. (Shall we call him or her X, and shall we say X is intelligent, good looking, and has a good sense of humor.) Let's say you met this person at a convention, but you know neither the last name of this individual nor the city/town of his or her residence. All you know is that this individual does live somewhere in North America. Admittedly, the long distance telephone companies may (for a price) be able to work miracles in locating individuals, but even for them, this seems a tall order. This is a true test of the detective powers of the health professional, a true challenge for those followers of the great Holmes (not Oliver Wendell, although he might also have made a good shot at it). The question is where do you begin? Well, you may remember that at the convention, X was accompanied by several siblings, and they may be able to direct you to X. Indeed, under these circumstances, in the search for a disease gene, the one logical path is to find other family members because it is, indeed, possible that some of them will also carry the disease gene or manifest the disease.

This approach can be called **positional cloning** because you are trying to find markers within DNA that may lead you to the disease gene. These markers may be shared by family members carrying the gene. This is called **linkage analysis** because there is a good possibility that there may be characteristic inherited DNA sequences that are found in relatively close proximity to the disease gene. These markers lie outside the disease gene and may be shown by individual family members who have the disease gene. Thus, a search for a gene becomes a search for common DNA markers within a family.

RESTRICTION FRAGMENT LENGTH POLYMORPHISMS

Looking at DNA within a human population, it is apparent that individual genes can differ, existing as two or more alleles. Thus, genes can be polymorphic. It is also true that noncoding regions of DNA (although not detectable in expressed proteins) can also show polymorphisms. These polymorphisms within and outside the coding sequences are very common and can be shown by differences in base sequences. However, certain polymorphisms are more readily seen following restriction enzyme digestions. You will remember that restriction enzymes recognize specific sequences of bases in duplex DNA and cut the two DNA strands at specific sites, producing characteristic fragments of duplex DNA. If a DNA polymorphism leads to the loss of a restriction enzyme site, there will be a loss of DNA fragments of specific sizes and the presence of a larger fragment (Figure 8–21) made by the enzyme. Similarly, if a DNA polymorphism creates a new restriction site, a smaller DNA fragment will be generated by digestion. This can be seen by electrophoretic separation of fragments after restriction enzyme digestion and the Southern blotting procedure. Thus, DNA polymorphisms are noticeable by changes in the lengths of restriction fragments—hence the name restriction fragment length polymorphisms

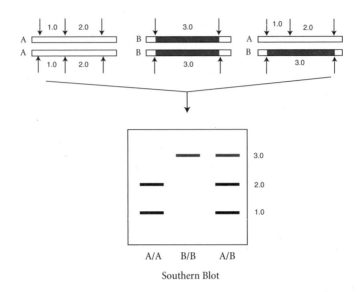

Figure 8–21 The absence of a polymorphic restriction site on chromosome B, but which is found on chromosome A, will lead to differences in the restriction fragments produced. As noted above, Southern blotting indicates the lack of the restriction site by the larger (3 kb) fragment in the B/B chromosome pair, the presence of the two smaller fragments (1 and 2 kb) in the A/A chromosome pair, and the presence of all three fragments in A/B.

(RFLPs). The basis for these polymorphisms may be mutations in DNA sequences, either by substitutions of individual nucleotides or deletions or insertions of DNA sequences.

Another way that differences in DNA fragment lengths may be produced lies in polymorphisms based on variable number of tandem repeats (VNTR) within a DNA sequence. Recall our discussion of repetitive DNA sequences. There can be variations in the length of minisatellites (20 to 70 bp long). Microsatellite repeat polymorphisms (2 to 4 bp) are also apparent within a population. These polymorphisms in tandem repeats are more useful as markers, as there is a greater degree of variability possible. More recently, single-nucleotide polymorphisms (SNPs, where one specific base shows variation among individuals) have been employed in positional cloning. Polymorphisms are inherited and can be found close to disease genes that also have a characteristic mutation.

In certain cases, an RFLP may actually be caused by the mutation within the gene sequence itself, and this is the case for the globin gene in sickle cell anemia, where a single nucleotide mutation is responsible for the disease. In this case, the gene mutation causes a change in the site for the restriction enzyme *MstII*, and those who have the sickle cell gene will show a larger RFLP following *MstII* digestion. The presence of this RFLP can be directly indicative of the disease and used diagnostically. In most other cases, mutations in restriction sites are not in the coding regions, but the resulting RFLPs can be used as potential markers for a disease gene. Thus, linkage studies involve the analysis of a number of family members who have the disease (e.g., for CF, these would be homozygous for the disease gene) or carriers of the disease gene (heterozygous in the case of CF). If one or more RFLPs can be identified in these individuals, then they may be markers for the disease gene (Figure 8–22). The use of RFLPs as markers has largely been replaced by the use of polymorphisms in tandem repeats (VNTRs), which are most useful now in these gene searches. For historical reasons, we will use the RFLP examples, as these were critical in the early searches for disease genes (e.g., CF).

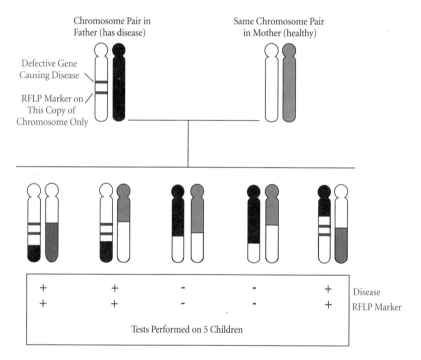

Figure 8–22 Genetic linkage analyses attempt to identify RFLP markers within the DNA of family members who may have, or be carriers for, a disease. It is possible that specific RFLP markers found within this familial population will flank a disease gene, as both the disease gene and the markers will be passed from parents to children within families. Large numbers of family members may need to be screened to accurately assess the validity of RFLP markers. The use of RFLPs in genetic linkage studies has been largely replaced by the use of other polymorphisms (e.g., microsatellites). Adapted from Alberts B, Bray D, Lewis J, et al. Molecular biology of the cell. 3rd ed. New York: Garland Publishing; 1994.

Chromosome Walking and Jumping

Once an RFLP is identified, what then? It's a little like finding a spot (say, the RFLP gas station) on a city's major roadway that is within 10 miles of a house you are seeking. Essentially, you have to walk along the DNA-chromosome road until you get to your destination. If an RFLP is identified, an oligonucleotide probe can be designed to identify DNA fragments that contain the RFLP. Thus, following a restriction digest, the probe may hybridize to one or more DNA fragments. Sequencing the largest fragment (recall the dideoxy method for DNA sequencing) may reveal the presence of a gene, but given the length of DNA, it is more likely that you will still be walking by the time you get to the end of this fragment. This DNA fragment can be used as a probe to identify an overlapping DNA fragment in the restriction enzyme digest, one that contains the next sequence of nucleotides in your linear search for the gene (Figure 8–23). This is somewhat like using a piece of roadway with a sequence of houses to pull up the next adjoining/overlapping piece in the roadway. In turn, after sequencing the second fragment, it can be used to probe for a third, and so on. Thus, overlapping fragments are used to walk along a DNA sequence, allowing you to pull out and follow a logical linear trail among the various DNA fragments within the digest.

If this is beginning to sound a little like "Pilgrim's Progress," you are, indeed, correct in thinking that there may be hazards (like the Slough of Despond or Vanity Fair) along the way. One is the finding of tandem repeats along the DNA road. These may serve as markers for a gene, but you can appreciate that a long stretch of tandem repeats may be difficult to follow using the walking method described. A little like finding a long repetitive sequence of 5 or 6 townhouses along our DNA highway. Under such

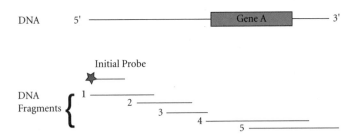

Figure 8–23 Chromosome walking along a DNA fragment involves the use of an RFLP or another marker to identify a fragment relatively close to a disease gene. When this fragment has been sequenced, it may, in turn, be used as a probe to identify an overlapping DNA fragment. In turn, this fragment (1) can be used to identify fragment 2, and so on. As shown above, the fourth and fifth fragments lie within or contain the gene. Adapted from Murray RK, Granner DK, Mayes PA, Rodwell VW. Harper's biochemistry. 25th. ed. Stamford (CT): Appleton and Lange; 2000.

circumstances, chromosome jumping may allow you to circumvent this sea of tandem repeats. In essence, you join the ends of the DNA fragment you are following (that contains the tandem sea at its middle) and cut the circular fragment at a new spot, hopefully placing you in front of a new nonrepetitive vista (Figure 8–24). This may get you closer to the gene destination so that you can resume "walking." A little like jumping to the end of a

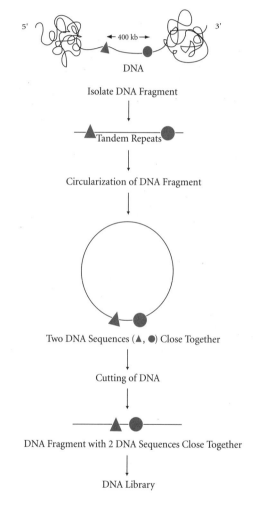

Figure 8–24 Chromosome jumping occurs when a DNA fragment is circularized and cut at a new location, in order to jump over an intervening sequence of DNA that may be difficult to "walk." This may allow two DNA sequences to be brought closer together and speed chromosome walking between the two regions. The new DNA fragment may be used to generate a jumping library of new DNA fragments. Adapted from Trent RJ. Molecular medicine. 2nd ed. London (UK): Churchill Livingstone; 1997.

mystery novel to find out who the murderer is. If the fragment is quite large, you may wish to generate a jumping library by cloning fragments from this new DNA segment. The hunt for disease genes is, indeed, an art form and a science within itself, and these brief descriptions of walking and jumping are only a small sampling of the techniques that are in use.

Nonetheless, one very valid question: as I "walk" or "jump" along the DNA highway, how do I know when I have arrived at the gene (or the house in our analogy)? It is possible that other markers will be found as you close in on the genetic sequence. As well, there are features that characterize a gene. For example, CpG islands (i.e., with the base sequence cytosine-guanine) can be found 5′ to a gene. There will also be promoter regions 5′ to the gene. Within the gene sequence, there should be an **open reading frame**, that is, an absence of stop codons (that are normally used to terminate the translation of mRNA sequences into protein). If you have found a gene, there should be mRNA sequences that correspond to the DNA sequence in cells where this gene is transcribed. If a similar gene is found in other species, cross-hybridization should be seen using the gene sequence and DNA from other sources. Of course, the ultimate test is the identification of a DNA mutation in comparison with controls, a mutation that is the basis for the genetic defect.

One useful correlative procedure was adopted in the hunt for the CF gene. mRNA from sweat gland was used to construct a cDNA library. It was considered likely that this tissue would manifest the genetic defect because abnormal sweat gland function is a hallmark of CF. Thus, it was predicted that the mutated mRNA would probably be present within the sweat gland mRNA population. When chromosome walking and jumping techniques were followed, the DNA fragments identified were tested against this sweat gland cDNA library. Ultimately, a DNA fragment that hybridized with an element of the library was found. Using this specific cDNA as a probe, a genomic library was used to identify the gene sequence. For CF, the gene was found to extend over about 250 kb, with 23 introns. The corresponding mature mRNA was 6,500 nucleotides long. This mRNA coded for a protein that was identified as a mutated form of a membrane-bound chloride channel and was called the cystic fibrosis transmembrane regulator (CFTR). Defective chloride transport has been related to the thick mucus secretions associated with CF. The position of the CF gene in human chromosome 7 is shown in Figure 8–25. The most frequently occurring mutation was also identified as a deletion of three nucleotides resulting in the loss of the amino acid phenylalanine. The positional cloning technique has also been described as an example of **reverse genetics**, in which you identify and localize putative markers for a disease, search for and identify the gene, clone and sequence the gene, identify the mutation, determine the amino acid sequence from the genetic sequence, and ultimately isolate the mutant protein.

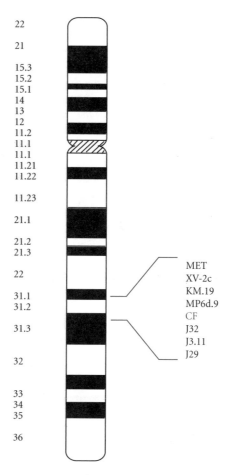

Figure 8–25 A genetic map of human chromosome 7, showing the CF gene locus, its surrounding region, and the chromosome bands. Adapted from Brock DJH. Molecular genetics for the clinician. Cambridge (UK): Cambridge University Press; 1993.

THE HUMAN GENOME PROJECT AND THE POSITIONAL CANDIDATE APPROACH

What is apparent in the search for disease genes is that a map would be helpful. Obviously, the 22 autosomal chromosomes and the X and Y chromosomes represent a vast expanse of DNA, and a map would certainly assist and accelerate research in the discovery of new genes. It has been estimated that if each nucleotide were a single letter, the human genome would be represented by some million pages of text (of which a small proportion is represented by genes). Thus, the Human Genome Project was initiated in numerous laboratories throughout the world in order to sequence the human genome. The dates for completing the project have been moved up as new technology developed, so that a draft sequence would be known by the summer of 2000 and a final draft of the 3 x 10⁹ base pairs ready by 2003. The sequence for chromosome 22, the second shortest of the chromosomes, was essentially completed in the fall of 1999. In February 2001, major sequences and features of the human genome were published in the journals Science and Nature. These two publications were the products of Celera Genomics and the International Human Genome Sequencing Consortium. For each chromosome, mapping involves the generation of a genetic map (genetic markers like RFLPs and microsatellites), a cytogenetic map (the chromosomal banding pattern), the physical map (ultimately the complete sequence), the restriction map (sites for restriction enzyme activity), the sequence tagged sites (STS) map (areas of DNA sequence already known and expanding daily), and the contig map (overlapping DNA fragments) (see Figure 8–26). A map for chromosome 7

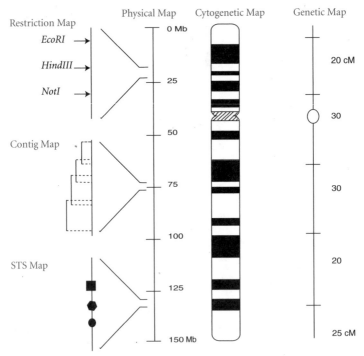

Figure 8–26 A comparison of various maps that can be constructed for a chromosome, including the genetic map, the cytogenetic map (including chromosome bands), the physical map that will eventually include the complete base sequence, the restriction map with restriction enzyme digestion sites, the contig map of established overlapping, DNA fragments, and the STS map of sequenced areas within the chromosome. Adapted from Murray RK, Granner DK, Mayes PA, Rodwell VW. Harper's biochemistry. 25th ed. Stamford (CT): Appleton and Lange; 2000.

is also shown in Figure 8–25, indicating the bands and regions of interest, including the CF gene. Some chromosomes can be divided into regions on the basis of the two parts of the chromosome, divided by the constriction seen at the centromere. The smaller arm of the chromosome is designated "p" for petit, while the larger arm is designated "q." We suppose that puns about molecular biologists minding their p's and q's would not be appreciated. The developing genetic maps for the various human chromosomes can be accessed online at www.ncbi.nlm.nih. gov/omim/.

The completion of genetic maps will assist in disease gene location by what is a **positional candidate approach.** Having information at hand about gene mapping within chromosomes can speed connections between disease genes and dysfunctional proteins. For example, the disease gene for Marfan syndrome (a connective tissue disorder) was mapped to the q-arm of chromosome 15 at about the time that the gene for the protein fibrillin was also localized to this area. Indeed, fibrillin is the dysfunctional protein in this disease.

It is possible to find the disease gene, identify a protein, but still be unsure as to the function of the protein. In this case, the genetic sequence for the protein may be introduced into an appropriate DNA vector and a bacterial expression vector selected so that the protein can be cloned. Antibodies can be raised to this unknown protein to identify cells, tissues, or subcellular sites that may contain the protein (and provide clues to its function). Similarly, and more rapidly, the protein sequence can be searched using databases for identification with a known protein.

RELATED rDNA TECHNOLOGIES

While we don't have the space to describe all the interesting recombinant technologies, some of these are outlined below:

1. Gene therapy: While it is one thing to identify a gene mutation and the corresponding dysfunctional protein, it is quite another to try to correct the problem. Theoretically, this could be accomplished by gene replacement (replacement of the mutated gene with a normal gene), gene correction (replace the specific mutation in the native gene with a correct nucleotide sequence), or gene augmentation (introduction of an extra functional gene to compensate for the impaired gene). At present, gene augmentation technologies and trials are being pursued, using modified retroviral vectors to deliver correct gene sequences into cells. One potential danger inherent in this technique is the disabling of a functional native gene by insertion of this new gene.
2. Gene knock-outs: The importance of a particular gene and its protein may be tested by breeding mice with a single gene mutation. Cross-

breeding can produce mice that are homozygous for the defective gene so that function or dysfunction in the absence of a specific protein may be assessed. It is possible that proteins with similar functions may be encoded by more than one gene, and it is not always appropriate to extrapolate from results with murine studies to the importance of corresponding proteins in humans.

3. Transgenic animals: A gene may be injected into a fertilized mouse ovum so that the gene is incorporated into the genome of somatic and germ cells. This newly acquired gene will be passed on to progeny and, thus, can be inherited. Using this approach, it is possible to introduce a mutated gene into animal cells. For example, a transgenic CF mouse, which is homozygous for CFTR (the mutated chloride channel), shows defects in intestinal and respiratory cell functions. This mouse can be used in studies of tissue abnormalities in CF, as well as the effectiveness of drugs designed to alleviate symptoms of the disease.

4. Site-directed mutagenesis: Using the gene for a specific protein, a specific mutation can be introduced into the gene and the gene inserted into a bacterial host using vectors. The mutated protein so produced by the bacteria can differ from the normal protein by a single amino acid. Thus, it is possible to evaluate the importance of single amino acids within the enzymes, transporters, receptors, and other proteins. It is also possible to truncate a genetic sequence so that a portion of the protein is missing, in order to evaluate the function of a particular amino acid sequence or protein domain.

5. High-density DNA arrays: As many genetic diseases can be characterized by very specific gene mutations, it is possible to generate oligonucleotide probes specific for the mutated sequence and, thus, for the presence of the disease. Naturally, there can be ethical considerations in the use of such diagnostic procedures. For example, CF can be caused by the mutation that we have described earlier in this chapter, but there are other mutations to the CF gene that will bring about the disease. Thus, there is the possibility of a false-negative result, if an individual harbors a rare or undescribed mutation for the CF gene. This is certainly an ethical issue associated with this molecular diagnosis, as probes to all mutations associated with a disease may not be available. This limitation must be considered in any prenatal screening technique, if parents consider their unborn child at risk for a disease gene they may be carrying.

Given the growing number of genetic diseases whose mutations are known, Gene Chips (a type of DNA array) have been designed with a large number of small squares, each bearing an oligonucleotide probe for a particular genetic sequence. A Chip, 1 cm square, can have 100,000 such probes. A child suspected of having a genetic disorder may be tested by constructing cDNA from a cellular mRNA pool. The cDNA may be labeled fluorescently and exposed to the various probes arrayed on the Gene Chip. Hybridization of specific probes to DNA can be assessed as the chip is scanned by a laser and the fluorescent squares located and recorded with the help of a computer. This can assist in the diagnosis of a large number of genetic diseases. The Chips can also be used in research to identify the expression of certain proteins. For example, during ischemia, when the blood supply to the cells is compromised, there can be an inflammatory response leading to the synthesis of cyclooxygenase 2 (COX-2). This is found in heart attack and stroke. This enzyme participates in the pathway that leads to the synthesis of a number of eicosanoids (e.g., prostaglandins, thromboxanes) that bring about inflammation (Chapter 4). The COX-2 gene is upregulated during cell injury with a corresponding increase in the production of its mRNA by transcription. If a cDNA library is constructed from the cells known to be at risk, this library could be tested using the Chips for the presence of a variety of proteins known to be expressed during ischemia. At present, these commercial gene chips are quite expensive and can be used only once; however, there are initiatives to promote the development of the hardware needed to produce such chips within individual laboratories, at considerably less cost.

FUTURE DIRECTIONS

The information provided by the **Human Genome Project** (HGP) has been compared to a "library of life." It will have a tremendous impact on biology in general and medicine in particular.

With respect to **biology** in general, the field of comparative genomics (i.e., the systematic determination of the entire genomes of many species and their comparisons) will expand astronomically. This will undoubtedly shed further light on evolution and the origins of all species, including humans. In particular, determination of the mouse genome will have great impact on studies of the human genome. This is because of the general similarities of these two genomes, the ability to construct complex genetic backgrounds in mice, and the ability to do gene knock-out studies in the mouse, thus helping to reveal gene function. New scientific fields are already gearing up to take advantage of the novel information. These include bioinformatics and proteomics. The former includes the development of appropriate computer systems to accommodate the nucleic acid and protein databases that are burgeoning as new information floods in. Proteomics, which, in its broadest sense, covers the study of all the proteins encoded by the genomes of species, is poised to explode its boundaries. This will become an even larger field than genomics because of the complexities of protein structures, the existence of alternative splicing and numerous post-translational modifications, the variations in amounts of proteins during the development and life of cells, and the numerous interactions of proteins with each other.

With regard to **medicine**, the most immediate pay-off is likely to be in the revelation of newly discovered genes that may be responsible for or be involved in the causation of various diseases. This, in turn, will lead to new diagnostic tests based on gene probes or measurements of specific proteins. As further advances are made, there will be an increase in the gene-based methods of assessing the likelihood of disease development in individuals, and this will hopefully allow the early start of appropriate preventive measures. The investigation of the genetic basis of complex diseases, in which many genes interact, will be promoted as new markers (e.g., single-nucleotide polymorphisms or SNPs) revealed by the HGP are used. Knowledge of entire areas, such as human development and behavior, will expand markedly as new genes involved in them are uncovered. Oncology (the branch of medicine dealing with the diagnosis and treatment of tumors) will benefit from this as gene-expression profiles (involving measurements of mRNAs and proteins) for individual tumors are collected and specific targets for therapy are selected on the basis of this information. The application of the new genetic information to pharmacology has catalyzed the development of the new field of pharmacogenomics. For example, precise knowledge of individual genes and their variants encoding drug-metabolizing enzymes will hopefully lead to the development of tailor-made drugs based on this information; this should help diminish the adverse effects that many individuals experience when taking certain medications.

In short, the overall implications of the HGP are enormous and are likely to affect all species. At the human level, our knowledge of both health and disease will advance immeasurably. Considering the progress made in the last decade, who can predict accurately the situation 10 or 20 years down the road?

Index